Practical Manual of Gastroesophageal Reflux Disease

Practical Manual of Gastroesophageal Reflux Disease

EDITED BY

Marcelo F. Vela

MD, MSCR

Director of GI Motility
Gastroenterology Section
Baylor College of Medicine & Michael E. DeBakey VA Medical Center
Houston, TX, USA

Joel E. Richter

MD, MACG, FACP

Hugh Culverhouse Professor of Medicine
Director, Division of Digestive Diseases and Nutrition
Director, Joy M. Culverhouse Center for Esophageal Diseases
University of South Florida
Tampa, FL, USA

John E. Pandolfino

MD, MSCI

Professor of Medicine
Feinberg School of Medicine
Northwestern University
Chicago, IL, USA

WILEY-BLACKWELL

A John Wiley & Sons, Ltd., Publication

This edition first published 2013, © 2013 by John Wiley & Sons, Ltd

Wiley-Blackwell is an imprint of John Wiley & Sons, formed by the merger of Wiley's global Scientific, Technical and Medical business with Blackwell Publishing.

Registered Office
John Wiley & Sons, Ltd, The Atrium, Southern Gate, Chichester, West Sussex, PO19 8SQ, UK

Editorial Offices
9600 Garsington Road, Oxford, OX4 2DQ, UK
The Atrium, Southern Gate, Chichester, West Sussex, PO19 8SQ, UK)
111 River Street, Hoboken, NJ 07030-5774, USA

For details of our global editorial offices, for customer services and for information about how to apply for permission to reuse the copyright material in this book please see our website at www.wiley.com/wiley-blackwell.

Library of Congress Cataloging-in-Publication Data

Manual of gastroesophageal reflux disease / edited by Marcelo F. Vela, Joel E. Richter, John A. Pandolfino.
    p. cm.
    Includes bibliographical references and index.
    ISBN 978-0-470-65626-6 (pbk. : alk. paper) – ISBN 978-1-118-44478-8 (obook) – ISBN 978-1-118-44479-5 (mobi) – ISBN 978-1-118-44480-1 (epub) – ISBN 978-1-118-44482-5 (ebook/epdf)   1. Gastroesophageal reflux–Handbooks, manuals, etc.   I. Vela, Marcelo F. II. Richter, Joel E.   III. Pandolfino, John E.
    RC815.7.M368 2013
    616.3′24–dc23
                                        2012030222

A catalogue record for this book is available from the British Library.

Wiley also publishes its books in a variety of electronic formats. Some content that appears in print may not be available in electronic books.

Cover design by Andrew Magee Design Ltd

Set in 9.5/13pt Meridien by SPi Publisher Services, Pondicherry, India
Printed in Singapore by Ho Printing Singapore Pte Ltd

1 2013

Contents

Color plate section can be found facing page 118

List of Contributors

Sami R. Achem, MD, FACP, FACG, AGAF, FASGE
Professor of Medicine
Division of Gastroenterology
Mayo Clinic Florida
Jacksonville, FL, USA

Cristina Almansa, MD, PhD
Assistant Professor of Medicine
Division of Gastroenterology
Mayo Clinic Florida
Jacksonville, FL, USA

Albert J. Bredenoord, MD
Department of Gastroenterology
Academic Medical Centre
Amsterdam, The Netherlands

Stanislas Bruley des Varannes
Institut des Maladies de l'Appareil Digestif
Centre Hospitalier Universitaire de Nantes
Nantes, France

Donald O. Castell, MD
Director, Esophageal Disease Program
Medical University of South Carolina
Charleston, SC, USA

Gary W. Falk, MD, MS
Professor of Medicine
Division of Gastroenterology
Perelman School of Medicine at the University
of Pennsylvania
Philadelphia, PA, USA

Ronnie Fass, MD, FACP, FACG
Division of Gastroenterology and Hepatology
MetroHealth Medical Center
Case Western Reserve University
Cleveland, Ohio, USA

Jean-Paul Galmiche
Institut des Maladies de l'Appareil Digestif
Centre Hospitalier Universitaire de Nantes
Nantes, France

David Y. Graham, MD
Professor of Medicine
Gastroenterology Section
Baylor College of Medicine
Michael E. DeBakey VA Medical Center
Houston, TX, USA

Tiberiu Hershcovici, MD
Neuroenteric Clinical Research Group
Section of Gastroenterology
Department of Medicine
Southern Arizona VA Health Care System and
University of Arizona School of Medicine
Tucson, AZ, USA

Ikuo Hirano, MD
Professor of Medicine
Northwestern University
Feinberg School of Medicine
Department of Medicine
Division of Gastroenterology
Chicago, IL, USA

David A. Johnson, MD, FACG, FASGE
Professor of Medicine and Chief of
Gastroenterology
Eastern Virginia School of Medicine
Norfolk, VA, USA

Peter J. Kahrilas, MD
Professor, Division of Gastroenterology
Northwestern University
Chicago, IL, USA

Robert T. Kavitt, MD
Division of Gastroenterology, Hepatology,
and Nutrition
Vanderbilt University Medical Center
Nashville, TN, USA

Boudewijn F. Kessing, MD
Department of Gastroenterology and
Hepatology
Academic Medical Center
Amsterdam, The Netherlands

Kumar Krishnan, MD
Northwestern University
Feinberg School of Medicine
Department of Medicine
Division of Gastroenterology
Chicago, IL, USA

Maria Pina Dore, MD, PhD
Professor of Gastroenterology
Clinica Medica – Dipartimento di Medicina
Clinica e Sperimentale
University of Sassari
Sassari, Italy
Baylor College of Medicine
Houston, TX, USA

Sabine Roman
Digestive Physiology
Claude Bernard Lyon I University and Hospices
Civils de Lyon
Lyon, France

Ryuichi Shimono, MD
Wingate Institute for Neurogastroenterology
Barts and the London School of Medicine and
Dentistry
Research Fellow at GI Physiology Unit,
Royal London Hospital
London, UK

Daniel Sifrim, MD, PhD
Professor of Gastrointestinal Physiology
Wingate Institute for Neurogastroenterology
Barts and the London School of Medicine and
Dentistry
Director GI Physiology Unit,
Royal London Hospital
London, UK

Erick R. Singh, MD
Department of Medicine
Section of Gastroenterology and Hepatology
Georgia Health Sciences University
Augusta, GA, USA

André J.P.M. Smout, MD, PhD
Department of Gastroenterology and
Hepatology
Academic Medical Center
Amsterdam, The Netherlands

Jianmin Tian, MD
Barrett's Esophagus Unit
Mayo Clinic
Rochester, MN, USA

Michael F. Vaezi, MD, PhD, MSc(Epi)
Division of Gastroenterology, Hepatology, and
Nutrition
Vanderbilt University Medical Center
Nashville, TN, USA

Nimish Vakil, MD, FACP, FACG, AGAF, FASGE
University of Wisconsin School of Medicine
and Public Health
Madison, WI, USA

Nicolas A. Villa
Gastroenterology Section
Baylor College of Medicine
& Michael E. DeBakey VA Medical Center
Houston, TX, USA

Kenneth K. Wang, MD
VanCleve Professor of Gastroenterology
Research
Director, Advanced Endoscopy
Director, Barretts Esophagus Unit
Mayo Clinic
Rochester, MN, USA

Pim W. Weijenborg, MD
Department of Gastroenterology and
Hepatology
Academic Medical Center
Amsterdam, The Netherlands

Etsuro Yazaki, PhD, MAGIP
Wingate Institute for Neurogastroenterology
Barts and the London School of Medicine and
Dentistry
Manager GI Physiology Unit,
Royal London Hospital
London, UK

Frank Zerbib
Département de Gastroentérologie
CHU de Bordeaux
Centre Hospitalier Saint André de Bordeaux
Bordeaux, France

Preface

Gastroesophageal reflux disease (GERD) is a very common clinical problem and a frequent reason for consultation. Many patients have a typical presentation of heartburn and regurgitation, and a good response to treatment with acid suppressive medication, such as a proton pump inhibitor (PPI). However, the evaluation and management of GERD has become more challenging for several reasons. The spectrum of clinical presentations attributed to GERD has moved beyond the typical esophageal symptoms of heartburn and regurgitation, and now incorporates various extraesophageal manifestations including laryngeal symptoms, cough, and even disordered sleep. Furthermore, we are facing an increasing number of patients in whom symptoms, either typical or atypical, persist despite acid suppression with a PPI. Some of these patients with refractory symptoms have persistent reflux due to treatment failure and require alternative therapeutic approaches, while in others the reported symptoms may be due to causes other than GERD, including functional disorders; in the latter, a negative evaluation for GERD can direct the diagnostic and treatment efforts toward other causes. Finally, how concomitant conditions such as eosinophilic esophagitis and *Helicobacter pylori* gastritis affect GERD management is not always clear, and a lucid perspective about these issues is needed in daily practice.

Practical Manual of Gastroesophageal Reflux Disease, as it name indicates, is meant to serve as a practical manual to aid the clinician in managing GERD. The first section of the book presents an overview of pathophysiology, epidemiology, diagnostic tools and treatment options of GERD. Whole chapters are devoted to the potential side effects of medical and surgical therapy, a highly relevant topic in routine practice. In the second section, the evaluation and management of specific clinical presentations in GERD (refractory heartburn, functional heartburn, chest pain, laryngitis, cough, sleep disorders, belching, and dysphagia) are discussed and a management algorithm is suggested for each clinical entity. In addition, further chapters focus on the role of eosinophilic esophagitis and *Helicobacter pylori* in GERD patients. A third section is devoted to Barrett's esophagus, to help the clinician deal with the challenges of screening for, diagnosing, and treating this complication of GERD.

We are fortunate and thankful for the participation of the many recognized experts from around the world who agreed to write the chapters that make up this book. Our hope is that this book will provide a first-line reference for clinicians who deal with this common and often challenging problem of GERD.

Marcelo F. Vela
Houston, TX

PART 1

Gastroesophageal Reflux Disease Overview

CHAPTER 1

Gastroesophageal Reflux Disease: Pathophysiology

Pim W. Weijenborg, Boudewijn F. Kessing, and André J.P.M. Smout

Department of Gastroenterology and Hepatology, Academic Medical Center, Amsterdam, The Netherlands

---

Key points

- The anti-reflux barrier does not solely consist of the intrinsic pressure generated by the lower esophageal sphincter, but is complemented by the extrinsic pressure exerted by the crural diaphragm and the presence of the flap valve.
- Transient lower esophageal sphincter relaxations constitute the main mechanism of reflux in gastroesophageal reflux disease patients and healthy subjects.
- The presence of a hiatal hernia increases the severity of esophageal acid exposure, and changes the position of the acid pocket.
- The severity of gastroesophageal reflux disease-related symptoms is not predicted by the severity of esophageal acid exposure and is dependent on factors influencing the perception of reflux.
- Dilated intercellular spaces are more frequently present in non-erosive reflux disease patients and possibly contribute to symptom generation.

Introduction

Over the past decades, considerable changes in our understanding of gastroesophageal reflux disease (GERD) have taken place. In the era before widespread application of endoscopy, when radiography was the only diagnostic tool available, the diagnosis of GERD was more or less synonymous with hiatal hernia. After the introduction of flexible esophagogastroduodenoscopy, mucosal lesions in the distal esophagus became the most important characteristic of the disease. Nowadays, we know that reflux symptoms can be present in the absence of reflux esophagitis. This subset of the disease is labeled non-erosive reflux disease (NERD). In addition, extraesophageal symptoms and signs, such

---

Practical Manual of Gastroesophageal Reflux Disease, First Edition.
Edited by Marcelo F. Vela, Joel E. Richter and John E. Pandolfino.
© 2013 John Wiley & Sons, Ltd. Published 2013 by John Wiley & Sons, Ltd.

as laryngitis, gastric asthma and chronic cough, were recognized. The Montreal definition encompasses all of these elements of the disease by stating that it is characterized by either bothersome symptoms and/or lesions caused by reflux of gastric contents. This gradual broadening of our understanding of what GERD is has led to an expansion of our concepts of the pathophysiology of the disease [1]. Whilst the factors that determine the exposure of the esophageal mucosa to gastric contents are still relevant to the pathophysiology of GERD, factors that affect the sensitivity of the esophagus have become recognized as equally important. This chapter aims to summarize the many factors that are presently seen as important in the pathophysiology of GERD.

Mechanisms leading to gastroesophageal reflux

Anti-reflux barrier

In the early days after the advent of esophageal manometry, the lower esophageal sphincter (LES) was conceptually prominent in the pathophysiology of GERD. A LES able to maintain a sufficiently high pressure at the esophagogastric junction (EGJ) was considered to be the most important factor preventing gastroesophageal reflux. Nowadays, the anti-reflux barrier is thought to consist of intrinsic LES pressure, extrinsic compression of the LES by the crural diaphragm, and the "flap valve" constituted by an acute angle of His.

Lower esophageal sphincter

The LES is a 3–4 cm segment of tonically contracted smooth muscle at the EGJ. Normally, the LES is surrounded by the crural diaphragm. When a sliding hiatus hernia is present, the LES is proximal to the crural diaphragm (Figure 1.1). Resting LES tone, best measured during end-expiration, varies among normal individuals from 10 to 30 mmHg relative to intragastric pressure. Within a subject, LES pressure varies considerably during the day. The highest pressure occurs during phase III of the migrating motor complex, during which it may exceed 80 mmHg. Immediately after a meal, LES pressure typically decreases. The genesis of LES tone is a property of both the smooth muscle itself and of its extrinsic innervation.

Lower esophageal sphincter pressure is affected by myogenic factors, intraabdominal pressure, gastric distension, peptides, hormones, various foods, and many medications.

Crural diaphragm

The opening in the diaphragm through which the esophagus reaches the abdomen (hiatus esophagei) is shaped like a teardrop. In the absence of a

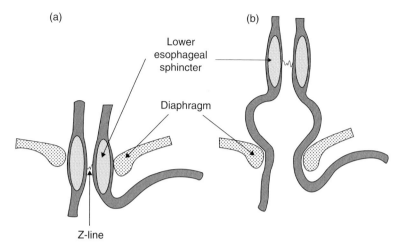

Figure 1.1 Position of the LES with respect to the crural diaphragm. (a) Normal morphology. (b) Hiatus hernia.

hiatal hernia, the LES is surrounded at this point by the crural diaphragm, i.e. the right diaphragmatic crus. Especially during inspiration, the crural diaphragm contributes to the maintenance of EGJ competence. For this reason, the crural diaphragm is often referred to as the extrinsic sphincter, the smooth muscle of the LES being the intrinsic sphincter. This situation resembles that of the internal and external sphincters surrounding the anal canal.

Flap valve

A third component of the anti-reflux barrier at the EGJ is constituted by the so-called flap valve, formed by a musculomucosal fold created by the entry of the esophagus into the stomach along the lesser curvature. With this anatomical arrangement, increased intraabdominal or intragastric pressure compresses the subdiaphragmatic portion of the esophagus. This is supposed to prevent EGJ opening and reflux during periods of abdominal straining. Hill and colleagues proposed a grading scheme based on the endoscopic appearance of the gastroesophageal flap valve during retroflexion (Plate 1.1).

Mechanisms of reflux

Current thinking is that there are three dominant reflux mechanisms: transient LES relaxations, LES hypotension, and anatomical distortion of the EGJ, e.g. hiatus hernia. Transient LES relaxations (TLESRs), constituting the most important reflux mechanism in healthy subjects and in a large subset of GERD patients, will be discussed in greater detail in the next paragraph.

When diminished LES pressure is present (either with or without anatomical abnormality), short-lived increases in intraabdominal pressure caused by straining are often the precipitating factor of the reflux. Manometric data suggest that this rarely occurs when the LES pressure is greater than 10 mmHg [2]. It is also a rare occurrence in patients without hiatus hernia [3]. Free reflux is characterized by a fall in intraesophageal pH without an identifiable change in either intragastric pressure or LES pressure. Episodes of free reflux are observed only when the LES pressure is lower than 5 mmHg.

It is important to realize that EGJ relaxation as measured manometrically does not equate to EGJ opening or EGJ compliance, which are likely to be more relevant to the occurrence of reflux. EGJ compliance can be assessed with a water-filled balloon straddling the EGJ and measurement of the diameter of the balloon at various levels of filling. In patients with hiatus hernia, the compliance of the EGJ is increased but even patients without hiatus hernia may have increased EGJ compliance. In the latter, defects not readily detectable with imaging techniques, such as an abnormal gastroesophageal flap valve, defects in the LES musculature or a wide diaphragmatic hiatus, are thought to be present. Subtle differences in EGJ opening and compliance are likely to explain the discriminatory function of the EGJ: large volumes of gas can be vented from the stomach while at the same time fluid is largely contained within the stomach.

Transient lower esophageal sphincter relaxations
Function and definition
Lower esophageal sphincter relaxations are common and occur mainly during swallows to allow passage of a bolus into the stomach [4]. In addition, the LES can relax during the so-called TLESR which occurs less frequently, about 3–6 times per hour [5,6]. TLESRs are considered the physiological mechanism which enables venting of gas from the stomach, also known as belching [7]. This belching reflex acts as a protective mechanism which prevents excess amounts of gas accumulating in the stomach. Since the discovery of TLESRs in the early 1980s, it has become increasingly clear that most reflux episodes occur during TLESRs [8]. Other mechanisms which can induce reflux episodes include straining, coughing, and free reflux. However, these mechanisms only become important – relatively and absolutely – in patients with severe reflux disease associated with hiatal hernia.

A TLESR is currently defined as an abrupt decline in pressure at the position of the LES which is not induced by swallowing [9]. Additional criteria which could be helpful but are not needed for the identification of TLESRs are crural diaphragm inhibition and a prominent after-contraction [10]. Since the definition of TLESR is based solely on the esophageal pressure profile, the gold standard by which to measure TLESRs is esophageal manometry (Plate 1.2).

Pharyngeal stimulation can also result in an LES relaxation which resembles a TLESR [4]. However, LES relaxations induced by pharyngeal stimulation are rarely associated with inhibition of the crural diaphragm and acid reflux [6]. Furthermore, esophageal reflux was found only when an LES relaxation was associated with diaphragm inhibition [6].

Mechanisms of transient lower esophageal sphincter relaxation

The primary stimulus which triggers a TLESR is gastric distension, often resulting from accumulation of gastric air or consumption of a meal. Distension in any part of the stomach can trigger a TLESR. However, the subcardiac region of the stomach showed the lowest threshold for triggering TLESRs [11]. While still under debate, several studies suggest that tension receptors in the stomach appear to be more relevant than pressure receptors as the stimulus for transient LES relaxation [12,13].

Transient LES relaxations are characterized by four different events. The concerted action of these events results in complete relaxation of the EGJ. The first and most prominent event during a TLESR is relaxation of the inner part of the LES [14]. The second event is relaxation of the crural diaphragm [15]. The third event is suppression of esophageal peristalsis [14] and the fourth is a contraction of the distal esophageal longitudinal muscle leading to esophageal shortening [16]. It has been hypothesized that the longitudinal muscle contraction of the distal esophagus may be the primary motor event leading to LES relaxation [17] but this hypothesis remains to be proven.

Relaxation of the EGJ during a TLESR is terminated by primary peristalsis or, more commonly, by secondary peristalsis [18]. Swallow-induced primary peristalsis is characterized by upper esophageal sphincter (UES) relaxation with pharyngeal contraction and esophageal peristalsis progressing along the entire esophagus. Secondary peristalsis is defined as a wave in the esophagus which is not associated with UES relaxation and is a result of esophageal distension, often arising from gastroesophageal reflux.

The rate of TLESRs can vary greatly during the day. The postprandial period is characterized by a four- to fivefold increase in the rate of TLESRs and an increase in the proportion of TLESRs accompanied by reflux [19]. Body position can also influence the rate of TLESRs since the incidence of TLESRs, as well as the incidence of reflux-associated TLESRs, is higher in the right recumbent position compared to the left recumbent position [20]. Furthermore, the rate of TLESRs is greatly decreased during the night [18]. This is in accordance with the observation that reflux episodes occur less often during the night than during the day [8]. Despite this nocturnal decrease in the rate of TLESRs, a subset of GERD patients still shows substantial acid exposure during the night. Therefore, in patients with pathological nocturnal reflux, additional mechanisms are involved, such as free reflux through a mechanically incompetent sphincter [21].

The reflex pathway of the TLESR is a vagovagal reflex which commences with activation of gastric receptors primarily in the subcardiac region [11]. Sensory signals from the stomach are projected to the brain through afferent sensory fibers of the vagus [22] and its terminating synapses are located in the nucleus tractus solitarius (NTS) [23]. Signals from the NTS do not provide signals to the EGJ directly but are relayed to the caudal part of the dorsal motor nucleus of the vagus [24,25]. This central pathway which modulates TLESRs is shared by both the LES and crural diaphragm [26]. Furthermore, the crural diaphragm is innervated not only through efferent vagal endings but also by the phrenic nerve [27]. The brainstem sites responsible for this dual innervation are yet to be defined. Efferent motor function signals from the brain to the LES and crural diaphragm are conducted through the motor tract of the vagus [28]. Finally, motor signals are relayed through the myenteric plexus from where they are further distributed to the esophageal body and LES [28].

Many excitory and inhibitory neurotransmitters and receptors, including nitric oxide, opioids, anticholinergic agents and the neuropeptide CCK, have been found to play a role in the neuromodulation of TLESRs [29]. Among these neurotransmitters, the gamma-aminobutyric acid (GABA) and metabotropic glutamate receptors (mGluR), and the cannabinoid receptor 1 (CBR1) are of particular interest as potential targets for therapeutic interventions. The most extensively investigated neurotransmitter in the TLESR pathway is GABA-B. GABA-B acts as an inhibitory neurotransmitter, and its receptors are located at both central and peripheral sites in the TLESR reflex arch [30,31]. Metabotropic glutamate receptors are also present throughout the central and peripheral nervous system. The most extensively investigated metabotropic glutamate receptor is mGluR5 which has an excitatory function, mainly with a periperal site of action [32, 33]. The CBR1 has only recently been investigated with regard to TLESRs. Its site of action is believed to be the central nervous system [34].

Despite the importance of the TLESR in the pathophysiology of GERD, most of our knowledge regarding the neural pathways involved in the reflex arc of the TLESRs is derived from animal studies. However, it is assumed that TLESRs in humans follow similar pathways.

Association between gastroesophageal reflux and transient lower esophageal sphincter relaxations

Transient LES relaxations are considered to be the main mechanism leading to gastroesophageal reflux in GERD patients. However, the majority of the studies show a similar rate of TLESRs in healthy subjects and GERD patients [35,36]. This means that in GERD patients, there is a higher percentage of TLESRs which not only vent air but are also associated with gastroesophageal reflux. Therefore, a different underlying mechanism is necessary which results in this loss of discrimination between air and liquid by the LES.

In GERD patients, a slightly higher transsphincteric pressure gradient is present before and during a TLESR when compared to healthy subjects [37]. More importantly, the pressure gradient is greater during TLESRs accompanied by acid reflux compared to TLESRs without acid reflux. Another proposed contributing factor is EGJ compliance, also known as EGJ distensibility. GERD patients are characterized by an increase in EGJ compliance which could explain the loss of discrimination between air and liquids [38]. Furthermore, EGJ compliance in GERD patients with hiatal hernia is increased compared to GERD patients without hiatal hernia [39]. Obesity is associated with an increased rate of TLESRs as well as with an increased association of TLESRs with gastroesophageal reflux [40]. In addition, a higher pressure gradient has been measured during TLESRs in obese subjects compared to normal-weight subjects. The influence of different nutritional factors on the association of TLESRs and reflux as well as the rate of TLESRs has been extensively studied. However, no correlation between reflux-associated TLESRs or an influence on the rate of TLESRs has been demonstrated.

Hiatal hernia

In 1971, Cohen and Harris published a paper in which they reported that reflux symptoms correlated with low LES pressure, rather than with presence of a hiatus hernia [41]. From then on, the emphasis in studies on GERD pathophysiology was on basal LES pressure. Another change took place when the phenomenon of TLESR was found to play a pivotal role [42]. The sleeve sensor that was required to record TLESRs did not allow recognition of the two distinct components of the high-pressure zone, i.e. LES and crural diaphragm. Awareness of the importance of hiatal hernia for the pathophysiology of GERD emerged again around the turn of the century. It is clear that esophageal acid exposure is greater in patients with hiatus hernia [3,43–45]. In addition, the severity of esophageal acid exposure increases with increasing size of the hernia [45,46] and esophagitis is more severe with more severe acid exposure [47]. Patients with Barrett's esophagus have the highest prevalence of hiatus hernia [48].

Hiatus hernia is not an all-or-nothing phenomenon. The so-called physiological hernia (also known as phrenic ampulla) is only present during swallowing when the esophageal shortening leads to displacement of the Z-line to a site proximal to the diaphragm. This displacement is <2 cm. A reducing hiatal hernia is a hernia which is greater than 2 cm but which is only seen during a swallow; between swallows, the Z-line is at the level of the diaphragm. A non-reducing hiatal hernia is defined as a hernia greater than 2 cm in which the Z-line does not return to its normal position between swallows. At moments at which a hiatus hernia is present, the anti-reflux effect of the crural diaphragm is exerted at the wrong spot, i.e. distal to the LES, and the effect is weakened because the hiatus is usually wider than normal. Using pull-through manometry and three-dimensional representation of the pressure profiles, Kahrilas and co-workers demonstrated in hiatus hernia patients that there are distinct intrinsic sphincter and hiatal canal pressure components, with each one exerting pressure of lower magnitude than normal. Simulating reduction of the hernia by repositioning the intrinsic sphincter back within the hiatal canal and arithmetically summing superimposed pressures resulted in calculated EGJ pressures which were practically indistinguishable from those of the control subjects [49]. Prolonged manometric studies have also made clear that mechanisms other than TLESR play a more prominent role when a hiatus hernia is present. These other mechanisms include low LES pressure, straining-induced reflux and swallow-associated reflux [3].

Even within the same patient, the mechanisms leading to reflux vary from time to time, depending on the reduced or non-reduced status of the hiatus hernia [50]. Another mechanism by which the presence of a hiatus hernia is associated with excessive esophageal acid exposure is characterized by superimposed reflux from the hiatal sac during swallowing-induced LES relaxation. This can be seen in non-reducing hiatus hernias [51, 52].

Gastric factors
Total gastric emptying
It is tempting to speculate that delayed gastric emptying is an important factor in the pathogenesis of GERD. However, the evidence for this hypothesis appears to be controversial.

Numerous studies have observed delayed gastric emptying in a proportion of GERD patients compared to healthy controls [53] and only a few studies reported no difference. However, no correlation between esophageal acid exposure time and delayed gastric emptying could be proven [54]. Furthermore, acceleration of gastric emptying by cisapride was not associated with a decrease in esophageal acid exposure or with the number of reflux events [55]. Studies investigating the association between gastroesophageal reflux and gastric emptying are limited by measuring acidic reflux episodes only. To our knowledge, no study has been published which assesses the influence of gastric emptying on weakly acidic reflux episodes.

Emptying of the proximal stomach

Over the last few decades, the role of the proximal stomach in the pathogenesis of GERD has gained much attention since TLESRs are triggered by distension of the proximal stomach and the refluxate is located in the proximal stomach as well. The motor response of the proximal stomach to a meal is characterized by a relaxation followed by a gradual recovery of gastric tone. It has been found that GERD patients are characterized by a delayed recovery of proximal gastric tone after a meal compared to healthy controls [56]. Furthermore, emptying from the proximal stomach, but not the distal stomach, was significantly delayed in GERD patients compared to healthy controls.

Slow proximal emptying shows a correlation with increased esophageal acid exposure time [57]. Furthermore, the number of acidic reflux episodes correlates with proximal gastric retention [58]. Thus, in contrast to gastric emptying of the whole stomach, delayed emptying of the proximal stomach appears to be a factor in the pathogenesis of GERD. In theory, delayed emptying of the proximal stomach could cause an altered position of the postprandial acid pocket (see below) and influence the association of TLESRs with reflux. However, this hypothesis remains to be proven.

Acid pocket

Until recently it was assumed that gastric acid secreted after a meal is instantly mixed with the ingested food into one homogeneous mixture. The buffering effect of many food constituents leads to a postprandial increase in gastric pH. However, Fletcher *et al.* observed that the pH in the body of the stomach was markedly higher (pH 4.7) than the pH of the esophageal refluxate (pH 1.6) [59]. In subsequent pull-through pH studies, they identified a pocket of unbuffered gastric acid which lies on top of a homogenized fatty meal. This so-called acid pocket extends from the cardia to the distal esophagus [59].

The position of the acid pocket in GERD patients differs from healthy controls, i.e. a supradiaphragmatic localization of the pocket was more frequent in patients with GERD, especially those with a large HH (Plate 1.3) [60]. Localization of the acid pocket strongly correlates with the occurrence of acid reflux. When the acid pocket is located above the diaphragm, 70–85% of all TLESRs are accompanied by acid reflux [60]. In contrast, when the acid pocket is located below the diaphragm, only 7–20% of TLESRs are accompanied by an acidic reflux episode. Even during reflux episodes which are caused by mechanisms other than TLESRs, the position of the acid pocket is still of major importance.

Effect of posture on reflux

Body position does not affect the acidity in the gastric cardia and corpus. However, the right recumbent position is associated with an increase in acid exposure time in the distal esophagus compared to the left recumbent position [61]. This is due to an increase in reflux episodes, TLESRs and TLESRs associated with reflux [20]. The duration of reflux episodes is not affected by body position.

Obesity

Overall, the weight of the evidence suggests that obesity and GERD are related. When dissected to individual aspects of the disease, there are areas of controversy. For instance, the results of studies on esophageal acid exposure – as measured with 24-h pH monitoring – in obesity are not entirely unequivocal [40,62–72]. Recent data indicate that the proximal esophageal extent of the refluxate is higher in obese subjects [73]. It is likely that, in the obese, waist circumference is a more important determinant of excessive reflux [65,66].

There are relatively few studies on LES function in the obese. The limited data available suggest that basal LES pressures in the morbidly obese are similar to those of ideal body weight [74]. However, obesity is associated with an increased incidence of TLESRs, the association being present for increased Body Mass Index (BMI) as well as waist circumference [40].

Hiatal hernia is found more often in patients with obesity than in subjects with a normal BMI [75,76]. Increased intragastric pressure may promote the development of hiatus hernia by applying an axial pressure strain through the diaphragm [77].

Apart from promoting the development of hiatus hernia, the increased intragastric pressure found in the obese tends to promote reflux. Especially during inspiration, increased intragastric pressure and the gastroesophageal pressure gradient are correlated with increased BMI. The changes noted above are more strongly correlated with waist circumference.

In summary, obese subjects are more likely to have a high incidence of TLESRs, a hiatal hernia, increased intragastric pressure, and an increased gastroesophageal pressure gradient. These factors all facilitate reflux. A positive association between reflux symptoms and BMI was found in more than a dozen studies. Two metaanalyses incorporating these studies confirmed the existence of such an association and found the risk of having reflux symptoms in the overweight and obese to be 43–94% higher than in normal-weight subjects [66,78]. In a study in women, a BMI $> 30\,\mathrm{kg/m^2}$ was associated with a threefold increase in the odds of having frequent reflux symptoms [79].

Despite the equivocal nature of the evidence for increased gastroesophageal reflux in the obese, a metaanalysis showed a statistically significant increase in the risk for esophageal lesions with increasing weight. A BMI greater than $25\,\mathrm{kg/m^2}$ had an odds ratio of 1.76 for erosive esophagitis and 2.02 for esophageal adenocarcinoma, compared with patients with normal weight [78]. Four prospective multicenter, randomized, double-blind trials comparing esomeprazole and other proton pump inhibitors found a weak but statistically significant increased risk for Los Angeles grades C and D esophagitis, but not grades A and B, in the obese [80]. In a case–control study that evaluated cases with Barrett's esophagus and two control groups (normal-weight patients and patients with GERD but without Barrett's esophagus), abdominal diameter was found to be an independent risk factor for Barrett's esophagus. There was no association between Barrett's esophagus and BMI [66].

Studies on the effect of weight loss obtained by non-surgical methods on reflux symptoms, endoscopic findings or pH monitoring have yielded somewhat disappointing results [81,82]. However, when studies describing surgically achieved weight loss are also taken into account, a positive conclusion can be drawn [83].

Mechanisms involved in perception of reflux

With the development of new techniques it has become clear that esophageal acid exposure is not the only factor involved in the generation of reflux symptoms, and that mechanisms altering the perception of gastroesophageal reflux must have an effect.

The addition of ambulatory pH measurement to the diagnostic armamentarium made it possible to not only quantify the severity of esophageal acid exposure, but also to assess the temporal relation between symptoms and acid reflux episodes. In order to describe this relationship between gastroesophageal reflux and symptoms, several tools have been developed. The one considered to have the fewest shortcomings is the Symptom Association Probability (SAP), proposed by Weusten *et al*. [84]. To calculate the SAP, the 24-h pH measurement is divided into 2-min time frames and the occurrence of reflux in these periods and in the 2-min time frame preceding the moments of symptom onset is noted. Thereafter the probability that symptoms are associated with reflux is calculated. The SAP is considered to be positive once it is >95%.

Using the SAP, it has become apparent that esophageal acid exposure is not closely related with the number of reflux symptoms experienced by the patient and that acid exposure and positive symptom-reflux associations are largely independent phenomena [85]. This is in contrast to the finding that as the severity of esophageal acid exposure increases, this is accompanied by an increasing severity of erosions [47]. When a patient's esophagus is exposed to physiological acid reflux and there is no correlation between symptoms and the reflux episodes (negative SAP), he or she is classified as having "functional heartburn." When physiological reflux is present and bothersome reflux symptoms appear to be correlated with that reflux, the patient is considered to have a "hypersensitive esophagus." In patients with pathological esophageal acid reflux, the distribution between those with a positive and a negative SAP is not different from the distribution in patients with physiological esophageal acid exposure, suggesting that symptom generation is mostly independent of the severity of the reflux [85].

Intraluminal factors influencing perception and thereby symptom generation include several reflux characteristics. First, reflux episodes preceded by a higher cumulative acid exposure time are more likely to be perceived. The difference in cumulative acid exposure time between symptomatic and asymptomatic reflux episodes is apparent for up to 75 min [86]. Furthermore, symptomatic reflux episodes have a higher median proximal extent and a longer median duration [87]. However, it must be considered that there is an overlap in proximal extent between symptomatic and asymptomatic reflux episodes and therefore an individual threshold above which a reflux episode will always be symptomatic cannot be established.

Non-acid reflux

The introduction of combined pH and impedance monitoring broadened the spectrum of gastroesophageal reflux since the technique allows further characterization of reflux episodes according to acidity and composition (liquid or mixed liquid-gas). By the addition of impedance, reflux episodes without a pH drop that would have been missed with a conventional ambulatory pH measurement can be detected. Thereby the new phenomenon of non-acid reflux emerged. Whereas it was long felt to be unlikely that non-acid reflux can provoke symptoms, results of a perfusion study carried out two decades ago had indicated that non-acid solutions with pH up to 6 exacerbate symptoms in around 50% of subjects [88]. We now know that esophageal exposure to non-acid gastric content is a possible explanation for the persistence of symptoms after adequate acid-suppressive therapy.

Using impedance measurement, it has been shown that acid suppression with a proton pump inhibitor (PPI) reduces neither the total number of reflux events nor their proximal extent. Rather, PPI treatment decreases the number of acid reflux in favor of weakly acidic (nadir pH between 4 and 7) and alkaline (nadir pH > 7) reflux [89].

Non-acid reflux proved to be responsible for 15% of symptomatic reflux episodes in patients off PPI [86]. In patients on PPI therapy presenting with persistent reflux symptoms, 37% of subjects showed a positive Symptom Index (SI) for non-acid reflux. This emphasizes the possible role of impedance measurement in identifying this subgroup of patients who could benefit from additional therapy aimed at reducing the absolute number of reflux events (TLESR inhibitors, fundoplication) [90]. The most interesting finding made with impedance monitoring is that the majority of patients with persisting symptoms under PPI therapy show a negative symptom index for acid and non-acid reflux, suggesting an erroneous initial diagnosis and supporting the possibility of stopping PPI therapy.

As mentioned, the composition of the refluxate differs, with about half of total reflux episodes being completely liquid and half having a gaseous component, which is similar in GERD patients and healthy volunteers. However, the reflux episodes causing symptoms in NERD patients more often contain a gaseous component [91].

Dilated intercellular spaces

The mechanical barrier that lies between luminal acid gastric content and esophageal nociceptors is the esophageal epithelium. The human esophageal epithelium is a stratified squamous epithelium consisting of three layers: the upper layer is the stratum corneum or so-called functional layer, below which lies the stratum spinosum or prickle cell layer. Finally, on the serosal side of the epithelium, the stratum basale is located. A functional epithelial barrier function is maintained by desmosomes and tight junctions. Desmosomes enable strong cell-to-cell adhesion by linking cell surface adhesion proteins to intracellular keratin cytoskeletons. They are present throughout the three layers of esophageal epithelium but are most frequently located in the prickle cell layer [92]. In addition, tight junctions seal the intercellular space and prevent the paracellular diffusion of fluid and small molecules.

Several histopathological changes in the esophageal epithelium of GERD patients have been described, such as thickening of the basal cell layer, elongation of mucosal papillae [93] and dilated intercellular spaces (DIS) [94]. Since Tobey *et al.* first described DIS in NERD patients [95], the phenomenon has been extensively studied and proposed as a possible key mediator of symptom generation in GERD patients. DIS can be seen as a dysfunction of the epithelial barrier function, enabling the diffusion of fluid and acid molecules into the intercellular space and allowing them to reach and activate chemosensitive nociceptors in the underlying layers [96].

Several studies have assessed DIS in human esophageal biopsy samples, some of which used transmission electron microscopy (TEM), allowing accurate measurement of the intercellular space (Figure 1.2) [95,97,98]. These studies found that the mean diameter of intercellular spaces in NERD patients (1.0–2.2 μm) is at least twice that in healthy controls (0.45–0.56 μm) [99]. This suggests that DIS measurement by TEM in biopsies is a useful tool to confirm the otherwise difficult diagnosis of NERD. However, TEM is expensive and time-consuming and therefore it does not seem

(a)   (b)

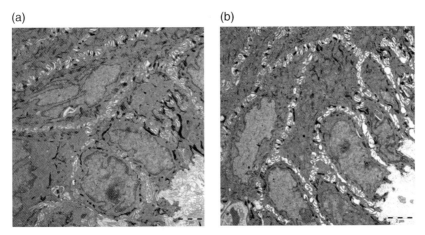

Figure 1.2 Transmission electron microscopy image of the basal layer of rat esophageal mucosa. (a) Normal morphology. (b) Dilated intercellular spaces in a rat treated with a moderate stressor.

easily applicable in clinical practice. Multiple studies have tried to measure intercellular space diameters using the more accessible technique of light microscopy (LM) [100,101]. However, the results regarding the variability between TEM and LM are conflicting and the correlation between measurements performed by the two techniques does not seem to be very promising [102,103].

The exact mechanism responsible for the generation of DIS has not been elucidated. Since exposure of esophageal mucosa to gastric contents was the first logical explanation, *in vitro* and *in vivo* studies have primarily focused on their relation with DIS.

Exposure of rabbit esophagus to an acidic solution with pH 1.1 causes no macroscopic erosions but shows clear DIS under TEM, which is accompanied by a drop in epithelial resistance and an increase of esophageal permeability to small molecules [104]. The addition of pepsin to an acidic solution further increased the rate of DIS, but the effect was only present with pH <3 [105]. Besides acid and pepsin, bile acids are other potentially harmful erosive components of gastric content. Exposure of rabbit esophageal mucosa to bile acids can cause the generation of DIS in both acidic and weakly acidic conditions [106]. This is in contrast to the earlier finding that biopsies of GERD patients with and without duodenal reflux exposure show a similar amount of DIS [97].

The concept of DIS generation in response to acid and acid-pepsin proved to hold *in vivo*, in a model where infusion of acid and acid-pepsin solutions in the distal esophagus was followed by the direct assessment of DIS in biopsy samples by TEM [107]. The concept of acid exposure generating DIS is corroborated by the fact that DIS recovered after 3 months of acid suppressive therapy [108]. Subsequently, the effect of weakly acidic solutions and bile salts on DIS was studied and proved to be present in a similar *in vivo* model [106]. An interesting finding in this study is that although these solutions provoked DIS, the majority of subjects did not experience heartburn. This supports the hypothesis that symptom generation is multifactorial and DIS is not the only determinant of symptoms.

Next to luminal effects, there are indications that systemic factors play a role in the generation of DIS. The predominant location of DIS in the basal layer of the epithelium, and the less pronounced presence in the more directly exposed prickle cell and functional layers, suggests that circulating agents such as cytokines exert a systemic effect, possibly in response to the aggressive luminal contents. Furthermore, it has been shown that acute stress increases the perception of heartburn in GERD patients [109] and acute stress enhances the effect of acid-pepsin on DIS and the permeability to small molecules in a rat model [110].

Visceral hypersensitivity

Visceral hypersensitivity is an established concept in inflammatory and functional gastrointestinal disorders, where patients have a heightened perception of various stimuli in the gastrointestinal tract [111]. This reduced pain threshold to mechanical, chemical, thermal or electrical stimuli is considered to be caused by a combination of peripheral sensitization, central sensitization and interactions between the neural and immune systems [112]. The previously mentioned finding that stress influences patients' heartburn perception suggests a similar role for visceral hypersensitivity in the pathophysiology of GERD. Peripheral nociceptors in the esophagus express several cation channels, of which the most relevant for GERD are cation channels sensitive to a low pH, like acid-sensitive ion channels (ASICs) 1–3, ionotropic purinergic (P2X) receptors and the transient receptor potential (TRP) channels. TRPV1, a member of the TRP family, has been shown to be upregulated in the esophageal mucosa of patients with esophagitis and NERD [113,114]. Sensitization of peripheral neurons occurs once the signaling threshold of these channels reduces in response to continuous noxious stimulation. A possible mechanism of sensitization in GERD is through direct contact of these channels with H+ by the presence of DIS and subsequent acidification of the intercellular space or via indirect signaling by cytokines released in response to the exposure of epithelium to aggressive gastric contents.

Central sensitization occurs once repetitive firing from the peripheral neurons leads to triggering of intercellular changes in the spinal dorsal horn neurons responsible for central signal transduction of nociceptors. This in turn leads to amplified responses to peripheral stimuli and also to triggering of adjacent spinal neurons, giving rise to hypersensitivity of more remote areas such as the chest wall [115].

Sustained esophageal contractions

Another mechanism proposed as a mediator in the perception of reflux episodes is the phenomenon of sustained esophageal contractions (SEC). Using high-frequency endoscopic ultrasonography, intermittent thickening of the esophageal wall can be observed, representing a sustained contraction of the longitudinal muscle. SECs preceded 70% of heartburn symptoms during ambulatory ultrasonography combined with a pH measurement and accompanied 75% of provoked heartburn symptoms during a Bernstein test [116]. SECs were also found to correlate with symptoms in patients with unexplained chest pain [117]. The findings suggest a role of SECs in the pathophysiology of esophageal pain perception, although it should be noted that all findings were obtained in a small number of patients. Furthermore, the concept cannot explain the entire spectrum of symptom generation since the majority of SECs do not cause symptoms and 30% of heartburn symptoms are not accompanied by a SEC [116].

Genetic factors

The observation that reflux symptoms are often clustered in families prompted a search for genetic factors that might play a role in GERD. An association was found between GERD and the heterozygous genotype of the C825T allele of the G-protein B3 subunit, coding for a receptor frequently present in the neural brain-gut axis which is associated with intracellular cell transduction [118]. The polymorphism had previously been associated with visceral hypersensitivity in functional dyspepsia. The association was specifically present in patients with a "hypersensitive esophagus," suggesting a genetic predisposition to visceral hypersensitivity in GERD.

Summary

Gastroesophageal reflux disease is a multifactorial disorder and although many aspects of the pathophysiology have been described, parts remain to be elucidated. The pathophysiology comprises factors that determine the exposure of the esophageal mucosa to gastric contents, and factors that influence the esophageal sensitivity and thereby alter the perception of reflux. The esophageal exposure to gastric contents is dependent on reflux mechanisms as TLESRs, LES hypotension and the presence of an anatomical disruption of the normal anti-reflux barrier, i.e. a hiatal hernia. Additionally, reflux is facilitated by gastric factors such as delayed emptying of the proximal stomach and an altered position of the acid pocket. Obesity leads to an increased severity of gastroesophageal reflux by influencing several of these mechanisms.

The fact that esophageal acid exposure and symptom generation are mainly independent phenomena has led to the understanding that sensitivity of the esophagus and perception of reflux are equally important in the pathophysiology of GERD. Characteristics of the reflux episode itself, such as proximal extent, duration and the composition of the refluxate, can lead to increased perception. Suggested changes at the esophageal level contributing to an increased perception of reflux are the presence of dilated intercellular spaces and visceral hypersensitivity. Lastly, genetic mutations could predispose to visceral hypersensitivity and thereby to reflux perception in GERD.

References

1 GI Motility online. Available from: www.nature.com/gimo/index.html.
2 Sloan S, Rademaker AW, Kahrilas PJ. Determinants of gastroesophageal junction incompetence: hiatal hernia, lower esophageal sphincter, or both? Ann Intern Med 1992;117(12):977–82.
3 Van Herwaarden MA, Samsom M, Smout AJ. Excess gastroesophageal reflux in patients with hiatus hernia is caused by mechanisms other than transient LES relaxations. Gastroenterology 2000;119(6):1439–46.
4 Pouderoux P, Verdier E, Kahrilas PJ. Patterns of esophageal inhibition during swallowing, pharyngeal stimulation, and transient LES relaxation. Lower esophageal sphincter. Am J Physiol Gastrointest Liver Physiol 2003;284(2):G242–7.
5 Schoeman MN, Holloway RH. Integrity and characteristics of secondary oesophageal peristalsis in patients with gastro-oesophageal reflux disease. Gut 1995;36(4):499–504.
6 Mittal RK, Chiareli C, Liu J, Shaker R. Characteristics of lower esophageal sphincter relaxation induced by pharyngeal stimulation with minute amounts of water. Gastroenterology 1996;111(2):378–84.
7 Wyman JB, Dent J, Heddle R, Dodds WJ, Toouli J, Downton J. Control of belching by the lower oesophageal sphincter. Gut 1990;31(6):639–46.
8 Dent J, Dodds WJ, Friedman RH, *et al.* Mechanism of gastroesophageal reflux in recumbent asymptomatic human subjects. J Clin Invest 1980;65(2):256–67.
9 Holloway RH, Penagini R, Ireland AC. Criteria for objective definition of transient lower esophageal sphincter relaxation. Am J Physiol 1995;268(1 Pt 1):G128–33.
10 Holloway RH, Boeckxstaens GE, Penagini R, Sifrim D, Smout A, Ruth M. T1229 objective definition and detection of transient lower esophageal relaxation revisited: is there room for improvement? Gastroenterology 2009;136(5, Suppl 1):A-527.
11 Franzi SJ, Martin CJ, Cox MR, Dent J. Response of canine lower esophageal sphincter to gastric distension. Am J Physiol 1990;259(3 Pt 1):G380–5.
12 Straathof JWA, van Veen MM, Masclee AAM. Provocation of transient lower esophageal sphincter relaxations during continuous gastric distension. Scand J Gastroenterol 2002;37(10):1140–3.

13 Scheffer RCH, Akkermans LMA, Bais JE, Roelofs JMM, Smout AJPM, Gooszen HG. Elicitation of transient lower oesophageal sphincter relaxations in response to gastric distension and meal ingestion. Neurogastroenterol Motil 2002;14(6):647–55.

14 Mittal RK, Holloway RH, Penagini R, Blackshaw LA, Dent J. Transient lower esophageal sphincter relaxation. Gastroenterology 1995;109(2):601–10.

15 Mittal RK, Fisher MJ. Electrical and mechanical inhibition of the crural diaphragm during transient relaxation of the lower esophageal sphincter. Gastroenterology 1990;99(5):1265–8.

16 Shi G, Pandolfino JE, Joehl RJ, Brasseur JG, Kahrilas PJ. Distinct patterns of oesophageal shortening during primary peristalsis, secondary peristalsis and transient lower oesophageal sphincter relaxation. Neurogastroenterol Motil 2002;14(5):505–12.

17 Babaei A, Bhargava V, Korsapati H, Zheng WH, Mittal RK. A unique longitudinal muscle contraction pattern associated with transient lower esophageal sphincter relaxation. Gastroenterology 2008;134(5):1322–31.

18 Kuribayashi S, Massey BT, Hafeezullah M, et al. Terminating motor events for TLESR are influenced by the presence and distribution of refluxate. Am J Physiol Gastrointest Liver Physiol 2009;297(1):G71–5.

19 Holloway RH, Kocyan P, Dent J. Provocation of transient lower esophageal sphincter relaxations by meals in patients with symptomatic gastroesophageal reflux. Dig Dis Sci 1991;36(8):1034–9.

20 Van Herwaarden MA, Katzka DA, Smout AJ, Samsom M, Gideon M, Castell DO. Effect of different recumbent positions on postprandial gastroesophageal reflux in normal subjects. Am J Gastroenterol 2000;95(10):2731–6.

21 Freidin N, Fisher MJ, Taylor W, et al. Sleep and nocturnal acid reflux in normal subjects and patients with reflux oesophagitis. Gut 1991;32(11):1275–9.

22 Martin CJ, Patrikios J, Dent J. Abolition of gas reflux and transient lower esophageal sphincter relaxation by vagal blockade in the dog. Gastroenterology 1986; 91(4):890–6.

23 Kalia M, Mesulam MM. Brain stem projections of sensory and motor components of the vagus complex in the cat: II. Laryngeal, tracheobronchial, pulmonary, cardiac, and gastrointestinal branches. J Comp Neurol 1980;193(2):467–508.

24 Rinaman L, Card JP, Schwaber JS, Miselis RR. Ultrastructural demonstration of a gastric monosynaptic vagal circuit in the nucleus of the solitary tract in rat. J Neurosci 1989;9(6):1985–96.

25 Rossiter CD, Norman WP, Jain M, Hornby PJ, Benjamin S, Gillis RA. Control of lower esophageal sphincter pressure by two sites in dorsal motor nucleus of the vagus. Am J Physiol 1990;259(6 Pt 1):G899–906.

26 Niedringhaus M, Jackson PG, Evans SRT, Verbalis JG, Gillis RA, Sahibzada N. Dorsal motor nucleus of the vagus: a site for evoking simultaneous changes in crural diaphragm activity, lower esophageal sphincter pressure, and fundus tone. Am J Physiol Regul Integr Comp Physiol 2008;294(1):R121–31.

27 Young RL, Page AJ, Cooper NJ, Frisby CL, Blackshaw LA. Sensory and motor innervation of the crural diaphragm by the vagus nerves. Gastroenterology 2010;138(3):1091–101.

28 Yuan S, Costa M, Brookes SJ. Neuronal pathways and transmission to the lower esophageal sphincter of the guinea pig. Gastroenterology 1998;115(3):661–71.

29 Kessing BF, Conchillo JM, Bredenoord AJ, Smout AJPM, Masclee AAM. Review article: the clinical relevance of transient lower oesophageal sphincter relaxations in gastro-oesophageal reflux disease. Aliment Pharmacol Ther 2011;33(6):650–61.

30 Yuan CS, Liu D, Attele AS. GABAergic effects on nucleus tractus solitarius neurons receiving gastric vagal inputs. J Pharmacol Exp Ther 1998;286(2):736–41.

31 Blackshaw LA, Smid SD, O'Donnell TA, Dent J. GABA(B) receptor-mediated effects on vagal pathways to the lower oesophageal sphincter and heart. Br J Pharmacol 2000;130(2):279–88.

32 Cartmell J, Schoepp DD. Regulation of neurotransmitter release by metabotropic glutamate receptors. J Neurochem 2000;75(3):889–907.

33 Young RL, Page AJ, O'Donnell TA, Cooper NJ, Blackshaw LA. Peripheral versus central modulation of gastric vagal pathways by metabotropic glutamate receptor 5. Am J Physiol Gastrointest Liver Physiol 2007;292(2):G501–11.

34 Van Sickle MD, Oland LD, Ho W, *et al.* Cannabinoids inhibit emesis through CB1 receptors in the brainstem of the ferret. Gastroenterology 2001;121(4):767–74.

35 Bredenoord AJ, Weusten BLAM, Timmer R, Smout AJPM. Gastro-oesophageal reflux of liquids and gas during transient lower oesophageal sphincter relaxations. Neurogastroenterol Motil 2006;18(10):888–93.

36 Sifrim D, Holloway R. Transient lower esophageal sphincter relaxations: how many or how harmful? Am J Gastroenterol 2001;96(9):2529–32.

37 Frankhuisen R, van Herwaarden MA, Scheffer RC, Hebbard GS, Gooszen HG, Samsom M. Increased intragastric pressure gradients are involved in the occurrence of acid reflux in gastroesophageal reflux disease. Scand J Gastroenterol 2009;44(5):545–50.

38 Pandolfino JE, Shi G, Curry J, Joehl RJ, Brasseur JG, Kahrilas PJ. Esophagogastric junction distensibility: a factor contributing to sphincter incompetence. Am J Physiol Gastrointest Liver Physiol 2002;282(6):G1052–8.

39 Pandolfino JE, Shi G, Trueworthy B, Kahrilas PJ. Esophagogastric junction opening during relaxation distinguishes nonhernia reflux patients, hernia patients, and normal subjects. Gastroenterology 2003;125(4):1018–24.

40 Wu JCY, Mui LM, Cheung CMY, Chan Y, Sung JJY. Obesity is associated with increased transient lower esophageal sphincter relaxation. Gastroenterology 2007;132(3):883–9.

41 Cohen S, Harris LD. Does hiatus hernia affect competence of the gastroesophageal sphincter? N Engl J Med 1971 13;284(19):1053–6.

42 Dodds WJ, Dent J, Hogan WJ, *et al.* Mechanisms of gastroesophageal reflux in patients with reflux esophagitis. N Engl J Med 1982;307(25):1547–52.

43 Kasapidis P, Vassilakis JS, Tzovaras G, Chrysos E, Xynos E. Effect of hiatal hernia on esophageal manometry and pH-metry in gastroesophageal reflux disease. Dig Dis Sci 1995;40(12):2724–30.

44 Mattioli S, d'Ovidio F, di Simone MP, *et al.* Clinical and surgical relevance of the progressive phases of intrathoracic migration of the gastroesophageal junction in gastroesophageal reflux disease. J Thorac Cardiovasc Surg 1998;116(2):267–75.

45 Jones MP, Sloan SS, Jovanovic B, Kahrilas PJ. Impaired egress rather than increased access: an important independent predictor of erosive oesophagitis. Neurogastroenterol Motil 2002;14(6):625–31.

46 Patti MG, Goldberg HI, Arcerito M, Bortolasi L, Tong J, Way LW. Hiatal hernia size affects lower esophageal sphincter function, esophageal acid exposure, and the degree of mucosal injury. Am J Surg 1996;171(1):182–6.

47 Berstad A, Weberg R, Frøyshov Larsen I, Hoel B, Hauer-Jensen M. Relationship of hiatus hernia to reflux oesophagitis. A prospective study of coincidence, using endoscopy. Scand J Gastroenterol 1986;21(1):55–8.

48 Cameron AJ. Barrett's esophagus: prevalence and size of hiatal hernia. Am J Gastroenterol 1999;94(8):2054–9.

49 Kahrilas PJ, Lin S, Chen J, Manka M. The effect of hiatus hernia on gastro-oesophageal junction pressure. Gut 1999;44(4):476–82.

50 Bredenoord AJ, Weusten BLAM, Timmer R, Smout AJPM. Characteristics of gastro-esophageal reflux in symptomatic patients with and without excessive esophageal acid exposure. Am J Gastroenterol 2006;101(11):2470–5.

51 Mittal RK, Lange RC, McCallum RW. Identification and mechanism of delayed esophageal acid clearance in subjects with hiatus hernia. Gastroenterology 1987;92(1):130–5.

52 Sloan S, Kahrilas PJ. Impairment of esophageal emptying with hiatal hernia. Gastroenterology 1991;100(3):596–605.

53 McCallum RW, Berkowitz DM, Lerner E. Gastric emptying in patients with gastro-esophageal reflux. Gastroenterology 1981;80(2):285–91.

54 Shay SS, Eggli D, McDonald C, Johnson LF. Gastric emptying of solid food in patients with gastroesophageal reflux. Gastroenterology 1987;92(2):459–65.

55 Carmagnola S, Fraquelli M, Cantù P, Conte D, Penagini R. Relationship between acceleration of gastric emptying and oesophageal acid exposure in patients with endoscopy-negative gastro-oesophageal reflux disease. Scand J Gastroenterol 2006;41(7):767–72.

56 Penagini R, Mangano M, Bianchi PA. Effect of increasing the fat content but not the energy load of a meal on gastro-oesophageal reflux and lower oesophageal sphincter motor function. Gut 1998;42(3):330–3.

57 Stacher G, Lenglinger J, Bergmann H, et al. Gastric emptying: a contributory factor in gastro-oesophageal reflux activity? Gut 2000;47(5):661–6.

58 Herculano JRL Jr, Troncon LE, Aprile LR, et al. Diminished retention of food in the proximal stomach correlates with increased acidic reflux in patients with gastro-esophageal reflux disease and dyspeptic symptoms. Dig Dis Sci 2004;49(5):750–6.

59 Fletcher J, Wirz A, Young J, Vallance R, McColl KE. Unbuffered highly acidic gastric juice exists at the gastroesophageal junction after a meal. Gastroenterology 2001;121(4):775–83.

60 Beaumont H, Bennink RJ, de Jong J, Boeckxstaens GE. The position of the acid pocket as a major risk factor for acidic reflux in healthy subjects and patients with GORD. Gut 2010;59(4):441–51.

61 Katz LC, Just R, Castell DO. Body position affects recumbent postprandial reflux. J Clin Gastroenterol 1994;18(4):280–3.

62 Wajed SA, Streets CG, Bremner CG, DeMeester TR. Elevated body mass disrupts the barrier to gastroesophageal reflux; discussion 1018-9. Arch Surg 2001;136(9):1014–18.

63 Hong D, Khajanchee YS, Pereira N, Lockhart B, Patterson EJ, Swanstrom LL. Manometric abnormalities and gastroesophageal reflux disease in the morbidly obese. Obes Surg 2004;14(6):744–9.

64 Suter M, Dorta G, Giusti V, Calmes JM. Gastro-esophageal reflux and esophageal motility disorders in morbidly obese patients. Obes Surg 2004;14(7):959–66.

65 El-Serag HB, Ergun GA, Pandolfino J, Fitzgerald S, Tran T, Kramer JR. Obesity increases oesophageal acid exposure. Gut 2007;56(6):749–55.

66 Corley DA. Obesity and the rising incidence of oesophageal and gastric adenocar-cinoma: what is the link? Gut 2007;56(11):1493–4.

67 Crowell MD, Bradley A, Hansel S, et al. Obesity is associated with increased 48-h esophageal acid exposure in patients with symptomatic gastroesophageal reflux. Am J Gastroenterol 2009;104(3):553–9.

68 Räihä I, Impivaara O, Seppälä M, Knuts LR, Sourander L. Determinants of symptoms suggestive of gastroesophageal reflux disease in the elderly. Scand J Gastroenterol 1993;28(11):1011–14.

69 Chang CS, Poon SK, Lien HC, Chen GH. The incidence of reflux esophagitis among the Chinese. Am J Gastroenterol 1997;92(4):668–71.

70 Jaffin BW, Knoepflmacher P, Greenstein R. High prevalence of asymptomatic esophageal motility disorders among morbidly obese patients. Obes Surg 1999;9(4):390–5.

71 Lagergren J, Bergström R, Nyrén O. No relation between body mass and gastro-oesophageal reflux symptoms in a Swedish population based study. Gut 2000;47(1):26–9.

72 Talley NJ, Howell S, Poulton R. Obesity and chronic gastrointestinal tract symptoms in young adults: a birth cohort study. Am J Gastroenterol 2004;99(9):1807–14.

73 Blondeau K, van Oudenhove L, Farré R, et al. T1682 increasing body weight is associated with a higher incidence and proximal extent of reflux in patients with GERD Both 'on' and 'off' PPI therapy. Gastroenterology 2010;138(5, Suppl 1):S-556.

74 O'Brien TF Jr. Lower esophageal sphincter pressure (LESP) and esophageal function in obese humans. J Clin Gastroenterol 1980;2(2):145–8.

75 Stene-Larsen G, Weberg R, Frøyshov Larsen I, Bjørtuft O, Hoel B, Berstad A. Relationship of overweight to hiatus hernia and reflux oesophagitis. Scand J Gastroenterol 1988;23(4):427–32.

76 Wilson LJ, Ma W, Hirschowitz BI. Association of obesity with hiatal hernia and esophagitis. Am J Gastroenterol 1999;94(10):2840–4.

77 Pandolfino JE, El-Serag HB, Zhang Q, Shah N, Ghosh SK, Kahrilas PJ. Obesity: a challenge to esophagogastric junction integrity. Gastroenterology 2006;130(3):639–49.

78 Hampel H, Abraham NS, El-Serag HB. Meta-analysis: obesity and the risk for gastroesophageal reflux disease and its complications. Ann Intern Med 2005 2; 143(3):199–211.

79 Jacobson BC, Somers SC, Fuchs CS, Kelly CP, Camargo CA Jr. Body-mass index and symptoms of gastroesophageal reflux in women. N Engl J Med 2006;354(22):2340–8.

80 El-Serag HB, Johanson JF. Risk factors for the severity of erosive esophagitis in Helicobacter pylori-negative patients with gastroesophageal reflux disease. Scand J Gastroenterol 2002;37(8):899–904.

81 Kjellin A, Ramel S, Rössner S, Thor K. Gastroesophageal reflux in obese patients is not reduced by weight reduction. Scand J Gastroenterol 1996;31(11):1047–51.

82 Mathus-Vliegen EMH, van Weeren M, van Eerten PV. Los function and obesity: the impact of untreated obesity, weight loss, and chronic gastric balloon distension. Digestion 2003;68(2–3):161–8.

83 De Groot NL, Burgerhart JS, van de Meeberg PC, de Vries DR, Smout AJPM, Siersema PD. Systematic review: the effects of conservative and surgical treatment for obesity on gastro-oesophageal reflux disease. Aliment Pharmacol Ther 2009;30(11–12):1091–102.

84 Weusten BL, Roelofs JM, Akkermans LM, van Berge-Henegouwen GP, Smout AJ. The symptom-association probability: an improved method for symptom analysis of 24-hour esophageal pH data. Gastroenterology 1994;107(6):1741–5.

85 Colas-Atger E, Bonaz B, Papillon E, et al. Relationship between acid reflux episodes and gastroesophageal reflux symptoms is very inconstant. Dig Dis Sci 2002;47(3):645–51.

86 Bredenoord AJ, Weusten BLAM, Curvers WL, Timmer R, Smout AJPM. Determinants of perception of heartburn and regurgitation. Gut 2006;55(3):313–18.

87 Weusten BL, Akkermans LM, van Berge-Henegouwen GP, Smout AJ. Symptom perception in gastroesophageal reflux disease is dependent on spatiotemporal reflux characteristics. Gastroenterology 1995;108(6):1739–44.

88 Smith JL, Opekun AR, Larkai E, Graham DY. Sensitivity of the esophageal mucosa to pH in gastroesophageal reflux disease. Gastroenterology 1989;96(3):683–9.

89 Hemmink GJM, Bredenoord AJ, Weusten BLAM, Monkelbaan JF, Timmer R, Smout AJPM. Esophageal pH-impedance monitoring in patients with therapy-resistant reflux symptoms: "on" or "off" proton pump inhibitor? Am J Gastroenterol 2008;103(10):2446–53.

90 Mainie I, Tutuian R, Shay S, *et al.* Acid and non-acid reflux in patients with persistent symptoms despite acid suppressive therapy: a multicentre study using combined ambulatory impedance-pH monitoring. Gut 2006;55(10):1398–402.

91 Emerenziani S, Sifrim D, Habib FI, *et al.* Presence of gas in the refluxate enhances reflux perception in non-erosive patients with physiological acid exposure of the oesophagus. Gut 2008;57(4):443–7.

92 Logan KR, Hopwood D, Milne G. Cellular junctions in human oesophageal epithelium. J Pathol 1978;126(3):157–63.

93 Ismail-Beigi F, Horton PF, Pope CE. Histological consequences of gastroesophageal reflux in man. Gastroenterology 1970;58(2):163–74.

94 Hopwood D, Milne G, Logan KR. Electron microscopic changes in human oesophageal epithelium in oesophagitis. J Pathol 1979;129(4):161–7.

95 Tobey NA, Carson JL, Alkiek RA, Orlando RC. Dilated intercellular spaces: a morphological feature of acid reflux-damaged human esophageal epithelium. Gastroenterology 1996;111(5):1200–5.

96 Barlow WJ, Orlando RC. The pathogenesis of heartburn in nonerosive reflux disease: a unifying hypothesis. Gastroenterology 2005;128(3):771–8.

97 Calabrese C, Fabbri A, Bortolotti M, *et al.* Dilated intercellular spaces as a marker of oesophageal damage: comparative results in gastro-oesophageal reflux disease with or without bile reflux. Aliment Pharmacol Ther 2003;18(5):525–32.

98 Caviglia R, Ribolsi M, Gentile M, *et al.* Dilated intercellular spaces and acid reflux at the distal and proximal oesophagus in patients with non-erosive gastro-oesophageal reflux disease. Aliment Pharmacol Ther 2007;25(5):629–36.

99 Van Malenstein H, Farré R, Sifrim D. Esophageal dilated intercellular spaces (DIS) and nonerosive reflux disease. Am J Gastroenterol 2008;103(4):1021–8.

100 Villanacci V, Grigolato PG, Cestari R, *et al.* Dilated intercellular spaces as markers of reflux disease: histology, semiquantitative score and morphometry upon light microscopy. Digestion 2001;64(1):1–8.

101 Zentilin P, Savarino V, Mastracci L, *et al.* Reassessment of the diagnostic value of histology in patients with GERD, using multiple biopsy sites and an appropriate control group. Am J Gastroenterol 2005;100(10):2299–306.

102 Solcia E, Villani L, Luinetti O, *et al.* Altered intercellular glycoconjugates and dilated intercellular spaces of esophageal epithelium in reflux disease. Virchows Arch 2000;436(3):207–16.

103 Cui R, Zhou L, Lin S, *et al.* The feasibility of light microscopic measurements of intercellular spaces in squamous epithelium in the lower-esophagus of GERD patients. Dis Esophagus 2011;24(1):1–5.

104 Tobey NA, Hosseini SS, Argote CM, Dobrucali AM, Awayda MS, Orlando RC. Dilated intercellular spaces and shunt permeability in nonerosive acid-damaged esophageal epithelium. Am J Gastroenterol 2004;99(1):13–22.

105 Tobey NA, Hosseini SS, Caymaz-Bor C, Wyatt HR, Orlando GS, Orlando RC. The role of pepsin in acid injury to esophageal epithelium. Am J Gastroenterol 2001;96(11):3062–70.

106 Farré R, Fornari F, Blondeau K, *et al.* Acid and weakly acidic solutions impair mucosal integrity of distal exposed and proximal non-exposed human oesophagus. Gut 2010;59(2):164–9.

107 Bove M, Vieth M, Dombrowski F, Ny L, Ruth M, Lundell L. Acid challenge to the human esophageal mucosa: effects on epithelial architecture in health and disease. Dig Dis Sci 2005;50(8):1488–96.

108 Calabrese C, Bortolotti M, Fabbri A, *et al*. Reversibility of GERD ultrastructural alterations and relief of symptoms after omeprazole treatment. Am J Gastroenterol 2005;100(3):537–42.

109 Fass R, Naliboff BD, Fass SS, *et al*. The effect of auditory stress on perception of intraesophageal acid in patients with gastroesophageal reflux disease. Gastroenterology 2008;134(3):696–705.

110 Farré R, de Vos R, Geboes K, *et al*. Critical role of stress in increased oesophageal mucosa permeability and dilated intercellular spaces. Gut 2007;56(9):1191–7.

111 Anand P, Aziz Q, Willert R, van Oudenhove L. Peripheral and central mechanisms of visceral sensitization in man. Neurogastroenterol Motil 2007;19(1 Suppl):29–46.

112 Knowles CH, Aziz Q. Visceral hypersensitivity in non-erosive reflux disease. Gut 2008;57(5):674–83.

113 Bhat YM, Bielefeldt K. Capsaicin receptor (TRPV1) and non-erosive reflux disease. Eur J Gastroenterol Hepatol 2006;18(3):263–70.

114 Guarino MPL, Cheng L, Ma J, *et al*. Increased TRPV1 gene expression in esophageal mucosa of patients with non-erosive and erosive reflux disease. Neurogastroenterol Motil 2010;22(7):746–51.

115 Sarkar S, Aziz Q, Woolf CJ, Hobson AR, Thompson DG. Contribution of central sensitisation to the development of non-cardiac chest pain. Lancet 2000;356(9236):1154–9.

116 Pehlivanov N, Liu J, Mittal RK. Sustained esophageal contraction: a motor correlate of heartburn symptom. Am J Physiol Gastrointest Liver Physiol 2001;281(3):G743–51.

117 Balaban DH, Yamamoto Y, Liu J, *et al*. Sustained esophageal contraction: a marker of esophageal chest pain identified by intraluminal ultrasonography. Gastroenterology 1999;116(1):29–37.

118 De Vries DR, ter Linde JJM, van Herwaarden MA, Smout AJPM, Samsom M. Gastroesophageal reflux disease is associated with the C825T polymorphism in the G-protein beta3 subunit gene (GNB3). Am J Gastroenterol 2009;104(2):281–5.

CHAPTER 2

Gastroesophageal Reflux Disease: Epidemiology, Impact on Quality of Life, and Health Economic Implications

Nimish Vakil

University of Wisconsin School of Medicine and Public Health, Madison, WI, USA

Key points

- Gastroesophageal reflux disease is defined as a condition which develops when the reflux of stomach contents causes troublesome symptoms and/or complications.
- Gastroesophageal reflux disease may present with many discrete syndromes defined by unique attributes or symptom complexes.
- Quality of life decreases in gastroesophageal reflux disease when heartburn occurs two or more times a week and is moderate in severity.
- Gastroesophageal reflux disease is associated with significant costs related to treatment and delivery of healthcare.
- Gastroesophageal reflux disease reduces work productivity and is associated with significant indirect costs to society.
- Treatment of gastroesophageal reflux disease is cost-effective and restores quality of life and decreases the cost of the disease.

Potential pitfalls

- Epidemiology studies are generally based on identifying patients who have heartburn once a week. These may not be patients who present in clinical practice.
- Cost-effectiveness studies on medical therapy for gastroesophageal reflux disease predate the availability of generic proton pump inhibitors.
- Cost-effectiveness studies comparing surgery and medical therapy have several limitations (costs of generic drugs not considered, long-term failure of surgery not considered, ill effects of surgery underestimated).
- Many work productivity studies are based on self-report of absenteeism and presenteeism.

Practical Manual of Gastroesophageal Reflux Disease, First Edition.
Edited by Marcelo F. Vela, Joel E. Richter and John E. Pandolfino.
© 2013 John Wiley & Sons, Ltd. Published 2013 by John Wiley & Sons, Ltd.

Introduction

A global consensus group has developed a definition of gastroesophageal reflux disease (GERD) called the Montreal definition of reflux disease [1]. The Montreal definition is the basis of guidelines and regulatory guidance for the management of GERD and is simple enough for use in clinical practice [2]. GERD is defined as a condition which develops when the reflux of stomach contents causes troublesome symptoms and/or complications [1]. Patients with typical symptoms can be diagnosed based on symptoms alone [1,2]. To aid in making a clinical diagnosis in primary care settings, simple questionnaires have been developed that can identify patients with GERD with an accuracy that is similar to that achieved by consultation with a gastroenterologist [3].

Individual reflux syndromes

A disease may have many symptoms. Symptom clusters can provide clinical syndromes with which patients may be identified. These syndromes can overlap with each other. The Montreal classification recognizes two groups of syndromes: esophageal and extraesophageal syndromes.

Esophageal and extraesophageal syndromes (Figure 2.1)

The spectrum of GERD has expanded from a primarily esophageal disorder into a group of syndromes that mirror the different manifestations of reflux disease. These are conveniently divided into esophageal and extraesophageal syndromes [1].

Esophageal syndromes: symptomatic

There are two symptomatic reflux syndromes.

1 *Typical reflux syndrome.* The typical reflux syndrome is defined by the presence of troublesome heartburn and/or regurgitation. Heartburn is defined as a burning sensation in the retrosternal area (behind the breastbone). Regurgitation is defined as the perception of flow of refluxed gastric content into the mouth or hypopharynx. The typical reflux syndrome can be diagnosed on the basis of the characteristic symptoms, without diagnostic testing.

2 *Reflux chest pain syndrome.* Gastroesophageal reflux can cause episodes of chest pain that resemble coronary ischemia. The chest pain can be indistinguishable from ischemic cardiac pain and may not be accompanied by heartburn or regurgitation.

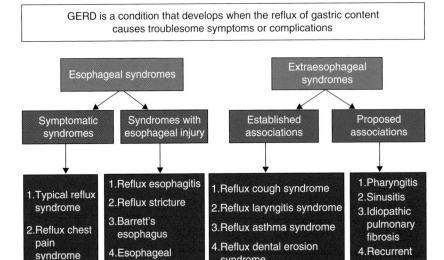

Figure 2.1 The Montreal definition and classification of GERD. Reproduced from Vakil *et al.* [1] with permission from Blackwell Publishing.

Syndromes with esophageal injury: reflux esophagitis

Reflux esophagitis is defined endoscopically by visible breaks of the distal esophageal mucosa. In clinical practice, endoscopic evidence of esophagitis is seen in less than half of patients with typical GERD symptoms. Reflux esophagitis is the most common manifestation of esophageal injury.

Syndromes with esophageal injury: Barrett's esophagus and esophageal adenocarcinoma

The Montreal group addressed two difficult areas in the definition and classification of suspected and proven Barrett's esophagus. It simplified the definition of Barrett's esophagus by stating that when biopsies of endoscopically suspected esophageal metaplasia show columnar epithelium, it should be called Barrett's esophagus and the presence or absence of intestinal-type metaplasia specified, acknowledging possible differences between the risk of cancer in patients with intestinal and gastric metaplasia. Esophageal adenocarcinoma is the most serious complication of chronic reflux disease.

Extraesophageal gastroesophageal reflux disease

The Montreal Consensus group recognized significant associations between chronic cough, chronic laryngitis, asthma, and GERD but also recognized that these disorders are usually multifactorial processes and gastroesophageal reflux may be a co-factor rather than a cause. An understanding of the various syndromes of GERD is essential for epidemiological studies in GERD.

Epidemiology of gastroesophageal reflux disease

Studies of the epidemiology of GERD have been limited by the lack of consensus as to when symptoms of heartburn or regurgitation become troublesome enough to constitute a disease. Population-based studies suggest that when symptoms of moderate intensity occur twice a week or moderate symptoms occur once a week, quality of life drops, suggesting that the symptoms become troublesome at these thresholds [1,4]. Unfortunately, epidemiological studies have used other thresholds for measurement, usually weekly symptoms of heartburn, making it difficult to extrapolate these studies to patients presenting with symptoms in clinical practice. There are geographic differences in the prevalence of reflux disease.

Two recent systematic reviews have evaluated the prevalence of reflux disease in different regions of the world [5,6]. The prevalence of GERD (as defined by heartburn and/or acid regurgitation at least weekly) in North America (19.8–20%) is similar to that in Europe (9.8–18%) [6]. The prevalence of GERD is lower in Asia (2.5–4.8%) [6]. In a UK database, the incidence of GERD is estimated to be 4–5 per 1000 patient-years [7]. Obesity, increasing age and smoking were significant risk factors. Patients who had a diagnosis of GERD had a higher incidence of a subsequent diagnosis of esophageal adenocarcinoma, esophageal stricture, chronic cough, sinusitis, and sleep problems. In this study, the mortality of subjects with a diagnosis was higher in the first year after diagnosis but not in subsequent years. An association with chronic obstructive airway disease has also been reported in other studies of the same database [7].

Children with reflux and reflux-related problems are a growing problem in many countries. A UK database found that the incidence of GERD in children was 0.84 per 1000 patient-years [8]. The incidence decreases from the age of 1 year to the age of 12 years, after which it increases again, reaching a maximum prevalence at age 16–17 years of age [8]. Children with reflux disease often continue to have symptoms as an adult [9]. A pediatric definition and classification of GERD has recently been published that should help simplify epidemiological studies [10].

Population-based studies have suggested that differences may exist between different ethnic groups with regard to the prevalence of GERD. There is a higher prevalence of reflux symptoms in Hispanic subjects compared to Caucasian subjects [11]. In a multiracial population in Malaysia, Indian ethnicity was consistently associated with reflux disease [12]. Other risk factors that have been identified in a number of studies include the presence of a hiatus hernia, a family history of reflux disease, smoking, obesity, pregnancy, and increasing age [6].

Obesity is a major risk factor for the development of reflux disease and its complications. Truncal obesity raises intragastric pressure and compromises the esophagogastric junction, increasing the likelihood of reflux in patients predisposed to this disorder [13]. In a large epidemiological study in Norway, increasing Body Mass Index (BMI) was associated with increasing GERD symptoms [14]. There was a dose–response relationship between increasing BMI and reflux symptoms in both men and women, with a significantly stronger association in women. Compared with those with a BMI less than 25, the risk of reflux was increased significantly among those with a BMI >35: men (odds ratio (OR) 3.3, 95% confidence interval (CI) 2.4–4.7) and women (OR 6.3, 95% CI 4.9–8.0).

A US case–control study showed that waist circumference but not BMI was associated with Barrett's esophagus [15]. Measures of visceral adiposity correlate best with the risk of cancer in Barrett's esophagus. Patients with a high waist-hip ratio have approximately twice the rate of developing adenocarcinoma [16]. In a recent study of the risk of cancer in Barrett's esophagus, the adjusted odds ratios for the development of cancer was 2.4 (95% CI 1.4–3.9) for all cases, 2.8 (95% CI 1.5–5.1) for visible Barrett's esophagus, and 4.3 (95% CI 1.9–9.9) for long segment Barrett's esophagus [16].

The epidemiology of extraesophageal syndromes and their relationship with reflux disease are more difficult to assess. Studies are based on associations between asthma, laryngitis, chronic obstructive airway disease and symptoms of GERD but a causal relationship between reflux disease and the extraesophageal syndrome cannot be inferred from such studies. Patients with a diagnosis of chronic obstructive pulmonary disease (COPD) are more likely to have a diagnosis of GERD compared with individuals with no COPD diagnosis [17]. In this study, 1628 patients in the UK general practice database were identified with a first diagnosis of chronic obstructive airway disease and compared to 4391 patients with a first diagnosis of GERD. Over a 5-year follow-up, the relative risk of having GERD diagnosed among patients with a diagnosis of COPD was 1.46 (95% CI 1.19–1.78) [17].

A systematic review found a strong association between dental erosions and reflux disease, particularly in children [18]. The median prevalence of dental erosions in patients with GERD was 24% (range 5–47.5%), and 17% (range 14–87%) in children. A study of 1980 children with GERD between ages 2 and 18 showed that compared to healthy controls, children with GERD had a significant risk for extraesophageal complications of GERD. GERD was a significant risk factor for sinusitis (adjusted OR 2.3,

95% CI 1.7–3.2, $P<0.0001$), laryngitis (OR 2.6, 95% CI 1.2–5.6, $P=0.0228$), asthma (OR 1.9, 95% CI 1.6–2.3, $P<0.0001$), pneumonia (OR 2.3, 95% CI 1.8–2.9, $P<0.0001$), and bronchiectasis (OR 2.3, 95% CI 1.1–4.6, $P=0.0193$) [19].

A study that compared 8228 hospitalized patients with laryngeal cancers and 1912 with pharyngeal cancers to controls reported that GERD was a significant risk factor for the development of these cancers [20]. For outpatients, GERD was associated with an adjusted OR of 2.31 (95% CI 2.10–2.53) for laryngeal cancer and adjusted OR of 1.92 for pharyngeal cancer (95% CI 1.72–2.15).

Health-related quality of life in gastroesophageal reflux disease

Health-related quality of life (HRQOL) is defined as the patient's subjective perception of the impact of their disease and its treatment on daily life, physical, psychological and social functioning and well-being. Health-related quality of life can be measured by general scales such as the Short Form (SF)-36 and the Psychological General Well-Being Scale (PGWS). Quality of life measured by generic quality of life instruments such as the SF-36 and the PGWS is significantly reduced in patients with GERD [4,21]. There is a relationship between symptom severity and general quality of life scales [4,22]. Figure 2.2 shows the relationship between symptom severity and general quality of life as measured by the PGWS. Symptom frequency is also related to decreases in quality of life. A recent population-based study of patients with reflux symptoms found that 6% of subjects reported reflux symptoms (heartburn and/or regurgitation) daily, 14% weekly and 20% less than weekly during the previous 3 months [23]. Compared to patients with no reflux symptoms, a clinically relevant impairment of health-related quality of life ($\geq$5 points) was seen in all eight SF-36 dimensions for patients with daily symptoms and in five dimensions for patients with weekly symptoms [23]. In a study of 1011 patients with GERD in Germany and Sweden, health-related quality of life was measured using the EUROQol5. Patients with GERD had a significant impairment in quality of life and the impairment was related to the severity of symptoms [24].

Disease-specific quality of life instruments have been developed for GERD and are helpful in assessing the response to treatment. Quality of life has been assessed using the QOLRAD, a disease-specific instrument developed for reflux disease. In adolescents with GERD, quality of life is impaired and treatment with a proton pump inhibitor improves all domains of quality of life [22]. Improvements in symptoms are associated with improvements in quality of life and overall satisfaction with treatment [22].

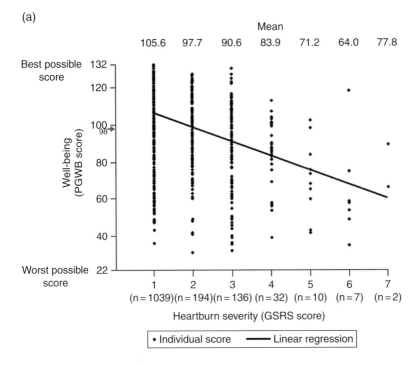

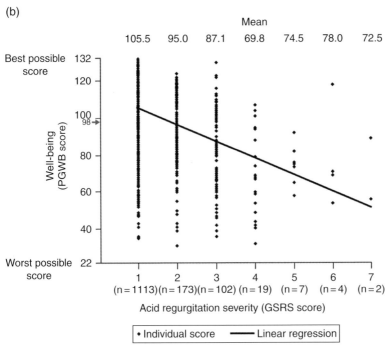

Figure 2.2 The relationship between the severity of heartburn (a) and acid regurgitation (b) measured by the score on the Gastrointestinal Symptoms Rating Scale (GSRS) and quality of life measured by the Psychological General Well-Being (PGWB) Scale. As symptom severity increases, well-being decreases. Normal values are 103 and a clinically relevant change is a decrease in 5 points to 98. Reproduced from Wiklund *et al.* [4] with permission from Blackwell Publishing.

Health economic implications

The Agency for Health Care Policy and Research has conducted a survey of the inpatient costs of treating GERD in the USA from 1998 to 2005 [25]. Hospitalizations with either a primary or secondary GERD diagnosis increased by 216% from 995,402 in 1998 to 3,141,965 in 2005. Adult hospitalizations with a primary GERD diagnosis decreased by 2.4% from 77,783 in 1998 to 75,888 in 2005. However, for pediatric GERD, stays with a primary GERD diagnosis increased by 42% for infants and by 84% for children age 2–17. Eight out of every 1000 hospitalizations with a GERD diagnosis had Barrett's esophagus. The average cost per hospital stay with a primary GERD diagnosis was $5616 in 1998 and $6545 in 2005. The total national hospital costs for all hospitalizations with a primary GERD diagnosis increased by 22% from $509 million in 1998 to $622 million in 2005 [22].

In Canada, in 2004–5, the Canadian healthcare system spent a mean of $6915 per patient for the 7554 patients who had a primary diagnosis of diseases of the esophagus and associated complications, for a total of $52,235,910 [26].

The outpatient costs of treating GERD are significant. Managed care organizations spend large amounts of money for the treatment of acid-related disorders. The IMS tracks the costs and trends of drug use in the USA [27]. In 2009, proton pump inhibitors were the third largest therapeutic class in sales. Proton pump inhibitors sales totaled $13.6 billion, and dispensed prescription volume for this therapeutic class rose 5% [27]. Treatment of GERD can reduce healthcare costs. A managed care study of 41,895 patients with GERD, conducted between 2000 and 2005, found that patients who were started on a proton pump inhibitor had a reduction in costs and patients who were compliant with proton pump inhibitor therapy had lower overall downstream costs than those who were non-compliant due to lower outpatient visits and hospital admissions [27,28].

Impact of gastroesophageal reflux disease on work productivity

A systematic review of the impact of GERD on work productivity was reported in 2006 [29]. The studies were conducted in seven countries and involved eight different study populations. The results of these studies show that absences from work related to GERD were infrequent and ranged from <1% to 7%. Presenteeism, which is defined as reduced work productivity while present at work, was much more common, ranging from 6% to 42%. Assuming a 40-h work week and average US wages for 2005, the mean productivity loss per employee with GERD is estimated to range from $62–430/week [29]. Treatment of GERD restores quality of life and work productivity (29).

Cost-effectiveness of medical therapy

Many patients with reflux disease stop and start treatment rather than taking it continuously. This form of therapy (on-demand therapy) may make sense in patients without esophagitis. In one study, 424 patients with endoscopy-negative reflux disease were randomized to placebo or proton pump inhibitor (omeprazole 20 mg or omeprazole 10 mg) on demand [29]. Of those patients randomized to on-demand therapy with omeprazole 20 mg a day, 83% were satisfactorily maintained over the 6-month time frame. The mean number of omeprazole capsules used per day was 0.43, suggesting that the total medication use was reduced by approximately 50%. In a study of esomeprazole therapy, 320 patients with endoscopy-negative reflux disease who had complete symptom resolution after 4 weeks of therapy with either esomeprazole 20 mg or omeprazole 20 mg were randomized to receive esomeprazole 20 mg on-demand or placebo on-demand for 6 months [30]. Medication intake was measured using electronic chips embedded in the caps of the medication containers. On average, esomeprazole was taken once every 3 days and 86% of patients were managed with on-demand therapy compared to 49% in the placebo group. These data suggest that on-demand therapy is effective and can substantially reduce costs of medical therapy [31].

Economics of medical versus surgical therapy

Several cost models have compared medical therapy to fundoplication. Bojke *et al.* evaluated the costs of laparoscopic fundoplication using a Markov model and UK cost estimates [32]. The incremental cost per additional quality-adjusted life-year (QALY) for surgery compared to medical therapy medical management was £180. The cost-effectiveness of surgery could not be demonstrated and the probability that surgery was cost-effective using a generally accepted threshold of £30,000 per QALY was only 60%. A study by Arguedas *et al.* [33] is interesting because the authors revised a previously published analysis that had suggested that surgery was cost-effective. When they reexamined the model which covered a 10-year time frame, using newly available data from randomized controlled trials and adding quality of life as an outcome measure, they found that medical therapy had a total per-patient cost of $8798 and 4.59 quality-adjusted life-years, while the surgical approach was more expensive at $10,475 and less effective 4.55 quality-adjusted life-years. Cost models are sensitive to the cost of the proton pump inhibitor, which has dropped significantly in many countries with the availability of low-cost generic proton pump inhibitors. They are also sensitive to the success rates assumed for surgery and medical therapy (effectiveness).

A recent randomized controlled trial suggests that newer proton pump inhibitors may be more effective than surgery at 5 years. Estimated remission rates at 5 years were 92% (95% CI 89–96%) in the esomeprazole group and 85% (95% CI 81–90%) in the fundoplication group ($P=0.048$) [34].

Evolution and natural progression of gastroesophageal reflux disease

The evolution and natural progression of GERD are unclear because longitudinal studies were not performed before acid inhibitory therapy became generally available. The natural history of GERD is influenced by changes in the populations being studied. For example, obesity has been increasing in Western populations and is increasing in some countries in Asia. A recent study evaluated healthy women in a longitudinal study in the USA [35]. Compared with women who had a BMI of 20.0–22.4, the multivariate odds ratio for frequent symptoms was 2.92 (95% CI 2.35–3.62) for a BMI of 30.0–34.9, and 2.93 (95% CI 2.24–3.85) for a BMI of 35.0 or more. An interesting aspect of this study was that symptoms of GERD regress if a substantial weight loss occurs. A recent systematic review examined the effects of age on the severity of reflux disease [36]. Age is associated with a decrease in GERD symptom prevalence but more severe patterns of acid reflux and more severe esophagitis.

An aspect of the natural history that remains controversial is the relationship between non-erosive reflux disease and reflux esophagitis. The ProGERD study, a naturalistic study that follows patients on treatment in Germany, suggests that patients may transition between non-erosive reflux disease and erosive esophagitis [37]. Twenty-five percent of patients who had non-erosive reflux disease at baseline progressed to Los Angeles Grade A or B esophagitis and 0.6% to Los Angeles Grade C or D; 1.6% of patients who had Los Angeles Grade A or B disease progressed to Los Angeles Grade C or D and 61% regressed to non-erosive reflux disease; 42% of patients who had Los Angeles Grade C or D disease regressed to Grade A or B disease and 50% regressed to non-erosive reflux disease. Patients with Grade C or D esophagitis were at greatest risk of developing Barrett's esophagus (5.8%) compared with patients with grade A and B disease (1.4%) and patients with non-erosive reflux disease (0.5%). Some complications such as esophageal strictures have declined in frequency in the last decade and this change corresponds with the availability of proton pump inhibitors [38].

Over the last 25 years there has been a remarkable change in the epidemiology of esophageal cancer in Western countries. The incidence of esophageal adenocarcinoma has been rising rapidly in some countries although the absolute annual risk of developing adenocarcinoma remains low at 0.4% [39]. Esophageal adenocarcinoma has been causally linked to GERD and is the final stage in the evolution of reflux disease. In a large epidemiological study in Sweden, the risk of esophageal adenocarcinoma was increased (OR 7.7) in patients suffering from long-standing reflux symptoms [40]. A higher frequency of symptoms (greater than three times per week) and a long duration (greater than 10–20 years) of symptoms increased the risk (OR 16–20).

Summary

Gastroesophageal reflux disease is widely prevalent throughout the world and its prevalence is increasing in Asia. GERD has a number of symptom associations, including esophageal adenocarcinoma, laryngeal and pharyngeal cancer, chronic obstructive airway disease and laryngitis. The cost of treating GERD poses an important economic burden to most healthcare organizations. GERD is associated with a marked impairment in quality of life. It is also associated with loss of work productivity and this is primarily due to decreased effectiveness while at work rather than absences from work. Treatment with proton pump inhibitors restores quality of life and improves work productivity.

References

1 Vakil N, van Zanten SV, Kahrilas P, Dent J, Jones R, Global Consensus Group. The Montreal definition and classification of gastroesophageal reflux disease:a global evidence-based consensus. Am J Gastroenterol 2006;101(8):1900–20.
2 Kahrilas PJ, Shaheen NJ, Vaezi MF, American Gastroenterological Association Institute. Technical review on the management of gastroesophageal reflux disease. Gastroenterology 2008;135(4):1392–413.
3 Dent J, Vakil N, Jones R, et al. Accuracy of the diagnosis of GORD by questionnaire, physicians ad a trial of proton pump inhibitor treatment:the Diamond study. Gut 2010;59(6):714–21.
4 Wiklund I, Carlsson J, Vakil N. Gastro-esophageal reflux symptoms and well-being in a random sample of the general population of a Swedish community. Am J Gastroenterol 2006;101(1):18–28.
5 Wong BC, Kinoshita Y. Systematic review on epidemiology of gastroesophageal reflux disease in Asia. Clin Gastroenterol Hepatol 2006;4(4):398–407.
6 Dent J, El-Serag H, Wallander M, Johansson S. Epidemiology of gastroesophageal reflux disease:a systematic review. Gut 2005;54:710–17.
7 Ruigómez A, García Rodríguez LA, Wallander MA, Johansson S, Graffner H, Dent J. Natural history of gastro-oesophageal reflux disease diagnosed in general practice. Aliment Pharmacol Ther 2004;20(7):751–60.

8 Ruigomez A, Wallander AM, Lundborg P, Johansson S, Garcia Rodriguez L. Gastroesophageal reflux disease in children and adults in primary care. Scand J Gastroenterol 2010;45:139–46.

9 El-Serag HB, Gilger M, Carter J, Genta RM, Rabeneck L. Childhood GERD is a risk factor for GERD in adolescents and young adults. Am J Gastroenterol 2004;99(5):806–12.

10 Sherman PM, Hassall E, Fagundes-Neto U, *et al.* A global, evidence-based consensus on the definition of gastroesophageal reflux disease in the pediatric population. Am J Gastroenterol 2009;104(5):1278–95.

11 Yuen E, Romney M, Toner RW, *et al.* Prevalence, knowledge and care patterns for gastro-esophageal reflux disease in United States minority populations Aliment Pharmacol Ther 2010;32(5):645–54.

12 Rosaida MS, Goh KL. Gastro-esophageal reflux disease, reflux esophagitis and non-erosive reflux disease in a multiracial Asian population: a prospective endoscopy based study. Eur J Gastroenterol Hepatol 2004;16(5):495–501.

13 Pandolfino JE, El-Serag HB, Zhang Q, Shah N, Ghosh SK, Kahrilas PJ. Obesity: a challenge to esophagogastric junction integrity. Gastroenterology 2006;130(3):639–49.

14 Nilsson M, Johnsen R, Ye W, Hveem K, Lagergren J. Obesity and estrogen as risk factors for gastroesophageal reflux symptoms. JAMA 2003 2;290(1):66–72.

15 Corley DA, Kubo A, Levin TR, *et al.* Abdominal obesity and body mass index as risk factors for Barrett's esophagus. Gastroenterology 2007;133(1):34–41.

16 Edelstein ZR, Farrow DC, Bronner MP, Rosen SN, Vhan TL. Central adiposity and risk of Barrett's esophagus. Gastroenterology 2007;133(2):403–11.

17 García Rodríguez LA, Ruigómez A, Martín–Merino E, Johansson S, Wallander MA. Relationship between gastroesophageal reflux disease and COPD in UK primary care. Chest 2008;134(6):1223–30.

18 Pace F, Pallotta S, Tonini M, Vakil N, Bianchi Porro G. Systematic review: gastro-esophageal reflux disease and dental lesions. Aliment Pharmacol Ther 2008; 27(12):1179–86.

19 El-Serag HB, Gilger M, Kuebeler M, Rabeneck L. Extraesophageal associations of gastroesophageal reflux disease in children without neurologic defects. Gastroenterology 2001;121(6):1294–9.

20 El-Serag HB, Hepworth EJ, Lee P, Sonnenberg A. Gastroesophageal reflux disease is a risk factor for laryngeal and pharyngeal cancer. Am J Gastroenterol 2001;96(7):2013–18.

21 Revicki DA, Wood M, Maton PN, Sorensen S. The impact of gastroesophageal reflux disease on health-related quality of life. Am J Med 1998;104(3):252–8.

22 Revicki DA, Zodet MW, Joshua-Gotlib S, Levine D, Crawley JA. Health-related quality of life improves with treatment-related GERD symptom resolution after adjusting for baseline severity. Health Qual Life Outcomes 2003;1:73.

23 Ronkainen J, Aro P, Storskrubb T, *et al.* Gastro-oesophageal reflux symptoms and health-related quality of life in the adult general population – the Kalixanda study. Aliment Pharmacol Ther 2006;23(12):1725–33.

24 Jones R, Horbach S, Sander P, Rydén-Bergsten T. Heartburn in patients with gastro-oesophageal reflux disease in Germany and Sweden: a study on patients' burden of disease. Pharmacoeconomics 2003;21(15):1091–102.

25 Zhao Y, Encinosa W. *Gastroesophageal reflux disease (GERD) hospitalizations in 1998 and 2005: Statistical Brief #44.* Washington, DC: Agency for Health Care Policy and Research, 2006.

26 Fedorak RN, Veldhuyzen van Zanten S, Bridges R. Canadian Digestive Health Foundation Public Impact Series: gastro-esophageal reflux disease in Canada: incidence, prevalence, and direct and indirect economic impact. Can J Gastroenterol 2010;24(7):431–4.

27 Anonymous. Cost of drugs. Available at: www.imshealth.com/portal/site/ims/menu-item.d248e29c86589c9c30e81c033208c22a/?vgnextoid=d690a27e9d5b7210VgnVC M100000ed152ca2RCRD&vgnextfmt=default.

28 Gosselin A, Luo R, Lohoues H, *et al*. The impact of proton pump inhibitor compliance on health-care resource utilization and costs in patients with gastroesophageal reflux disease. Value Health 2009;12(1):34–9.

29 Wahlquist P, Reilly M, Barkun A. Systematic review: the impact of gastro-esophageal reflux on work productivity. Aliment Pharmacol Ther 2006;24:259–72.

30 Lind T, Havelund T, Lundell L, *et al*. On demand therapy with omeprazole for the long-term management of patients with heartburn without esophagitis – a placebo-controlled randomized trial. Aliment Pharmacol Ther 1999;13:907–14.

31 Talley N, Lauritsen K, Tunturi-Hihnala H, *et al*. Esomeprazole 20 mg maintains symptom control in endoscopy-negative GERD. A randomized placebo-controlled trial of on-demand therapy for 6 months. Aliment Pharmacol Ther 2001;15:347–54.

32 Bojke L, Hornby E, Sculpher M. A comparison of the cost effectiveness of pharmaco-therapy or surgery (laparoscopic fundoplication) in the treatment of GORD. Pharmacoeconomics 2007;25:829–41.

33 Arguedas MR, Heudebert GR, Klapow JC, *et al*. Re-examination of the cost-effectiveness of surgical versus medical therapy in patients with gastroesophageal reflux disease: the value of long-term data collection. Am J Gastroenterol 2004;99:1023–8.

34 Galmiche JP, Hatlebakk J, Attwood S, *et al*., LOTUS Trial Collaborators. Laparoscopic antireflux surgery vs esomeprazole treatment for chronic GERD: the LOTUS randomized clinical trial. JAMA 2011;305(19):1969–77.

35 Jacobson BC, Somers SC, Fuchs CS, Kelly CP, Camargo CA Jr. Body mass index and symptoms of gastroesophageal reflux in women. N Engl J Med 2006;354(22):2340–8.

36 Becher A, Dent J. Systematic review: ageing and gastro-esophageal reflux disease symptoms, oesophageal function and reflux esophagitis. Aliment Pharmacol Ther 2011;33:442–54.

37 Labenz J, Nocon M, Lind T, *et al*. Prospective follow-up data from the ProGERD study suggest that GERD is not a categorial disease. Am J Gastroenterol 2006;101(11):2457–62.

38 Guda NM, Vakil N. Proton pump inhibitors and the time trends for esophageal dilation. Am J Gastroenterol 2004;99(5):797–800.

39 De Jonge PJ, van Blankenstein M, Looman CW, Casparie MK, Meijer GA, Kuipers EJ. Risk of malignant progression in patients with Barrett's oesophagus: a Dutch nation-wide cohort study. Gut 2010;59(8):1030–6.

40 Lagergren J, Bergström R, Lindgren A, Nyrén O. Symptomatic gastroesophageal reflux as a risk factor for esophageal adenocarcinoma. N Engl J Med 1999;340(11):825–31.

CHAPTER 3

Overview of the Tools for the Diagnosis of Gastroesophageal Reflux Disease

Nicolas A. Villa and Marcelo F. Vela

Section of Gastroenterology, Baylor College of Medicine, and Michael E. DeBakey
VA Medical Center, Houston, TX, USA

Key points

- Endoscopy is indicated when there are alarm features such as dysphagia, weight loss, and anemia.
- The presence of erosive esophagitis on endoscopy provides robust evidence of gastroesophageal reflux disease, but endoscopy is normal in the majority of patients.
- Ambulatory reflux monitoring is the gold standard for diagnosing gastroesophageal reflux disease.
- In some patients, the reported symptoms are due to non-gastroesophageal reflux disease causes; in this context, a negative evaluation for gastroesophageal reflux disease can direct the diagnostic and treatment efforts toward other causes.

Potential pitfalls

- Gastroesophageal reflux disease can be diagnosed by symptoms and a "positive proton pump inhibitor test" in some settings, but the limited sensitivity and specificity of this approach as a diagnostic intervention need to be kept in mind.
- Gastroesophageal reflux disease cannot be diagnosed by barium esophagram or esophageal manometry.
- A normal endoscopy does not exclude gastroesophageal reflux disease.

Introduction

Gastroesophageal reflux disease (GERD) is a very common clinical problem. Heartburn or acid regurgitation is experienced on a weekly basis by nearly 20% of the US population, with an annual prevalence of up to 59% [1].

Practical Manual of Gastroesophageal Reflux Disease, First Edition.
Edited by Marcelo F. Vela, Joel E. Richter and John E. Pandolfino.
© 2013 John Wiley & Sons, Ltd. Published 2013 by John Wiley & Sons, Ltd.

Diagnostic testing options for GERD include the assessment of symptoms (e.g. patient history or GERD questionnaires), the response to a trial of acid suppression (generally with a proton pump inhibitor – PPI), evaluation for acid-related damage to the esophageal mucosa (endoscopy), or determination of pathological reflux on prolonged ambulatory monitoring with pH or impedance pH. In clinical practice, a diagnosis of GERD is often made based upon symptom presentation along with a good response to a trial of PPI therapy. While the PPI trial is a reasonable and simple option in the appropriate setting (e.g. primary care), it is important to remember its limitations in terms of sensitivity and specificity.

Beyond taking a careful history for typical symptoms of GERD, a number of validated questionnaires are available including specific symptom scales, GERD-related quality of life scales, and combined instruments to assess both symptoms and quality of life. Questionnaires can be helpful but they generally have similar specificity and sensitivity compared to clinical examination by a gastroenterologist and therefore, to date, their role has often been limited to clinical trials.

Upper endoscopy is indicated when the clinical presentation includes alarm features such as dysphagia, bleeding or weight loss. Endoscopy provides a robust diagnosis of GERD when erosive esophagitis is present, but this is only found in approximately 30% of untreated patients [2] and even a smaller proportion of patients after treatment with a PPI. Random biopsies to look for evidence of GERD in those with normal endoscopy are not recommended because conventional histology has poor performance for a diagnosis of GERD.

Direct measurement of gastroesophageal reflux through pH monitoring (catheter based or wireless) can establish whether there is a pathological amount of acid reflux and if there is an association between symptoms and reflux episodes. Impedance-pH monitoring enables measurement of both acid and non-acid reflux (with a pH > 4); the latter may be clinically important in patients with persistent symptoms despite acid-suppressive therapy.

Evaluation should always begin with a careful history. A PPI trial is a reasonable option for diagnosing GERD in patients with typical symptoms. GERD cannot be diagnosed by barium esophagram or esophageal manometry. Endoscopy should be performed when alarm features are present. Objective documentation of GERD by endoscopy or reflux monitoring is mandatory before antireflux surgery. Evaluation by endoscopy and reflux monitoring is useful in patients with extraesophageal symptoms, and those in whom symptoms persist despite acid suppression. It is important to note that in some patients the reported symptoms may be due to causes other than GERD, including functional disorders; in these patients, endoscopy and reflux monitoring can be valuable tools to exclude GERD. The advantages, disadvantages, and clinical use of tests to diagnose GERD are discussed in

Table 3.1 Advantages and disadvantages of diagnostic tests for gastroesophageal reflux disease.

Test	Advantages	Disadvantages
Proton pump inhibitor test	• Simple • Widely available • Non-invasive	• PPI dose and duration not standardized • Definition of response not standardized • Low sensitivity and specificity
Endoscopy	• Provides robust diagnosis when erosive esophagitis is present • Can diagnose and treat complications such as stricture • Can exclude non-GERD disorders	• Invasive • Normal in two-thirds of GERD patients
Reflux monitoring		
Catheter-based pH	• Measures esophageal acid exposure, the gold standard for GERD diagnosis	• Catheter discomfort may limit activities • Cannot detect non-acid reflux • Study restricted to 24 h
Wireless pH	• Measures esophageal acid exposure, the gold standard for GERD diagnosis • Better tolerability • Prolonged monitoring (up to 96 h)	• More costly than catheter-based techniques • Requires endoscopy for placement • Cannot detect non-acid reflux
Impedance pH	• Measures esophageal acid exposure, the gold standard for GERD diagnosis • Can detect non-acid reflux	• Catheter discomfort may limit activities • Study restricted to 24 h • Analysis of tracings more laborious than pH alone

GERD, gastroesophageal reflux disease; PPI, proton pump inhibitor.

this chapter and summarized in Table 3.1. The approaches to diagnosing GERD in patients with non-cardiac chest pain, extraesophageal reflux presentations, dysphagia, and refractory symptoms are discussed in detail in other chapters.

Gastroesophageal reflux disease symptoms, questionnaires, and the proton pump inhibitor test

Heartburn and regurgitation are considered typical symptoms of GERD. Heartburn is defined as a burning sensation in the retrosternal area, and regurgitation is defined as the perception of flow of refluxed gastric contents into the pharynx or mouth [3]. Heartburn and regurgitation are the most reliable symptoms for making a history-based diagnosis of GERD but are far from perfect in this respect. When heartburn and regurgitation are the dominant symptoms, they have high sensitivity but poor specificity [4]. While heartburn is the most typical symptom of GERD, it may also be present in patients with other esophageal disorders such as eosinophilic esophagitis or achalasia. Furthermore, some patients may have no organic cause for heartburn, a condition that is termed "functional heartburn" that is discussed in detail in a later chapter. Dysphagia may be part of the clinical presentation in a patient with GERD and is considered to be an alarm symptom that warrants endoscopic evaluation to exclude a complication, including malignancy. Chest pain may also be experienced by GERD patients, but this symptom requires thorough evaluation for a cardiac cause before GERD is considered.

More recently, the spectrum of clinical presentations attributed to GERD has moved beyond the typical esophageal symptoms of heartburn and regurgitation, and now includes various extraesophageal manifestations that focus on respiratory and laryngeal symptoms. Several epidemiological studies have identified an association between GERD and asthma [5], chronic cough [6], and laryngitis [7]. However, causality cannot be inferred from these studies. Therefore, the Montreal Consensus recognized established associations between GERD and asthma, chronic cough, and laryngitis, while acknowledging that these disorders frequently have a multifactorial etiology and gastroesophageal reflux may be a co-factor rather than a cause. The Montreal Consensus also recognized the rarity of extraesophageal syndromes occurring in isolation without concomitant typical symptoms of GERD [3]. The evaluation of GERD in patients with non-cardiac chest pain, cough, and laryngitis is discussed in detail in later chapters.

A number of questionnaires have been developed for GERD. Available validated instruments include specific symptom scales, quality of life scales, and those which combine the two. A comprehensive review of these instruments is beyond the scope of this chapter, especially because they are not widely used in routine clinical practice. Questionnaires can be helpful, but have similar specificity and sensitivity as clinical examination by a gastroenterologist and therefore, to date, their role has been in screening large numbers of patients by non-specialists or as part of clinical trials [8].

Although, as noted above, the sensitivity and specificity of heartburn and regurgitation are not perfect for making a diagnosis of GERD, it is not necessary to conduct a diagnostic evaluation in all patients with typical symptoms and no alarm features. In this context, a 2–4-week trial of acid suppression with a PPI is a non-invasive, simple, and reasonable option for supporting a diagnosis of GERD. If the patient has a clear response to therapy, it can be assumed that GERD is present. That said, the potential shortcomings of this approach have to be kept in mind. The manner in which this "PPI test" is administered is not standardized. Studies evaluating this approach have used differing PPI doses (once versus twice daily), variable duration of treatment (from 1 to 4 weeks or even longer), and different definitions of what constitutes a positive test (for instance, 50% improvement as opposed to 100% improvement). In addition, a meta-analysis of several studies that evaluated the diagnostic capability of a short course (1–4 weeks) of PPI compared to other tests found a sensitivity of 78% and specificity of 54% for the PPI test [9].

Esophagram and esophageal manometry

Barium esophagram and esophageal manometry deserve a brief discussion because they are often used in the work-up of patients with symptoms suggestive of GERD. A diagnosis of GERD cannot be made based upon the results of an esophagram or esophageal manometry.

While a high-quality barium esophagram with double contrast can reveal signs of esophagitis, the overall sensitivity of this test for esophagitis is very low [10]. The finding of barium reflux from stomach to esophagus, with or without provocative maneuvers, may be absent in patients with GERD; furthermore, reflux of barium may be found with provocative maneuvers in some healthy subjects [11,12]. An esophagram can be helpful when a patient has dysphagia, as it may reveal a structural abnormality such as a stricture or ring. However, GERD cannot be diagnosed based upon esophagram.

Esophageal manometry will often reveal impaired peristalsis in GERD patients, and some but certainly not all GERD patients may have a hypotensive lower esophageal sphincter [13]. However, these findings are not specific and a diagnosis of GERD cannot be made based upon manometric findings. Manometry is useful to guide placement of transnasal pH or impedance pH catheters for ambulatory reflux monitoring. In addition, esophageal manometry should always be performed prior to antireflux surgery. While the presence of decreased peristalsis has not been found to reliably predict postfundoplication dysphagia [14], manometry should be performed to exclude aperistalsis due to a scleroderma-like esophagus or achalasia, as both of these conditions represent contraindications to fundoplication.

Endoscopy and esophageal biopsies

Upper endoscopy enables direct visualization of the esophageal mucosa in patients with symptoms suggestive of GERD. Endoscopy may reveal

---

Box 3.1 Los Angeles classification of esophagitis [15]

Grade A: one or more mucosal breaks no longer than 5 mm, that do not extend between the tops of two mucosal folds

Grade B: one or more mucosal breaks longer than 5 mm long that do not extend between the tops of two mucosal folds

Grade C: one or more mucosal breaks that are continuous between the tops of two or more mucosal folds but involve less than 75% of the esophageal circumference

Grade D: one or more mucosal breaks involving at least 75% of the esophageal circumference

---

erosive esophagitis, strictures or Barrett's esophagus. The finding of erosive esophagitis provides a robust diagnosis of GERD. The most widely used system for grading the severity of esophagitis is the Los Angeles classification (Box 3.1), which has been validated in terms of interobserver variability [15]. However, a normal endoscopy does not rule out GERD, and roughly two-thirds of patients with heartburn and regurgitation will have a negative endoscopy without erosions [16]. Alternatives to conventional endoscopy include ultra-thin endoscopes [17] and capsule endoscopy [18]; these avoid sedation and are thus generally safer and more efficient, but patient tolerance can be an issue with unsedated endoscopy and biopsies cannot be obtained during capsule esophagoscopy.

Histological findings suggestive of GERD include basal cell hyperplasia, increased papillary length, and infiltration with neutrophils or eosinophils. However, the diagnostic performance characteristics of these findings are rather poor as they are often absent in disease, while they may be present in healthy controls [19]. Therefore, obtaining random biopsies from the distal esophagus as a means of diagnosing GERD in a patient with normal endoscopy is not recommended [20]. That said, obtaining random distal and proximal esophageal biopsies may be useful in patients without a clear diagnosis because histology may be consistent with eosinophilic esophagitis (EoE), a condition with increasing prevalence that may present with symptoms that are similar to those experienced by GERD patients (heartburn, dysphagia, chest pain). Of note, while endoscopy will often reveal rings or linear furrows in EoE patients, the mucosa may appear normal in up to 10% of patients [21].

Ambulatory reflux monitoring

Ambulatory esophageal reflux monitoring is the most accurate means of confirming the diagnosis of GERD. This test quantifies reflux by measuring esophageal acid exposure or the number of reflux episodes, and it also enables an examination of the temporal relationship between reflux episodes and reported symptoms. Reflux monitoring was performed through catheter-based pH studies for many years. More recently, there have been two major developments in this field: the wireless pH capsule which allows catheter-free monitoring, and impedance pH measurement, a catheter-based technique that enables detection of acid and non-acid reflux (i.e. with pH >4). Additional techniques that will not be discussed in this chapter include esophageal bilirubin monitoring [22], which is not widely used in clinical practice, and a new transnasal catheter for pharyngeal monitoring that can measure pH in either liquid or aerosolized droplets [23]. Data to support the use of the latter are very limited and the test is not used routinely.

Catheter-based pH monitoring

Conventional ambulatory pH monitoring is performed by a transnasal catheter that records esophageal pH over a 24-h period, with a pH electrode positioned 5 cm above the proximal border of the lower esophageal sphincter. A reflux episode is defined by a drop in pH to below 4.0. Various measures can be derived from a pH monitoring study, including percent time with pH <4 (upright, recumbent, and total time), number of reflux episodes, number of reflux episodes longer than 5 min, and longest reflux episode [24]. Of these, the total percentage of time with pH <4 is felt to be the most useful indicator of pathological acid reflux [25]. A positive pH test can establish a diagnosis of GERD in a patient with normal endoscopy; it may also help to confirm or exclude GERD in patients who do not respond to PPI therapy, as explained in greater detail in Chapter 7. While the sensitivity and specificity of this test are above 90% in some studies [26,27], other data point to lower sensitivity [28]. Additional shortcomings of pH monitoring include the possibility of changes in patient behavior related to having a transnasal catheter, such as altered eating habits and decreased activity [29]. Finally, pH monitoring does not allow assessment of non-acid reflux (i.e. with pH >4), that may occur when the gastric contents are buffered (during pharmacological acid suppression, in the postprandial period or in patients with atrophic gastritis).

Bravo pH monitoring

A new technology has been developed recently to enable wireless monitoring of esophageal pH, obviating the need for a transnasal catheter. The system uses a small recording capsule that is endoscopically attached to the distal esophagus, and transfers pH data via radiofrequency signals to an external recording device. Wireless pH monitoring has similar and possibly improved accuracy compared to catheter-based pH monitoring [30]. In addition, it is better tolerated by patients [31], thus allowing for testing under more physiological conditions with fewer limitations on diet and activity [32]. An additional advantage of this approach is the capability for prolonged monitoring, with a standard study of 48 h that can be extended to up to 96 h [33]. In a study of 48-h wireless pH monitoring in 44 healthy subjects and 41 GERD patients, improved sensitivity in distinguishing controls from GERD patients was achieved by using the data from the worst of the 2 days [34].

The wireless pH monitoring system has some limitations, including early capsule detachment (an infrequent problem), chest pain or discomfort, increased cost and, like catheter-based pH monitoring, the inability to detect non-acid reflux, which may be clinically relevant in some patients.

Impedance-pH monitoring

Intraesophageal impedance, determined by measuring electrical conductivity across a pair of closely spaced electrodes within the esophageal lumen, is dependent on the conductivity of the material through which the current travels. By placing a series of conducting electrodes in a catheter that spans the length of the esophagus, changes in impedance can be recorded in response to movement of intraesophageal material in either antegrade or retrograde direction [35]. Because the esophageal mucosa, air, and any given bolus material (i.e. swallowed food, saliva, refluxed gastric contents) each produce a different change in impedance, the technique enables very detailed characterization of gastroesophageal reflux episodes, including composition (air, liquid or mixed), proximal extent (height), velocity, and clearance time.

Impedance-pH is currently the most accurate and detailed method for measuring gastroesophageal reflux [36]. During combined impedance and pH monitoring, impedance is used to detect retrograde bolus movement (i.e. reflux), while pH measurement establishes the acidity of the reflux episode (acid if pH <4.0, non-acid otherwise). Non-acid reflux may be further classified as either weakly acidic (pH ≥4 but <7) or weakly alkaline (pH ≥7). In this chapter, non-acid reflux refers to any reflux with pH ≥4. The main advantage of this method is the capability to detect non-acid reflux, which may be relevant in some patients, especially those with symptoms that persist despite PPI therapy. Examples of acid and non-acid reflux are shown in Figure 3.1.

Ambulatory-impedance-pH monitoring can be performed with different catheters that incorporate a varying number of impedance measuring segments and pH electrodes in different configurations. A typical catheter has a pH electrode positioned 5 cm above the manometrically determined lower esophageal sphincter (similar to conventional pH testing), along with six or more impedance-measuring segments (each composed of two metal ring electrodes usually spaced 2 cm apart) to detect impedance

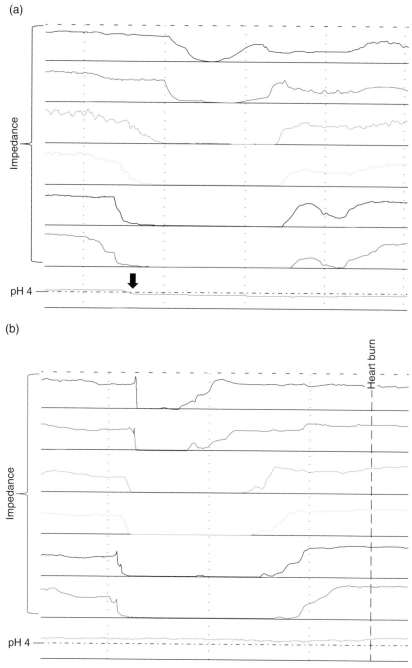

Figure 3.1 Acid and non-acid reflux detected by impedance-pH monitoring. Impedance changes in six measuring segments spanning the esophagus, and pH changes from a single sensor in the distal esophagus are shown. (a) Acid reflux: a typical impedance reflux pattern with sequential decreases in impedance starting in the distal esophagus and progressing upward in retrograde direction; this reflux episode is associated with a pH fall to below 4.0 (*arrow*). (b) Non-acid reflux: typical impedance reflux pattern; during this episode esophageal pH remains above 4. The patient reported heartburn during this reflux episode.

changes along variable lengths of the esophagus. Catheter placement is transnasal and thus similar to that of conventional pH monitoring. Ambulatory impedance-pH monitoring is conventionally performed over a 24-h period.

Assessment of reflux with impedance-pH is reproducible [37] and normal values for ambulatory 24-h impedance-pH monitoring are now well established [38,39]. While impedance pH is considered the most accurate method for reflux detection, the clinical indications for its use and its role in managing GERD patients are still evolving because the clinical relevance of non-acid reflux is awaiting confirmation by high-quality trials. Studies have shown that non-acid reflux can cause symptoms indistinguishable from those caused by acid reflux [40]. Furthermore, non-acid reflux can be treated by pharmacological inhibition of transient lower esophageal sphincter relaxations [41] or through fundoplication [42]. However, it is very important to note that there is a paucity of high-quality controlled studies examining the benefit of treating non-acid reflux. In addition, it must be remembered that non-acid reflux occurs predominantly in the postprandial period (when food buffers the stomach contents) or during pharmacological acid suppression. The potential relevance of non-acid reflux is discussed in greater detail in Chapter 7.

Impedance-pH monitoring has some limitations. It is catheter based which, like conventional pH testing, can result in patient discomfort and change in behavior on the day of testing. In addition to these catheter-based difficulties, low baseline impedance (seen in some patients with severe reflux) can make the tracing difficult to read. Finally, interpretation of impedance-pH tracings may be more time consuming compared to pH-metry.

Symptom association studies during reflux monitoring

As mentioned earlier, the total percentage of time with pH <4 is felt to be the most useful indicator of pathological acid reflux [25]. The number of reflux episodes detected by impedance can also serve as a measure of abnormal reflux, but the clinical utility of this approach is unclear and outcome studies proving that treating patients based upon this endpoint is beneficial are lacking.

Beyond establishing the presence of pathological reflux, ambulatory reflux monitoring with any of the available techniques (catheter or wireless pH, impedance-pH) may be used to determine whether the patient's symptoms are due to reflux. The two methods most commonly used to evaluate the temporal association between reflux episodes and symptoms are the Symptom Index (SI) [43] and the Symptom Association Probability (SAP) [44]. The SI is defined as the percentage of symptom events that are temporally related to a reflux episode (number of reflux-related symptom events/total number of symptom events×100%). An SI of 50% is considered positive, meaning that the symptom is related to reflux. Although this value was derived from receiver operating characteristic (ROC) curves that found this threshold to be sensitive and specific for heartburn [45], the SI is used to analyze any symptom that may be attributed to GERD. The SAP is calculated by dividing the pH or impedance-pH tracing in 2-min segments and determining whether a reflux episode and/or a symptom occurred in each 2-min segment. A 2×2 contingency table with the number of segments with and without symptoms and with and without reflux is built; the probability that a positive association between reflux and symptoms occurred by more than chance is evaluated through a modified chi-square test, with an SAP greater than 95% considered positive.

A detailed discussion of the advantages and disadvantages of the SI and the SAP is beyond the scope of this chapter, but both have methodological shortcomings that have been reviewed elsewhere [46]. Of note, both methods rely on precise and timely symptom recording by the patient, along with accurate reflux detection by the testing device. Furthermore, prospective data to validate the ability of these symptom association measures to predict response to treatment are scarce. Nevertheless, they are useful if their limitations are kept in mind, and they are commonly employed in clinical practice. In terms of patient management, a strongly positive SI or SAP may suggest the need for a therapeutic intervention and a negative result supports the notion that the patient's symptoms are unlikely to be due to reflux. However, these indices should not be used in isolation and other reflux monitoring parameters as well as the patient's presentation have to be incorporated into the decision-making process.

References

1 Locke GR III, Talley NJ, Fett SL *et al.* Prevalence and clinical spectrum of gastroesophageal reflux: a population-based study in Olmsted County, Minnesota. Gastroenterology 1997;112:1448–56.
2 Lind T, Havelund T, Carlsson R, *et al.* Heartburn without esophagitis: efficacy of omeprazole therapy and features determining therapeutic response. Scand J Gastroenterol 1997;32:974–9.
3 Vakil N, van Zanten SV, Kahrilas P, *et al.* The Montreal definition and classification of gastroesophageal reflux disease: a global evidence-based consensus. Am J Gastroenterol 2006;101:1900.
4 Klauser AG, Shcindelbeck NE, Muller-Lissner SA. Symptoms in gastro-oesophageal reflux disease. Lancet 1990;335:205.
5 Havemann BD, Henderson CA, El-Serag HB. The association between gastro-oesophageal reflux disease and asthma: a systematic review. Gut 2007;56:1654–64.
6 Irwin RS, Curley FJ, French CL. Chronic cough. The spectrum and frequency of causes, key components of the diagnostic evaluation, and outcome of specific therapy. Am Rev Respir Dis 1990;141:640–7.

7 El-Serag HB, Sonnenberg A. Comorbid occurrence of laryngeal or pulmonary disease with esophagitis in United States military veterans. Gastroenterology 1997;113:755–60.

8 Stanghellini V, Arsmtrong D, Monnikes H, Bardhan KD. Systematic review: do we need a new gastroesophageal diseases questionnaire? Digestion 2007;75(suppl 1):3–16.

9 Numans ME, Lau J, de Wit NK, Bonis PA. Short-term treatment with proton-pump inhibitors as a test for gastroesophageal reflux disease. Ann Intern Med 2004; 140:518–52.

10 Johnston BT, Troshinsky MB, Castell JA, et al. Comparison of barium radiology with esophageal pH monitoring in the diagnosis of gastroesophageal reflux disease. Am J Gastroenterol 1996;91:1181–5.

11 Thompson JK, Koehler RE, Richter JE. Detection of gastroesophageal reflux: value of barium studies compared with 24-hr pH monitoring. Am J Roentgenol 1994;162:621–6.

12 Richter JE, Castell DO. Gastroesophageal reflux. Pathogenesis, diagnosis, and therapy. Ann Intern Med 1982;97:93–103.

13 Savarino E, Gemignani L, Pohl D, et al. Oesophageal motility and bolus transit abnormalities increase in parallel with the severity of gastro-oesophageal reflux disease. Aliment Pharmacol Ther 2011;34:476–86.

14 Shaw J, Bornman PC, Callanan MD, Beckingham IJ, Metz DC. Long-term outcome of laparoscopic Nissen and laparoscopic Toupet fundoplication for gsatroesophageal reflux disease: a prospective, randomized trial. Surg Endosc 2010;24:924–32.

15 Lundell LR, Dent J, Bennett JR, et al. Endoscopic assessment of oesophagitis: clinical and functional correlates and further validation of the Los Angeles classification. Gut 1999;45:172–80.

16 Johnsson F, Joelsson B, Gudmundsson K, et al. Symptoms and endoscopic findings in the diagnosis of gastroesophageal reflux disease. Scand J Gastroenterol 1987; 22:714–18.

17 Mokhashi MS, Wildi SM, Glenn TF, et al. A prospective, blinded study of diagnostic esophagoscopy with a superthin, stand-alone, battery-powered esophagoscope. Am J Gastroenterol 2003;98:2383.

18 Eliakim R, Sharma VK, Yassin K, et al. A prospective study of the diagnostic accuracy of PillCam ESO esophageal capsule endoscopy versus conventional upper endoscopy in patients with chronic gastroesophageal reflux diseases. J Clin Gastroenterol 2005;39:572–8.

19 Nandurkar S, Talley NJ, Martin CJ, Ng T, Adams S. Esophageal histology does not provide additional useful information over clinical assessment in identifying reflux patients presenting for esophagogastroduodenoscopy. Dig Dis Sci 2000;45:217–24.

20 Tytgat G. The value of esophageal histology in the diagnosis of gastroesophageal reflux diseas in patients with heartburn and normal endoscopy. Curr Gastroenterol Rep 2008;10:231–4.

21 Prasad GA, Talley NJ, Romero Y, et al. Prevalence and predictive factors of eosinophilic esophagitis in patients presenting with dysphagia: a prospective study. Am J Gastroenterol 2007;102:2627.

22 Vaezi MF, Richter JE. Role of acid and duodenogastroesophageal reflux in gastroesophageal reflux disease. Gastroenterology 1996;111:1192–9.

23 Sun G, Muddana S, Slaughter JC, et al. A new pH catheter for laryngopharyngeal reflux: normal values. Laryngoscope 2009;119:1639–43.

24 Johnson LF, DeMeester TR. Twenty-four-hour pH monitoring of the distal esophagus. A quantitative measure of gastroesophageal reflux. Am J Gastroenterol 1974;62:325–32.

25 Pandolfino JE, Vela MF. Esophageal reflux monitoring. Gastrointest Endosc 2009;69:917–30.

26 Jamieson JR, Stein HJ, DeMeester TR, *et al.* Ambulatory 24-h esophageal pH monitoring: normal values, optimal thresholds, specificity, sensitivity, and reproducibility. Am J Gastroenterol 1992;87:1102–11.

27 Richter JE, Bradley LA, DeMeester TR, Wu WC. Normal 24-hr ambulatory esophageal pH values. Influence of study center, pH electrode, age, and gender. Dig Dis Sci 1992;37:849–56.

28 Schlesinger PK, Donahue PE, Schmid B, *et al.* Limitations of 24-hour intraesophageal pH monitoring in the hospital setting. Gastroenterology 1985;894:797–804.

29 Fass R, Hell R, Sampliner RE, *et al.* Effect of ambulatory 24-h esophageal pH monitoring on reflux-provoking activities. Dig Dis Sci 1999;44:2263–9.

30 Pandolfino J, Zhang Q, Schreiner M, *et al.* Acid reflux event detection using the Bravo™ wireless vs the Slimline™ catheter pH systems: why are the numbers so different? Gut 2005;54:1687–92.

31 Wenner J, Jonsson F, Johansson J, Oberg S. Wireless esophageal pH monitoring is better tolerated than the catheter-based technique: results from a randomized crossover trial. Am J Gastroenterol 2007;102:239–45.

32 Ward EM, Devault KR, Bouras EP, *et al.* Successful oesophageal pH monitoring with a catheter-free system. Aliment Pharmacol Ther 2004;19:449–54.

33 Hirano I, Zhang Q, Pandolfino JE, *et al.* Four-day Bravo pH capsule monitoring with and without proton pump inhibitor therapy. Clin Gastroenterol Hepatol 2005;3:1083–8.

34 Pandolfino JE, Richter JE, Ours T, *et al.* Ambulatory esophageal pH monitoring using a wireless system. Am J Gastroenterol 2003;984:740–9.

35 Vela MF. Non-acid reflux: detection by multichannel intraluminal impedance and pH, clinical significance and management. Am J Gastroenterol 2009;104:277–80.

36 Sifrim D, Castell D, Dent J, *et al.* Gastro-oesophageal reflux monitoring: reflux and consensus report on detection and definitions of acid, non-acid, and gas reflux. Gut 2004;53:1024–31.

37 Bredenoord AJ, Weusten BL, Timmer R, Smout AJ. Reproducibility of multichannel intraluminal electrical impedance monitoring of gastroesophageal reflux. Am J Gastroenterol 2005;100:265–9.

38 Shay S, Tutuian R, Sifrim D, *et al.* Twenty-four hour ambulatory simultaneous impedance and pH monitoring: a multicenter report of normal values from 60 healthy volunteers. Am J Gastroenterol 2004;99:1037–43.

39 Zerbib F, des Varannes SB, Roman S, *et al.* Normal values and day-to-day variability of 24-h ambulatory oesophageal impedance-pH monitoring in a Belgian-French cohort of healthy subjects. Aliment Pharmacol Ther 2005;22:1011–21.

40 Vela MF, Camacho-Lobato L, Srinivasan R, *et al.* Intraesophageal impedance and pH measurement of acid and non-acid reflux: effect of omeprazole. Gastroenterology 2001;96:647–55.

41 Vela MF, Tutuian R, Katz PO, *et al.* Baclofen decreases acid and non-acid post-prandial gastro-oesophageal reflux measured by combined multichannel intraluminal impedance and pH. Aliment Pharmacol Ther 2003;17:243–51.

42 Frazzoni M, Conigliaro R, Melotti G. Reflux parameters as modified by laparoscopic fundoplication in 40 patients with heartburn/regurgitation persisting despite PPI therapy: a study using impedance-pH moniotoring. Dig Dis Sci 2011;56:1099–106.

43 Wiener GJ, Richter JE, Copper JB, *et al.* The symptom index: a clinically important parameter of ambulatory 24-hour esophageal pH monitoring. Am J Gastroenterol 1988;83:358–61.

44 Weusten BL, Roelofs JM, Akkermans LM, *et al.* The symptom-association probability: an improved method for symptom analysis of 24-hour esophageal pH data. Gastroenterology 1994;107:1741–5.

45 Singh S, Richter JE, Bradley LA, Haile JM. The symptom index. Differential useful-
    ness in suspected acid-related copmlaints of heartburn and chest pain. Dig Dis Sci
    1993;34:309–16.
46 Connor J , Richter J. Increasing yield also increases false positives and best serves to
    exclude GERD. Am J Gastroenterol 2006;101:460–3.

CHAPTER 4

Overview of Gastroesophageal Reflux Disease Treatments

Sabine Roman and Peter J. Kahrilas

Division of Gastroenterology, Northwestern University, Chicago, IL, USA

Key points

- Proton pump inhibitors are the dominant treatment for gastroesophageal reflux disease.
- Proton pump inhibitors are progressively less effective in achieving the endpoints of healing esophagitis, relieving heartburn, treating regurgitation, and treating extraesophageal syndromes.
- The therapeutic gain with reflux inhibitors (gamma-amino butyric acid B agonists) is modest for typical gastroesophageal reflux disease symptoms.
- Reducing visceral hypersensitivity should be considered in patients with persistent heartburn or chest pain despite proton pump inhibitor treatment.

Potential pitfalls

- Indications for laparoscopic fundoplication must be balanced against its risks.
- In the absence of proton pump inhibitor response, an alternative diagnosis should be considered for suspected gastroesophageal reflux disease symptoms.

Introduction

Gastroesophageal reflux disease (GERD) is defined as "a condition which develops when the reflux of stomach contents causes troublesome symptoms and/or complications" [1]. Typical esophageal GERD symptoms include heartburn and regurgitation. Additional esophageal symptoms are dysphagia and chest pain. Extraesophageal or "atypical" symptoms with an established association with GERD on the basis of population-based studies are chronic cough, asthma, and laryngitis. However, these have potential etiologies other than GERD and in the absence of a concomitant

---

Practical Manual of Gastroesophageal Reflux Disease, First Edition.
Edited by Marcelo F. Vela, Joel E. Richter and John E. Pandolfino.
© 2013 John Wiley & Sons, Ltd. Published 2013 by John Wiley & Sons, Ltd.

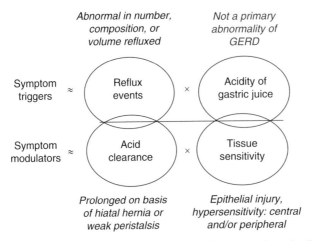

Figure 4.1 Conceptual model of the pathophysiology of gastroesophageal reflux disease (GERD). The most fundamental abnormality is in the number of reflux events as well as their composition and volume. The effect of reflux in eliciting symptoms is linked to the toxicity of gastric juice even though this factor is usually normal in GERD patients. Acid clearance and mucosal sensitivity modulate the effect of reflux events by prolonging the exposure of the esophageal mucosa to refluxate and making the mucosa fundamentally more sensitive. Each of these elements may be targeted by GERD treatments.

esophageal GERD syndrome, the causal role of GERD in extraesophageal symptoms remains controversial. GERD complications are mainly attributable to mucosal injury, the most common being reflux esophagitis. Peptic stricture, Barrett's metaplasia, and esophageal adenocarcinoma may also complicate GERD.

The pathogenesis of GERD symptoms and reflux esophagitis share some common elements but also have several independent determinants. Indeed, most patients with heartburn do not have esophagitis even prior to treatment [2] and this disconnect becomes more exaggerated with atypical GERD symptoms. Targeting individual elements of GERD pathophysiology is the basis of GERD treatments (Figure 4.1). Paradoxically, although gastric acid secretion is usually normal in GERD patients, the lethality of gastric juice to esophageal epithelial cells is a key event in the pathogenesis of esophagitis and, to a lesser degree, symptom occurrence.

Consequently, the dominant medical GERD treatments focus on inhibiting acid secretion. Reflux inhibition is an alternative GERD treatment strategy. Reflux inhibition can be achieved by reducing the number of transient lower esophageal sphincter relaxations (TLESRs) or by restoring an effective anti-reflux barrier with anti-reflux surgery or endoluminal treatment. Contact time between harmful refluxate content and esophageal mucosa is another primary element in GERD pathophysiology and may be attributable to the effects of a hiatal hernia or weak peristalsis [3]. Although pharmaceutical therapies have minimal effect in this domain, lifestyle modifications such as avoiding postprandial recumbency and anti-reflux surgery to eliminate hiatus hernia target this mechanism. Finally, visceral sensitivity is increasingly recognized as an important modulator of symptom severity and, when abnormal, should be considered as an alternative target for GERD treatment. The aim of this overview is to broadly consider alternative GERD treatments and their differential effectiveness in the context of varied GERD presentation and severity.

Lifestyle modifications

There are many recommendations regarding lifestyle modifications as GERD therapy. Generally, these fall into three categories:
- avoid food that may lead to reflux presumably by relaxing the lower esophageal sphincter (coffee, alcohol, chocolate, fatty foods)
- avoid acidic foods that may precipitate heartburn by a direct irritative effect on the esophageal mucosa (citrus, carbonated drinks, spicy foods)
- adopt behaviors that may reduce esophageal acid exposure by reducing the occurrence of reflux and/or enhancing the process of acid clearance (weight loss, smoking cessation, raising the head of bed, and avoiding recumbent position for 2–3 h after meals).

Although evidence supporting these recommendations is generally weak [4], they should be encouraged to the extent to which they seem relevant to the individual patient. For instance, patients with regurgitation and heartburn in the recumbent position should be advised to elevate the head of the bed and to avoid eating for the 2–3-h period before going to bed. Similarly, someone who consistently experiences heartburn after ingestion of alcohol, coffee or any specific food will benefit from avoidance of these items.

Obesity and weight control merit special attention because accumulating evidence suggests this to be one of the root causes of the GERD epidemic of the past two decades. Epidemiological data suggest a dose-dependent relationship between increasing Body Mass Index (BMI) and frequent reflux symptoms [5]. However, the benefit of weight loss on GERD symptoms has not been demonstrated in rigorous clinical trials [6–8]. Nonetheless, if the development of troublesome heartburn paralleled weight gain in an individual patient, it is very reasonable to propose weight loss as an intervention that may prevent the need for continuous acid suppressive therapy. This is particularly true in view of the added health benefits of weight loss beyond reflux disease and because obesity has been shown to be an independent risk factor for Barrett's esophagus and esophageal adenocarcinoma.

Acid suppression

Acid neutralization with antacid and pharmacologically inhibiting gastric acid secretion are cornerstones of GERD therapy. The most potent drugs are the proton pump inhibitors (PPIs), which covalently bind with gastric H+/K+ATPase to block the final common pathway for acid secretion. Histamine-2 receptor antagonists (H_2RA) competitively block histamine-stimulated acid secretion, making them less potent than PPIs and giving them a duration of action limited by their serum half-life. Antacids neutralize acid or acidic food without having any effect on subsequent acid secretion. It is well established that PPIs are more effective than H_2RAs in healing esophagitis and in relieving heartburn [9,10]. Similarly, H_2RAs are more effective than placebo in the same applications.

Returning to the principles of Figure 4.1, it follows that acid suppression in general and PPI therapy specifically do not "cure" reflux disease. Rather, PPIs treat GERD in an indirect fashion. It follows that PPI efficacy will vary widely across disease manifestations, dependent on the degree to which those manifestations are attributable to acid. The most responsive disease manifestation is esophagitis, in which case esophageal epithelial injury is directly attributable to gastric acid and eliminating acid facilitates mucosal healing with close to 100% effectiveness. Similarly, dysphagia, which is reported in about one-third of patients with esophagitis without stricture or malignancy, resolves in 83% with PPI therapy [11]. However, esophagitis is the best-case scenario for PPI efficacy. Heartburn is the next-best case, but already the therapeutic gain associated with PPI therapy is sharply reduced from that observed with esophagitis (Figure 4.2). Furthermore, there is a 10–20% difference in therapeutic gain for heartburn dependent on whether or not it occurs in the context of erosive esophagitis or non-erosive reflux disease. Conceptually, this is because the specificity of heartburn as an acid-induced symptom is less in the absence of esophagitis. This limitation is even more evident in the case of regurgitation wherein the therapeutic gain from PPI therapy is less than 20% [12]. Consequently, persistent regurgitation despite PPI therapy is a major contributor to treatment failure.

The linkage between PPI response and acid-mediated symptoms is particularly well illustrated in the case of the treatment of unexplained chest pain. A recent meta-analysis examined the responsiveness of chest pain to PPI therapy in randomized controlled trials that utilized pH monitoring as an objective means of distinguishing patients with or without abnormal acid reflux [13]. Based on the data from six randomized controlled trials, the therapeutic gain of >50% improvement with PPIs relative to placebo was achieved in 56–85% in GERD-positive patients and only 0–17% in

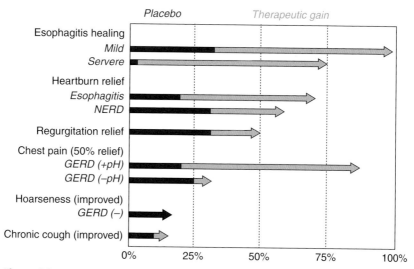

Figure 4.2 Summary of proton pump inhibitor (PPI) efficacy in randomized controlled trials for potential manifestations of GERD. In each case, data among trials are averaged to derive estimates of placebo effect and therapeutic gain (the degree to which the active therapy improved upon the benefit seen with placebo). The dark purple bars represent the placebo effect and the light purple bars the therapeutic gain beyond the placebo effect seen with PPI. No distinctions are implied between brands or doses of PPIs. In fact, the only disease manifestation in which a dose–response curve has been shown is in the healing of esophagitis, wherein higher doses or more potent PPIs are marginally more effective, especially in severe cases. In the case of hoarseness, controlled trial data are sparse and the only large trial (which was done in patients without objective evidence of GERD) failed to show any benefit of PPI versus placebo [48]. GERD, gastroesophageal reflux disease; NERD, non-erosive reflux disease.

GERD-negative patients [13]. Atypical or extraesophageal GERD manifestations remain a controversial topic in disease management. However, as shown in Figure 4.2, evidence supporting PPI therapy in this domain is very weak, showing little if any evidence of efficacy in randomized controlled trials. This despite usage of PPIs in twice-daily dosing for treatment periods of 3–4 months.

The example of chronic cough is particularly interesting, which was the topic of a recent Cochrane review exploring the efficacy of gastroesophageal treatment [14]. Nine adult studies were identified comparing PPI to placebo and included in a meta-analysis. No significant difference in effect was observed between PPI and placebo in total resolution of cough (odds ratio (OR) 0.46, 95% confidence interval (CI) 0.19–1.15). Patients on PPI did, however, exhibit a slight but significant improvement in cough scores after 2–3 months of PPI when data among studies were combined.

Finally, whatever the presentation of GERD, the likelihood of long-term spontaneous remission is low and maintenance therapy is usually required for continued symptom control. Maintenance therapy should be the lowest

PPI dose necessary for symptom relief. Regardless of physicians' instructions, most patients do this independently, adopting on-demand or intermittent dosing of PPIs as required for symptom control [4].

Reflux inhibition

Substantial experimental evidence suggests that TLESRs are the dominant mechanism of reflux in most GERD patients [15]. Increased compliance of the esophagagastric junction (EGJ), as occurs in GERD, is associated with increased opening and flow across the relaxed sphincter, making proximal reflux and regurgitation more likely. Consequently, pharmacological inhibition of TLESRs is an attractive therapeutic target for GERD and, conceptually, might be more effective than PPIs in treating regurgitation.

Baclofen, a GABA$_B$ agonist, inhibits the vagal pathway for TLESRs both centrally and peripherally [16]. However, since the drug crosses the blood–brain barrier, neurological side-effects (somnolence, dizziness, drowsiness) limit its use for GERD in clinical practice. Therefore, novel GABA$_B$ agonists have been developed in an attempt to limit these side-effects. Experimentally, arbaclofen placarbil, a pro-drug of the pharmacologically active R-isomer of balclofen, decreases the number of postprandial reflux events [17]. Similarly, lesogaberan, a novel GABA$_B$ agonist, has been shown to decrease postprandial TLESRs [18]. Preliminary studies have also shown GABA$_B$ agonists to be superior to placebo in controlling typical symptoms of GERD [17,19]. Nevertheless, larger scale studies have thus far failed to show significant improvement in heartburn or regurgitation with these drugs. In symptomatic GERD patients who failed to respond to PPI therapy, the proportion of patients who respond to reflux inhibition appeared modest and not specific for heartburn or regurgitation. In a recent randomized trial including 244 patients with persistent heartburn and/or regurgitation despite PPI therapy, lesogaberan, used as add-on therapy, increased the number of heartburn-free days by 14% and the number of regurgitation-free days by 13% compared to placebo [20]. As for the effect of GABA$_B$ agonists on extraesophageal symptoms of GERD, this may be difficult to evaluate. Baclofen inhibits cough via a central mechanism [21], making the role of reflux inhibition difficult to differentiate in chronic cough patients with GERD.

Enhancing acid clearance

Patients with symptomatic GERD exhibit longer volume and acid esophageal clearance times [22]. Mechanistically, this is attributable to both diminished peristaltic function and the effects of hiatus hernia. Of the two, the hiatus hernia effect is probably dominant, especially when in a supine posture [23,24]. Thus, limiting the contact time between the refluxate and the esophageal mucosa may be proposed to reduce the occurrence of symptoms. Lifestyle measures such as head of bed elevation and avoidance of recumbency after meals target this mechanism but it is also a key principal behind attempts at treating GERD with prokinetics and mucosal protectants.

Prokinetics

Ideally, a prokinetic would enhance esophageal clearance by enhancing peristalsis. Unfortunately, no such drugs are currently available. An alternative approach is to promote gastric emptying which may have the secondary consequence of reducing the occurrence of TLESR. Metoclopramide may improve gastric emptying [25], leading to its proposed use in GERD, especially if accompanied by measurably delayed gastric emptying. However, there are no high-quality data supporting the use of metoclopramide as either monotherapy or adjunctive therapy in esophageal or suspected extraesophageal GERD syndromes. Additionally, considering the toxicity profile of the drug, the current recommendation is against the use of metoclopramide in GERD because the potential risks exceed the potential benefits [4].

Mucosal protection

Decreasing esophageal mucosa permeability to luminal contents may reduce the toxic effect of the gastric refluxate on esophageal mucosa. Rebapimide has been shown to increase the gastric epithelial barrier [26]; it may also exert its effect on esophageal mucosa. Consistent with this hypothesis, the combination of rebamipide and lansoprazole 15 mg was more effective than lansoprazole 15 mg alone in maintaining long-term symptom relief in patients with Los Angeles Grade A and B esophagitis [27].

Stimulating secretion of mucosal protective factors may be another new therapy in GERD. Bicarbonates, mucin, epidermal growth factor (EGF), transforming growth factor alpha (TGF-alpha), and prostaglandin E2 are present in saliva and esophageal secretions; they may promote mucosal healing. Tegaserod, a serotonin 5-hydroxytryptamine 4 receptor agonist, has been shown to increase the volume of salivary and esophageal secretions in patients with GERD [28]. It particularly increased bicarbonate and EGF secretion. In a randomized trial including 88 patients with chronic constipation and GERD or dyspepsia, the combination of tegaserod plus esomeprazole induced complete relief of heartburn in 85% of patients versus 40% for esomeprazole alone and 47% for tegaserod alone ($P=0.012$) [29]. However, although these results seemed promising, tegaserod is no longer commercially available. Nonetheless, the serotonin pathway and stimulation of protective factor secretion may be a target for future therapy.

Visceral hypersensitivity

Some patients with erosive esophagitis and, especially, non-erosive reflux disease exhibit hypersensitivity to esophageal stimuli. This can be demonstrated by balloon distension in the esophagus or acid perfusion (Bernstein test). Hypersensitive patients have a diminished threshold for perceiving these stimuli and a reduced threshold for experiencing pain compared to healthy volunteers [30]. The same observations have been made in patients with functional chest pain [31]. In extreme cases, patients with hypersensitivity perceive the normal passage of food or fluid through the esophagus as uncomfortable.

Low-dose antidepressants

Antidepressants may modulate esophageal sensitivity at the central nervous system and/or sensory afferent level, potentially benefitting symptomatic patients. Low-dose tricyclic antidepressants have been shown to be effective in patients with chest pain after incomplete response to PPI [32]. Trazodone, a serotonin reuptake inhibitor, was more effective than placebo in patients with esophageal symptoms (chest pain, dysphagia, heartburn, and/or regurgitation) associated with esophageal contraction abnormalities [33]. Citalopram, another selective serotonin reuptake inhibitor, significantly increased the threshold for perception and discomfort after balloon distension in healthy volunteers [34]. It also prolonged the duration of esophageal acid perfusion required to induce heartburn. Consequently, these medications may be useful to alleviate esophageal discomfort and heartburn in the subset of GERD patients with hypersensitivity. A recent placebo-controlled trial of citalopram in patients with pH-impedance findings suggestive of hypersensitivity supports this concept [35]. However, thus far there are no large studies that evaluate antidepressants in GERD patients.

Acupuncture

In a series of 30 patients who failed PPI once daily, adding acupuncture was significantly better in controlling acid regurgitation and heartburn than doubling the PPI dose [36]. These results are promising and acupuncture may represent an alternative therapy in PPI non-responders.

Hypnotherapy

Response to PPI treatment can be modulated by the level of psychological distress [37]. Consequently, a therapy which reduces psychological distress may be beneficial in some patients who have an inadequate response to PPI. Hypnotherapy has been proposed as such an alternative therapy, especially for patients with atypical GERD symptoms. In a randomized trial including 28 patients with non-cardiac chest pain, patients treated with hypnotherapy experienced a global improvement in pain more frequently than did controls (80% versus 23%, $P=0.008$). Similarly, in a case series of patients with globus sensation, hypnotherapy appeared to be a beneficial intervention [38]. It remains to be determined if this alternative is effective in larger series of patients with GERD-associated functional symptoms.

Surgery and endoscopic treatment

Surgical fundoplication

High-quality evidence on the efficacy of anti-reflux surgery exists only for esophagitis and/or excessive distal acid exposure determined without ongoing PPI therapy [4]. Anti-reflux surgery is at least as effective as PPI therapy in controlling heartburn and acid regurgitation in controlled trials. The best illustration of this is the recently published LOTUS trial, a large randomized European trial comparing laparoscopic anti-reflux surgery with esomeprazole treatment for patients with chronic GERD. The diagnosis of GERD was established on the basis of typical symptoms and presence of esophageal mucosal breaks at endoscopy and/or a pathological pH monitoring study. Only patients with clinical response to esomeprazole during a 3-month run-in period were randomized. Over the first 3 years of follow-up, both laparoscopic fundoplication and PPI therapy were similarly effective in achieving complete symptom remission [39]. The estimated remission rates at 5 years were greater in the esomeprazole group than in the laparoscopic fundoplication group (92% versus 85%, $P=0.048$) [40]. However, differences were observed between treatments when analyzed by specific symptoms. Specifically, regurgitation was significantly worse in the medical group than in the surgical group (13% versus 2% respectively, $P<0.001$) while there was no significant difference between the groups in heartburn severity. Dysphagia, bloating, and flatulence were all significantly more common in the fundoplication group than in the PPI group.

Consequently the potential benefits of anti-reflux surgery should be weighed against the deleterious effect of new symptoms consequent upon surgery, particularly dysphagia, flatulence, an inability to belch, and post-surgery bowel symptoms (bloating, gas, diarrhea, abdominal pain). Another important requirement for anti-reflux surgery is the presence of some peristaltic activity in the esophagus. Although the precise cut-off remains uncertain, severe peristaltic dysfunction is a relative contraindication and complete absence of peristalsis an absolute contraindication for anti-reflux surgery [4]. Given this perspective, esophageal manometry should be done preoperatively to evaluate peristaltic function [41]. It also allows diagnosis of major esophageal motility disorders that may masquerade as GERD: achalasia and distal esophageal spasm.

Another practical limitation of anti-reflux surgery is that it is known to be highly operator dependent. Efficacy data from community practice reports [42] are widely divergent from those of the LOTUS trial, with as many as 30% of patients resuming PPI therapy within 5 years of anti-reflux surgery. Revision fundoplication surgery is also common, accounting for up to 50% of operations performed at some referral centers [43]. Hence, anti-reflux surgery should be recommended with restraint. Patients with esophagitis who are intolerant of PPIs will likely benefit from anti-reflux surgery. In contrast, patients with esophagitis who are well maintained on medical therapy have nothing to gain from anti-reflux surgery and incur added risk. Patients with esophageal GERD symptoms poorly controlled by PPIs may benefit from surgery, especially in the setting of persistent regurgitation. Even so, the indication must be balanced with the risk of surgery and patients need to be advised of potential dysphagia, inability to belch, flatulence, and the development of new bowel symptoms. There is currently no high-level evidence supporting the use of anti-reflux surgery in patients demonstrating only non-acid reflux on pH-impedance monitoring.

Novel procedural anti-reflux therapies

Recent years have seen many putative endoscopic reflux treatments come and go. As a group, they demonstrated minimal efficacy and an unacceptable incidence of adverse events, leading to poor acceptance and/or rapid withdrawal from the market. Currently, there are two procedural therapies, both designed to restore competency to the EGJ, that are still undergoing evaluation in clinical trials or the approval process: transoral incisionless fundoplication (TIF) with the EsophyX® device and the LINX® sphincter augmentation device.

Transoral incisionless fundoplication is done with the EsophyX® device (Endogastric Solutions, Inc., Redmond, WA), an instrument designed to be used in conjuction with an endoscope to create transmural plications in the region of the EGJ. With the TIF procedure, an omega-shaped, full-thickness gastroesophageal valve is created from inside the stomach [44]. In an early open label study, TIF was compared to laparoscopic fundoplication in patients with persistent heartburn or regurgitation despite PPI therapy [45]. TIF was significantly less effective than laparoscopic fundoplication in improving reflux parameters and symptoms even though more than half of the patients in the group who underwent endoscopic procedure were improved. Other reports also suggest that symptoms may be improved by the TIF procedure [46] and evaluation is continuing using a modified technique (TIF2) that more closely emulates the intragastric valve achieved by fundoplication [44].

LINX® is a recently developed sphincter augmentation device (LINX® Reflux Management System, Torax Medical, Shoreview, NM) [47]. The device consists of a miniature string of interlinked titanium beads with magnetic cores that is laparoscopically placed around the EGJ with or without surgical repair of the hiatus. The magnetic bond between adjacent beads augments sphincter competence by resisting opening and limiting distension. However, the beads do temporarily separate to allow swallowing, belching or vomiting. A recent open label report of 2 years follow-up after LINX® placement found significant symptomatic improvement in a series of 44 patients with typical GERD symptoms that had been at least partially responsive to PPI therapy. Furthermore, although all the patients had pathological esophageal acid exposure at baseline, 77% and 90% had normal esophageal acid exposure at 1 and 2 years. Early dysphagia was observed in 43% of patients, resolving spontaneously within 3 months in all but one who had the device removed at 1 month.

The eventual place of these novel procedures in GERD management remains to be determined, certainly awaiting a more comprehensive understanding of their effectiveness, limitations, and safety. In their favor, they are designed to be reversible and it is hoped that they will cause fewer adverse events than laparoscopic fundoplication, potentially representing a therapy intermediate between existing medical and surgical GERD approaches.

CASE STUDY

A 53-year-old woman was referred for heartburn and belching. Her previous medical history was remarkable for asthma and obesity (BMI 33 kg/m²). Her symptoms began several years before and progressively worsened. Rabeprazole 20 mg daily was sufficient to achieve complete heartburn relief but belching persisted. Because of the persistence of belching, an esophagogastroduodenoscopy was performed and was normal. A pH impedance study done while taking the rabeprazole revealed pathological esophageal acid exposure (esophageal pH <4 during 8.9% of the total time) with 65 reflux events in 24 h. During the recording, the patient reported 52 symptom-events (mainly belching) and the symptom association probability was 100%. Treatment with baclofen 10 mg twice daily was then added to the PPI therapy. This was effective in relieving the belching but the patient discontinued the treatment because the baclofen made her somnolent. Laparoscopic fundoplication was discussed as a possible alternative but after balancing of the potential benefit of treating belching against the risk of postoperative gas bloat syndrome, it was decided against. Instead, the patient attempted to modify her diet and lose weight; this was unsuccessful. Finally she was referred for behavioral therapy. After three sessions of diaphragmatic breathing and habit reversal training, the patient reported a significant improvement of her belching.

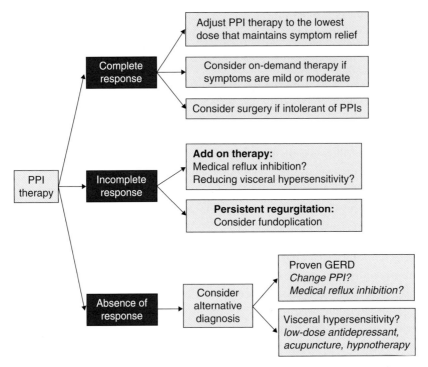

Figure 4.3 Management algorithm for GERD treatment. GERD, gastroesophageal reflux disease; PPI, proton pump inhibitor.

Management algorithm

A management algorithm for GERD treatment is presented in Figure 4.3. PPIs are the first-line therapy. The other alternative should be proposed when PPIs are not well tolerated or in case of incomplete response.

Conclusion

Reflux disease is caused by physiological dysfunction of the EGJ leading to excessive reflux of gastric secretions into the esophagus. Esophagitis is a direct consequence of this. Consequently, reducing gastric acid secretion with PPIs is very effective in esophagitis healing. However, PPIs do not eliminate reflux and the response of specific GERD symptoms to PPI therapy is dependent on the degree to which those symptoms are related to acid. PPIs are most effective for the symptom of heartburn but progressively less so for regurgitation, chest pain, and atypical symptoms. However, even in the case of heartburn, PPI efficacy is substantially less than for healing esophagitis. When the PPIs are not well tolerated or ineffective, alternative treatment should be tested. H₂RAs and antacids are alternatives with mild-to-moderate GERD symptoms. Reducing the occurrence of reflux is another important therapeutic target, especially in patients with persistent regurgitation on PPI therapy. Achieving this pharmacologically with TLESR inhibition raised expectations in this domain but thus far the therapeutic gain seems to be modest. Anti-reflux surgery is the main alternative in these patients if a clear relationship is established between persistent regurgitation and reflux. Finally, treating visceral hypersensitivity may be beneficial in the subset of GERD patients whose symptoms are driven by this mechanism.

References

1 Vakil N, van Zanten SV, Kahrilas P, Dent J, Jones R. The Montreal definition and classification of gastroesophageal reflux disease: a global evidence-based consensus. Am J Gastroenterol 2006;101(8):1900–20.
2 Sontag SJ, Sonnenberg A, Schnell TG, Leya J, Metz A. The long-term natural history of gastroesophageal reflux disease. J Clin Gastroenterol 2006;40(5):398–404.
3 Pandolfino JE, Kwiatek MA, Kahrilas PJ. The pathophysiologic basis for epidemiologic trends in gastroesophageal reflux disease. Gastroenterol Clin North Am 2008;37(4):827–43, viii.
4 Kahrilas PJ, Shaheen NJ, Vaezi MF, et al. American Gastroenterological Association Medical Position Statement on the management of gastroesophageal reflux disease. Gastroenterology 2008;135(4):1383–91.
5 Hampel H, Abraham NS, El-Serag HB. Meta-analysis: obesity and the risk for gastroesophageal reflux disease and its complications. Ann Intern Med 2005 2;143(3):199–211.
6 Kjellin A, Ramel S, Rossner S, Thor K. Gastroesophageal reflux in obese patients is not reduced by weight reduction. Scand J Gastroenterol 1996;31(11):1047–51.
7 Fraser-Moodie CA, Norton B, Gornall C, Magnago S, Weale AR, Holmes GK. Weight loss has an independent beneficial effect on symptoms of gastro-oesophageal reflux in patients who are overweight. Scand J Gastroenterol 1999;34(4):337–40.
8 Jacobson BC, Somers SC, Fuchs CS, Kelly CP, Camargo CA Jr. Body-mass index and symptoms of gastroesophageal reflux in women. N Engl J Med 2006; 354(22):2340–8.
9 Khan M, Santana J, Donnellan C, Preston C, Moayyedi P. Medical treatments in the short term management of reflux oesophagitis. Cochrane Database Syst Rev 2007;2:CD003244.
10 Van Pinxteren B, Sigterman KE, Bonis P, Lau J, Numans ME. Short-term treatment with proton pump inhibitors, H2-receptor antagonists and prokinetics for gastro-oesophageal reflux disease-like symptoms and endoscopy negative reflux disease. Cochrane Database Syst Rev 2010;11:CD002095.
11 Vakil NB, Traxler B, Levine D. Dysphagia in patients with erosive esophagitis: prevalence, severity, and response to proton pump inhibitor treatment. Clin Gastroenterol Hepatol 2004;2(8):665–8.

12 Kahrilas PJ, Howden CW, Hughes N. Response of regurgitation to proton pump inhibitor therapy in clinical trials of gastroesophageal reflux disease. Am J Gastroenterol 2011;106(8):1419–25.

13 Kahrilas PJ, Hughes N, Howden CW. Response of unexplained chest pain to proton pump inhibitor treatment in patients with and without objective evidence of gastro-oesophageal reflux disease. Gut 2011;60(11):1473–8.

14 Chang AB, Lasserson TJ, Gaffney J, Connor FL, Garske LA. Gastro-oesophageal reflux treatment for prolonged non-specific cough in children and adults. Cochrane Database Syst Rev 2011;1:CD004823.

15 Sifrim D, Holloway R, Silny J, Tack J, Lerut A, Janssens J. Composition of the postprandial refluxate in patients with gastroesophageal reflux disease. Am J Gastroenterol 2001;96(3):647–55.

16 Zhang Q, Lehmann A, Rigda R, Dent J, Holloway RH. Control of transient lower oesophageal sphincter relaxations and reflux by the GABA(B) agonist baclofen in patients with gastro-oesophageal reflux disease. Gut 2002;50(1):19–24.

17 Gerson LB, Huff FJ, Hila A, et al. Arbaclofen placarbil decreases postprandial reflux in patients with gastroesophageal reflux disease. Am J Gastroenterol 2010; 105(6):1266–75.

18 Boeckxstaens GE, Beaumont H, Mertens V, et al. Effects of lesogaberan on reflux and lower esophageal sphincter function in patients with gastroesophageal reflux disease. Gastroenterology 2010;139(2):409–17.

19 Ciccaglione AF, Marzio L. Effect of acute and chronic administration of the GABA B agonist baclofen on 24 hour pH metry and symptoms in control subjects and in patients with gastro-oesophageal reflux disease. Gut 2003;52(4):464–70.

20 Boeckxstaens GE, Beaumont H, Hatlebakk JG, et al. A novel reflux inhibitor lesogaberan (AZD3355) as add-on treatment in patients with GORD with persistent reflux symptoms despite proton pump inhibitor therapy: a randomised placebo-controlled trial. Gut 2011;60(9):1182–8.

21 Dicpinigaitis PV, Dobkin JB. Antitussive effect of the GABA-agonist baclofen. Chest 1997;111(4):996–9.

22 Bredenoord AJ, Weusten BL, Timmer R, Smout AJ. Characteristics of gastroesophageal reflux in symptomatic patients with and without excessive esophageal acid exposure. Am J Gastroenterol 2006;101(11):2470–5.

23 Sloan S, Kahrilas PJ. Impairment of esophageal emptying with hiatal hernia. Gastroenterology 1991;100(3):596–605.

24 Lin S, Ke M, Xu J, Kahrilas PJ. Impaired esophageal emptying in reflux disease. Am J Gastroenterol 1994;89(7):1003–6.

25 Durazo FA, Valenzuela JE. Effect of single and repeated doses of metoclopramide on the mechanisms of gastroesophageal reflux. Am J Gastroenterol 1993;88(10): 1657–62.

26 Matysiak-Budnik T, Heyman M, Megraud F. Review article: rebamipide and the digestive epithelial barrier. Aliment Pharmacol Ther 2003;18(Suppl 1): 55–62.

27 Yoshida N, Kamada K, Tomatsuri N, et al. Management of recurrence of symptoms of gastroesophageal reflux disease: synergistic effect of rebamipide with 15 mg lansoprazole. Dig Dis Sci 2010;55(12):3393–8.

28 Majewski M, Jaworski T, Sarosiek I, et al. Significant enhancement of esophageal pre-epithelial defense by tegaserod: implications for an esophagoprotective effect. Clin Gastroenterol Hepatol 2007;5(4):430–8.

29 Zeng J, Zuo XL, Li YQ, Wei W, Lv GP. Tegaserod for dyspepsia and reflux symptoms in patients with chronic constipation: an exploratory open-label study. Eur J Clin Pharmacol 2007;63(6):529–36.

30 Yang M, Li ZS, Chen DF, *et al.* Quantitative assessment and characterization of visceral hyperalgesia evoked by esophageal balloon distention and acid perfusion in patients with functional heartburn, nonerosive reflux disease, and erosive esophagitis. Clin J Pain 2010;26(4):326–31.

31 Nasr I, Attaluri A, Hashmi S, Gregersen H, Rao SS. Investigation of esophageal sensation and biomechanical properties in functional chest pain. Neurogastroenterol Motil 2010;22(5):520–6.

32 Prakash C, Clouse RE. Long-term outcome from tricyclic antidepressant treatment of functional chest pain. Dig Dis Sci 1999;44(12):2373–9.

33 Clouse RE, Lustman PJ, Eckert TC, Ferney DM, Griffith LS. Low-dose trazodone for symptomatic patients with esophageal contraction abnormalities. A double-blind, placebo-controlled trial. Gastroenterology 1987;92(4):1027–36.

34 Broekaert D, Fischler B, Sifrim D, Janssens J, Tack J. Influence of citalopram, a selective serotonin reuptake inhibitor, on oesophageal hypersensitivity: a double-blind, placebo-controlled study. Aliment Pharmacol Ther 2006;23(3): 365–70.

35 Viazis N, Keyoglou A, Kanellopoulos AK, *et al.* Selective serotonin reuptake inhibitors for the treatment of hypersensitive esophagus: a randomized, double-blind, placebo-controlled study. Am J Gastroenterol 2011; May 31 (epub ahead of print).

36 Dickman R, Schiff E, Holland A, *et al.* Clinical trial: acupuncture vs. doubling the proton pump inhibitor dose in refractory heartburn. Aliment Pharmacol Ther 2007; 26(10):1333–44.

37 Nojkov B, Rubenstein JH, Adlis SA, *et al.* The influence of co-morbid IBS and psychological distress on outcomes and quality of life following PPI therapy in patients with gastro-oesophageal reflux disease. Aliment Pharmacol Ther 2008; 27(6):473–82.

38 Kiebles JL, Kwiatek MA, Pandolfino JE, Kahrilas PJ, Keefer L. Do patients with globus sensation respond to hypnotically assisted relaxation therapy? A case series report. Dis Esophagus 2010;23(7):545–53.

39 Lundell L, Attwood S, Ell C, *et al.* Comparing laparoscopic antireflux surgery with esomeprazole in the management of patients with chronic gastro-oesophageal reflux disease: a 3-year interim analysis of the LOTUS trial. Gut 2008;57(9) :1207–13.

40 Galmiche JP, Hatlebakk J, Attwood S, *et al.* Laparoscopic antireflux surgery vs esomeprazole treatment for chronic GERD. The LOTUS randomized clinical trial. JAMA 2011;305(19):1969–77.

41 Pandolfino JE, Kahrilas PJ. AGA technical review on the clinical use of esophageal manometry. Gastroenterology 2005;128(1):209–24.

42 Vakil N, Shaw M, Kirby R. Clinical effectiveness of laparoscopic fundoplication in a U.S. community. Am J Med 2003;114(1):1–5.

43 Hunter JG, Smith CD, Branum GD, *et al.* Laparoscopic fundoplication failures: patterns of failure and response to fundoplication revision. Ann Surg 1999;230(4): 595–604; discussion 606.

44 Bell RC, Cadiere GB. Transoral rotational esophagogastric fundoplication: technical, anatomical, and safety considerations. Surg Endosc 2011;25(7):2387–99.

45 Frazzoni M, Conigliaro R, Manta R, Melotti G. Reflux parameters as modified by EsophyX or laparoscopic fundoplication in refractory GERD. Aliment Pharmacol Ther 2011;34(1):67–75.

46 Testoni PA, Corsetti M, di Pietro S, *et al.* Effect of transoral incisionless fundoplication on symptoms, PPI use, and ph-impedance refluxes of GERD patients. World J Surg 2010;34(4):750–7.

47 Bonavina L, DeMeester T, Fockens P, *et al.* Laparoscopic sphincter augmentation device eliminates reflux symptoms and normalizes esophageal acid exposure: one- and 2-year results of a feasibility trial. Ann Surg 2010;252(5):857–62.

48 Vaezi MF, Richter JE, Stasney CR, *et al.* Treatment of chronic posterior laryngitis with esomeprazole. Laryngoscope 2006;116(2):254–60.

Gastroesophageal Reflux Disease Treatment: Side-Effects and Complications of Acid Suppression

David A. Johnson

Department of Gastroenterology, Eastern Virginia School of Medicine, Norfolk, VA, USA

Key points

- Data suggesting relative "harm" for bone fracture and decreased clinical effectiveness of clopidogrel are found in retrospective studies with inferential "channeling bias".
- Bone fracture risks with proton pump inhibitors are not greater when patient risks are co-adjusted for other bone fracture relative risks.
- The only prospective randomized controlled trial of proton pump inhibitors (omeprazole) and clopidogrel evidenced no increased cardiovascular complications but demonstrable reduction (with proton pump inhibitor) in gastrointestinal bleeding.
- Hypomagnesemia and interstitial nephritis complications with proton pump inhibitors appear to be rare but real and are likely idiosyncratic.
- Data on proton pump inhibitor infectious risks remain questionable and controversial, in particular for enteric infections and diarrheal illness.

Potential pitfalls

- Retrospective studies should include nested cohorts of patients with achlorhydria to determine index risk for acid suppression-related harm.
- All studies with suggested harm implications have high potential for "channeling bias" which can suggest a risk for the event but be confounded by other more accountable risks.
- Continued use of proton pump inhibitors should always be questioned for explicit need and then risk/benefit ratios for continued use assessed.

Practical Manual of Gastroesophageal Reflux Disease, First Edition.
Edited by Marcelo F. Vela, Joel E. Richter and John E. Pandolfino.
© 2013 John Wiley & Sons, Ltd. Published 2013 by John Wiley & Sons, Ltd.

Introduction

Proton pump inhibitors (PPIs) are medications that are essentially ubiquitous in a gastroenterologist's practice. This class of medication has been available for commercial use for nearly 25 years and has supplanted the use of histamine-2 receptor antagonists for patients with moderate to severe gastric acid-related diseases as well as for prophylaxis of upper gastrointestinal (GI) injury, e.g. with non-steroidal antiinflammatory drugs (NSAIDs). The success of these drugs, with sales totaling approximately $13.6 billion worldwide in 2009 [1], is not just a result of their potency and effectiveness in improving symptoms and complications of acid-peptic diseases. Their safety among pharmacological agents has been unparalleled but although they are one of the safest classes of medication that gastroenterologists deal with, there have been emerging concerns with reports of potential adverse effects associated with use of PPIs. In the US, such reports have led the Food and Drug Administration to issue a number of broad-based product warnings, including all the available PPI drugs available either for prescription or over-the-counter purchase. The pathogenesis of these proposed associations is not clear in most cases and the evidence base to support a clear association for harm is extremely variable. These potential interactions have included altered absorption of vitamins and minerals, alteration of pharmacokinetics/pharmacodynamics of concomitant medications, infection risks, metabolic effects on bone density, and hypersensitivity responses with consequent organ damage.

This chapter will examine the proposed scientific basis for the adverse events and the evidence base surrounding these controversies.

Vitamin and mineral absorption effects

Long-term PPI therapy has been thought to be associated with micronutrient deficiencies, especially of iron, calcium, magnesium, and vitamin B_{12}.

Iron

Hydrochloric acid in the stomach assists in the dissociation of iron salts from food and the reduction of ferric iron to the more soluble ferrous iron. As non-heme (ferric) iron constitutes the majority of dietary iron requirements, there has been concern about impairment of iron absorption if the conversion to the more soluble ferrous iron is impaired. *In vivo* data have demonstrated that iron absorption was directly related to gastric juice release of ferric iron contained in food [2]. There is some evidence suggesting this may be more specifically related to the vitamin C which is released in gastric secretion [3]. There is also some evidence that PPIs may reduce the bioavailability of ingested vitamin C [4]. The long-term follow-up of patients taking chronic daily PPIs for up to 7 years has not shown iron absorption to be a clinically apparent problem [5].

Clinical summary

Despite the above theoretical considerations, there are relatively few data to indicate that proton pump inhibitor therapy causes iron deficiency. In fact, there is no report suggesting that proton pump inhibitor therapy under normal clinical circumstances results in the occurrence of iron deficiency. In patients with iron deficiency demanding increased iron absorption, it is conceivable that proton pump inhibitor therapy may reduce absorption of the non-heme iron and thereby retard replenishment of the iron pool. This, however, has not been well studied nor is it evident from widespread use in clinical practice.

Calcium

The solubilization of dietary calcium salts is thought to be essential for absorption of calcium. This is mediated through the release of ionized calcium from the insoluble calcium salts. It is believed that gastric acid mediates this solubilization of the dietary calcium and hence there is concern that reduction in gastric acid secretion may impair calcium absorption. However, the data linking hypochlorhydric states, including pharmacological hypocholorhyria induced by PPI therapy, have not shown consistent evidence of potential impaired calcium absorption. In fact, two high-quality studies have shown no adverse effect [6,7].

The clinical reports inferring potential harm from PPIs as an influence for bone fractures have been controversial but convincing enough to the FDA that a product label warning was issued for all PPIs. Most recently, this has been revised to release this warning from labels for over-the-counter products given that they are intended for short-term use (2 weeks) and for only up to three cycles/year [8]. The earlier published reports linking PPI use to development of hip fractures have been observational studies and case–control studies and thus have greater potential for bias and therefore less accurate estimates. Additionally, the strength of association in the PPI studies has been of low magnitude. The adjusted summary odds ratios (OR) were 1.18 (95% confidence interval (CI) 1.12–1.43), 1.44 (1.30–1.59), and 0.99 (0.90–1.11) but 1.92 (1.16–3.18) if 7 years of continuous PPI use [9–13]. Given that the estimates and even the upper bounds of most of the 95% CIs of the odds ratio were well below 2, there is a strong possibility that these differences could have been due to the channeling bias inherent in observational studies [14]. More recent cross-sectional, longitudinal and prospective observational reports do not support the reported association [15,16]. It is highly unlikely that randomized controlled clinical trials can be accurately done to further address the question of bone density loss and PPI therapy. The relative rarity of fracture across the population and the extent of potential confounding variables would make this an extremely difficult study to conduct.

It has also been demonstrated that there are proton pumps in osteo-clasts, the cells responsible for bone resorption. These vacuolar proton pumps are responsible for acidification at the ruffled border and facilitate the dissolution of bone matrix and subsequent resorption [17]. Accordingly, a PPI would be expected to impair this osteoclastic function of bone resorption, which should actually lead to an increase in bone density. Patients on PPIs have lower levels of urinary calcium and hydroxproline, suggesting a diminution of osteoclast activity. Furthermore, these patients have increased osteocalcin and tissue resistant alkaline phosphatase, suggestive of increased new bone formation [18].

Clinical summary

Overall, the studies suggest that calcium absorption is potentially nega-tively affected only in the setting of reduced acid secretion when ingested calcium carbonate is provided in the fasting state. As most dietary calcium is ingested either as a component of food or in supplements taken with meals, this calcium absorption issue is not likely to be of great clinical relevance. Furthermore, given that the biological plausi-bility is also not consistent for causality, it seems reasonable to conclude that, overall, it is unlikely that PPI use has a significant risk for bone density loss and related complications of osteoporotic fractures. Accordingly, the data on bone density loss/osteoporotic fractures would not suggest that PPI therapy be discontinued in patients taking PPIs for appropriate indications at appropriate doses. Clearly, adherence to osteo-porosis screening guidelines is recommended for all patients at risk, irrespective of the use of PPIs.

Magnesium

There have been several (total <50) cases of hypomagnesemia associated with long-term PPI use [19–21]. The patients generally presented with profound hypomagnesemia and typically required hospitalization. In approximately 25% of these cases, the patients had persistent hypomagne-semia despite supplements. Prompt resolution of magnesium levels was evident after discontinuance of PPIs, and in a few cases where the patients were rechallenged with a PPI, the hypomagesemia recurred, suggesting a PPI-related effect. None of the patients had identifiable GI wasting or renal loss etiologies. This prompted a recent alert by the FDA about PPI use and hypomagnesemia [22]. This alert suggested that healthcare providers should consider checking magnesium levels in patients who are anticipated to be on long-term PPIs.

The mechanism for the magnesium depletion is not known. The primary absorption of magnesium is through a passive pathway in the small intestine. There is some identifiable active transport, however, via transport channels (TRPM6 and 7) [23]. It is not known if PPIs may have some effect on this pathway but there are familial cases with mutations at this pathway who develop hypomagnesemia.

Clinical summary

Although omeprazole and esomeprazole were initially cited, other PPIs have now been included so this is likely a class effect. The FDA recommendation to consider checking magnesium levels before starting is not practical, in particular for the over-the-counter market. In patients who may be predisposed to present/ongoing magnesium loss, e.g. intestinal malabsorption or renal excretion/wasting, it may be reasonable to follow magnesium levels more closely and consider this association, particularly if a profound hypomagnesemia condition develops. Given the extreme rarity of the report and no controlled studies to delineate the mechanisms, it is important for healthcare providers to be aware of this but maintain PPI use where clinically justified, in their appropriate scope of practice.

Vitamin B$_{12}$

Gastric acid also facilitates the release of vitamin B$_{12}$ bound to proteins within ingested foodstuffs to permit binding to R-proteins for eventual absorption in the terminal ileum. This vitamin needs to be released from these proteins and subsequently bound to R-proteins and intrinsic factor in order to be absorbed in the terminal ileum. Gastric acid facilitates the proteolytic process involved in releasing the vitamin from the proteins in ingested food. Accordingly, there are theoretical reasons why the inhibition of gastric acid secretion by PPI therapy would reduce the bioavailability of of dietary vitamin B$_{12}$ [2].

Studies which have examined the potential association between long-term PPI use and vitamin B$_{12}$ have shown conflicting results [23]. Additionally, to date no studies have provided a longitudinal evaluation demonstrating alterations of specific metabolic intermediates (e.g. methylmalonate and homocysteine) which can accumulate with this deficiency.

Clinical summary

Despite the biological plausibility of this deficiency, there is currently little evidence to support a clinically relevant association to recommend a change in current practice.

Alteration of pharmacokinetics/pharmacodynamics

Proton pump inhibitors and related impairment of antiplatelet therapy (clopidogrel)

It is well known that PPIs are metabolized by the cytochrome p450 enzyme pathway, specifically CYP2C19 and CYP3A4. As clopidogrel is a pro-drug which requires active biotransformation via the cytochrome p450 pathway, it has been hypothesized that competition at CYP2C19 sites may result in reduced biological effects of clopidogrel when co-administered with PPIs. The concept of PPIs interfering with clopidogrel biotransformation stemmed from *in vitro* studies that demonstrated a pharmacodynamic interaction which was an attenuated antiplatelet effect as measured by adenosine diphosphate (ADP)-induced platelet aggregation and elevated platelet activity [24].

The inference in regard to PPIs and clopidogrel first arose from the combined use of clopidogrel and omeprazole, although several other PPIs have subsequently been found to be associated with a smaller or insignificant attenuation of the clopidogrel antiplatelet effect; these PPIs included pantoprazole, esomeprazole, and to a lesser degree lansoprazole [14,25]. However, these *in vitro* data were quickly extrapolated in several high-profile retrospective database evaluations that found higher cardiac event rates (stent thrombosis, myocardial infarct, and death) in patients who were taking clopidogrel with any PPI versus those on clopidogrel alone [26,27]. This physiological intermediary endpoint of attenuated effect led to a number of retrospective *post hoc* analyses and these suggested a potential clinical harm with adverse cardiovascular outcomes for patients taking clopidogrel and PPIs. Based on these data, the FDA issued a recommendation against the combined use of omeprazole and esomeprazole and clopidogrel [28]. In that statement the FDA also advised against the combined use of clopidogrel coupled with other potent inhibitors of the cytochrome p450 pathway such as cimetidine, as well as cautioning against use of other PPIs.

In fact, although consensus recommendations from the leading gastroenterology and cardiology national societies suggested that this combined use was appropriate for patients at significant increased risk for gastrointestinal bleeding [29], these recommendations were developed at the same time as the emerging controversy and the experts involved in the recommendations were in favor of combined use of PPI (as the preferred strategy over H2 receptor antagonists) plus clopidogrel for patients defined as being at risk of GI bleeding. Additionally, there were prospective randomized controlled studies emerging which showed no evidence of increased cardiovascular adverse events when patients had combined use of PPIs [30].

The most substantive data to date, supporting the lack of cardiovascular harm, come from a randomized prospective placebo-controlled trial comparing clopidogrel with or without omeprazole in patients who had coronary stents following an acute coronary syndrome [31]. In this study of 3761 patients, the *a priori* primary objectives were assessment of both cardiovascular and GI harm. There was no difference for cardiovascular adverse events between the placebo and omeprazole group. In all, 51 patients had a gastrointestinal event; the event rate was 1.1% with omeprazole and 2.9% with placebo at 180 days (hazard ratio (HR) with omeprazole, 0.34, 95% CI 0.18–0.63, $P < 0.001$). The rate of overt upper gastrointestinal bleeding was also reduced with omeprazole compared with placebo (HR 0.13, 95% CI 0.03–0.56, $P = 0.001$). Despite the published prospective randomized controlled data demonstrating no significant cardiovascular harm, but actually demonstrating increased GI harm when omeprazole was not used with clopidogrel, the FDA updated the warning in 2010, removing the other PPIs from the caution notice but reiterating the citation of omeprazole [32]. The safety of combined use of PPIs with clopidogrel has also been evident in patients following a stroke or transient ischemic event [33].

In light of all the controversy over the combined use of clopidogrel and PPIs, an expert consensus document was prepared and endorsed by the American College of Cardiology, the American College of Gastroenterology, and the American Heart Association [34]. The consensus recommendation was that if patients were deemed at significant risk of GI bleeding, then use of clopidogrel combined with PPIs was appropriate. Based on the extensive review of all available data, there was no evidence to suggest increased cardiovascular harm with this combined use.

What has become clearer in review of the retrospective analyses suggesting harm with PPI and clopidogrel combined usage is the high likelihood for channeling bias. In fact, the most recent *post hoc* database assessment (using the VA database) did suggest an apparent cardiovascular harm for combined usage, but when the authors used propensity-matched evaluations to correct for co-variate cardiovascular risks and medication compliance, they found no significant association between major cardiovascular events and use of clopidogrel with continuous, switched or discontinued PPIs [35].

It is not well understood that although clopidogrel is not an NSAID, there is significant risk for upper GI ulceration and related bleeding. Conventional wisdom suggests that clopidogrel should be a safer, non-ulcerogenic alternative for patients at high risk for aspirin-induced ulcers. However, Chan *et al.* reported on patients with NSAID-related ulcer disease who were randomized (after ulcer healing) to receive clopidogrel alone or esomeprazole plus aspirin [36]. After a 1-year follow-up period, the patients in the clopidogrel group had a significant increase in the rate of recurrent upper gastrointestinal bleeding from ulcers, compared with those in the group taking aspirin plus esomeprazole (8.6% versus 0.7%, $P=0.001$).

The impairment of ulcer healing by clopidogrel has not been widely appreciated. Platelet aggregation plays a critical role in healing, through the release of various platelet-derived growth factors that promote angiogenesis, which is essential for ulcer healing. ADP-receptor antagonists impair the healing of gastric ulcers by inhibiting the release by platelets of proangiogenic growth factors such as vascular endothelial growth factor, which promotes endothelial proliferation and accelerates the healing of ulcers [37]. Accordingly, although clopidogrel might not be the primary cause of gastrointestinal ulcers, the anti-angiogenic effects may impair the healing of background ulcers; when combined with the propensity to increase bleeding, these agents may convert small, silent erosions or ulcers into large ulcers that bleed. A recent prospective randomized controlled study involving patients with histories of peptic ulcer disease showed at 6 months that the combination of esomeprazole and clopidogrel had a 1.2% ulcer recurrence rate compared to 11.0% recurrence in patients receiving clopidogrel alone ($P=0.009$) [38].

Clinical summary

These results question the exact relationship between *ex vivo* platelet assays and clinical outcomes, especially with regard to the assessment of drug interactions. Platelet assays and observational data may be factual but are not always appropriate for extrapolation to clinical care, as evidenced by what we have seen during the last several months with the prescribing recommendations for PPI and clopidogrel usage. Platelet assays and observational data are not substitutes for randomized controlled trial data.

Appropriate use is the key consideration for any medication. Healthcare providers should be attuned to the need for PPI therapy in patients who exhibit signs or symptoms of acid-related disease, as well as in asymptomatic patients treated with NSAIDs or antiplatelet agents who meet risk stratification criteria to justify GI prophylaxis (co-therapy with a PPI).

Proton pump inhibitors and infection

As gastric acid creates a potential barrier to acid-sensitive spores and bacteria which may colonize the upper GI tract, there has been a concern about potential alteration of native GI flora and clinical consequences of bacterial overgrowth. Additionally, there are some data which suggest that PPIs may have a direct effect on white blood cell function with alterations of neutrophil chemotaxis and degranulation [39]. Specific infection risks have been cited for community- and hospital-acquired pneumonia, *Clostridium difficile* colitis, enteric infections, and spontaneous bacterial peritonitis.

Pneumonia

Several studies have suggested that PPI use may increase the risk for both community- and hospital-acquired pneumonia. In theory, when gastro-esophageal reflux occurs, gastric bacteria could be carried up to the hypo-pharynx where microaspiration into the lower airways could lead to pneumonia, especially in patients with compromised oropharyngeal protective reflexes, e.g. those on mechanical ventilation. In general, most of the studies assessing the relationship between PPIs and community-acquired pneumonia have revealed a modestly higher risk of community-acquired pneumonia in patients exposed to PPIs [40–42]. This risk was confirmed in a recent metaanalysis, which found a higher risk of community-acquired pneumonia with PPI use (OR 1.36, 95% CI 1.12–1.65). The authors refrained from drawing definitive conclusions from these data because of the significant heterogeneity between the studies [43]. Other studies from large database analyses, however, have not shown a significant increase in community-acquired pneumonia [44,45].

Clinical summary

Residual confounding may have complicated interpretation of these studies, suggesting an association of harm (increased pneumonia). These studies surprisingly showed that the association was weakest in current recipients who had been taking PPIs for the longest duration. If an associated risk of PPIs and pneumonia risk is in fact present, the relative risk is small and may be most likely accounted for by channeling bias.

Enteric infections

Alterations of the gastric pH and possible related changes in susceptibility to enteric infections have been a topic of long-standing debate. Although gastric hypochlorhydria is commonly listed as a risk factor for traveler's diarrhea [46], PPI exposure as a risk factor for enteric infections in travelers has not been formally studied. In fact, there is only one study evaluating acid reduction medication use and this study reported no significant association (OR 6.9, range 0.7–67.4) of travelers' diarrhea with antacids and H2 receptor antagonist use [47]. A metaanalysis of the diagnosis of enteric infections did identify an increased risk of acute bacterial infection associated with the usage of PPIs (OR 3.33, 95% CI 1.84–6.02) [48]. A recent comprehensive analysis of the data on PPI use and enteric infections concluded that there was no association of PPI use and viral or parasitic enteric infections [49]. The data on specific bacterial infections were generally supportive of no associated risk although there were a few specific case reports suggesting a remote causal association.

Previously, gastric acid was not believed to be important in protecting against *C. difficile* infection because acid-resistant spores were presumed to be the principal vector of transmission. Recently, this has been challenged, as several studies have found a higher risk of *C. difficile* infection in PPI users. In theory, PPIs may increase the risk of *C. difficile* infection by increasing the ability of the spore to convert to the vegetative form and to survive in the lumen of the GI tract. The data for community-acquired versus hospital-acquired infection have been variable and inconclusive for an associated risk of harm [49]. A recent metaanalysis of 11 papers, including nearly 127,000 patients, found a significant relationship between PPI use and *C. difficile* infection, with an odds ratio of 2.05 (95% CI 1.47–2.85) [48]. Further supporting the hypothesis of a direct causative association, a recent study found a significant dose–response relationship, with more aggressive acid suppression paired with higher odds association [50].

Other enteric infections have been found to be associated with PPIs [48,49]. A recent metaanalysis did suggest an increased risk of acute bacterial enteric infection with the use of PPIs, with a random effects model pooled risk OR of 3.33 (95% CI 1.84–6.02) [48]. Small intestinal bacterial overgrowth (SIBO), a condition associated with bloating, diarrhea, and malabsorption, has recently been associated with PPI use, although the significance of the association is uncertain [51]. In this report, SIBO was detected in 50% of patients using PPIs, 24.5% of patients with irritable bowel syndrome (IBS), and 6% of healthy control subjects. There was a statistically significant difference between patients using PPIs and those with IBS or healthy control subjects ($P < 0.001$). The prevalence of SIBO increased after 1 year of treatment with PPI. The reported eradication rate of SIBO (using rifaximin) was 87% in the PPI group and 91% in the IBS group.

Clinical summary
For community-acquired enteric infections including *C. difficile*, the reported odds ratios are low and difficult to evaluate fully beyond the potential for channeling bias of sicker patients. The situation is complex in hospitalized settings where drugs, such as PPIs, may be highly correlated with other variables, such as severity of illness and length of stay. The data for possible association with SIBO are extremely limited and will need further corroboration and validation before they can be considered applicable to current clinical use.

Spontaneous bacterial peritonitis
Recent reports have suggested that there is a relationship between PPI use and the development of spontaneous bacterial peritonitis in hospitalized cirrhotic patients with ascites [52,53]. One study found a strong association (OR 4.3, 95% CI 1.3–11.7) between PPIs and SBP [52] whereas another study found no significant association (OR 1.0, 95% CI 0.4–2.6) [53].

Clinical summary

The two studies on this association were small case–control studies of hospitalized patients and the data are conflicting as to a reported associated risk. At present, accordingly, no firm conclusion can be drawn about the relevance of this association.

Proton pump inhibitors and interstitial nephritis

Several case reports have implicated PPIs as a cause of acute interstitial nephritis [23]. This disorder is a humoral and cell-mediated hypersensitivity inflammatory reaction of the renal interstitium and tubules. A systematic review from 2007 found 64 cases documented in the literature, 12 of which were considered definitely associated and nine of which were probably associated [54]. Initial symptoms were non-specific and included nausea, malaise, and fever. With such extensive use worldwide as the denominator, the authors concluded that acute interstitial nephritis was a rare, idiosyncratic occurrence related to PPI use, but did not find enough evidence to support a causative relationship.

Clinical summary

Despite the extreme rarity of the syndrome, the association cannot be dismissed and a high level of clinical suspicion is necessary to detect acute interstitial nephritis early in its course, especially soon after the initiation of PPI therapy.

Conclusion

Although concerns have been raised about the long-term safety of PPIs, the majority of the evidence does not strongly support the deluge of reports citing a potential for significant adverse harm associated with PPI usage. When translating these studies into the routine management of patients, it is important to recall some very basic tenets of good patient care.

Obviously, no therapy is completely without risk, whether pharmacological, surgical or psychological. Consequently, no drug, procedure or treatment plan should be prescribed without a valid indication. Even with an appropriate indication for use, the risk/benefit ratio of every therapy prescribed should always be evaluated. If the indication for the PPI is weak or uncertain, then even a slight risk tips the balance away from the drug and the drug should be discontinued. Clearly, there are too many patients who receive continued PPI therapy without a valid need. When seeing patients in long-term care, the indication and necessity for continued usage for all drugs, including PPIs, should be reviewed and continually reevaluated.

CASE STUDY

A 75-year-old woman is seen in ongoing follow-up of her chronic gastroesophageal reflux disease (GERD). She has had prior relapsing symptoms of dysphagia with an endoscopy demonstrating Los Angeles Grade C erosive esophagitis and a distal esophageal stricture at the esophagogastric junction, which required endoscopic dilation. She had been well controlled over the last year, taking a daily proton pump inhibitor in the morning 30–60 min before breakfast. She recently saw a television broadcast which suggested that the use of PPIs was associated with an increased risk for bone fracture, in particular hip, neck, and wrist. She became frightened about her risks for fracture and therefore stopped her PPI. Since then, she has had recurrent heartburn on a daily basis and is now having increasing recurrent problems with solid food dysphagia. Despite her recurrent symptoms, she is very concerned about restarting the PPI medication which alleviated her GERD symptoms.

References

1 Gatyas G. IMS Health Reports 2009. Available at: www.imshealth.com.

2 Bezwoda W, Charlton R, Bothwell T, *et al.* The importance of gastric hydrochloric acid in the absorption of nonheme food iron. J Lab Clin Med 1978;92:108–16.

3 Conrad ME, Schade SG. Ascorbic acid chelates in iron absorption: a role for hydrochloric acid and bile. Gastroenterology 1968;55:35–43.

4 McColl KE. Effect of proton pump inhibitors on vitamins and iron. Am J Gastroenterol 2009;104(Suppl 2):S5–S9.

5 Koop H. Review article: metabolic consequences of long-term inhibition of acid secretion by omeprazole. Aliment Pharmacol Ther 1992;6:399–406.

6 Wright MJ, Sullivan RR, Gaffney-Stomberg E, *et al.* Inhibiting gastric acid production does not affect intestinal calcium absorption in young, healthy individuals: a randomized, crossover, controlled clinical trial. J Bone Miner Res 2010;25:2205–11.

7 Hansen KE, Jones AN, Lindstrom JM, *et al.* Do proton pump inhibitors decrease calcium absorption? J Bone Miner Res 2010;25:2510–19.

8 www.fda.gov/drugs/drugsafety/postmarketdrugsafetyinformationforpatientsand providers/ucm213206.htm

9 Vestergaard P, Rejnmark L, Mosekilde L. Proton pump inhibitors, histamine H2 receptor antagonists, and other antacid medications and the risk of fracture. Calcif Tissue Int 2006;79:76–83.

10 Yang YX, Lewis JD, Epstein S. *et al.* Long-term proton pump inhibitor therapy and risk of hip fracture. JAMA 2006;296:2947–53.

11 Targownik LE, Lix LM, Metge CJ, *et al.* Use of proton pump inhibitors and risk of osteoporosis-related fractures. CMAJ 2008;179:319–26.

12 Corley DA, Kubo A, Zhao W, Quesenberry C. Proton pump inhibitors and histamine-2 receptor antagonists are associated with hip fractures among at-risk patients. Gastroenterology 2010;139:93–101.

13 Laine L. Proton pump inhibitors and bone fractures? Am J Gastroenterol 2009; 104:S21–S26.

14 Johnson DA. Safety of proton pump inhibitors: current evidence for osteoporosis and interaction with antiplatelet agents. Curr Gastroenterol Rep 2010;12:167–74.

15 Targownik LE, Lix LM, Leung S, Leslies WD. Proton-pump inhibitor use is not associated with osteoporosis or accelerated bone mineral density loss. Gastroenterology 2010;138:896–904.

16 Gray SL, LaCroix AZ, Larson J, *et al*. Proton pump inhibitor use, hip fracture, and change in bone mineral density in postmenopausal women: results from the Women's Health Initiative. Arch Intern Med 2010;170:765–71.

17 Jefferies KC, Cipriano DJ, Forgac M. Function structure and regulation of the vacuolar (H+) ATPases. Arch Biochem Biophys 2008;476:33–42.

18 Mizunashi K, Furukawa Y, Katano K, Abe K. Effect of omeprazole, an inhibitor of H+, K+, ATPase on bone resorption in humans. Calcif Tissue Int 1993;53:21–5.

19 Epstein M, McGrath S, Law F. Proton pump inhibitors and hypomagesemic hyopparathyroidism. N Engl J Med 2006;355:1834–6.

20 Broeren MAC, Geerdink EAM, Vader HL, *et al*. Hyopmagnesmia induced by several proton pump inhibitors. Ann Intern Med 2009;151:755–6.

21 MacKay JD, Bladon PT. Hypomagesemia due ot proton pump inhibitor therapy: a clinical case series. Q J Med 2010;103(6):387–95.

22 www.fda.gov/Safety/MedWatch/SafetyInformation/SafetyAlertsforHumanMedical Products/ucm245275.htm

23 Yang YX, Metz DC. Safety of proton pump inhibitor exposure. Gastroenterology 2010;139:1115–27.

24 Gilard M, Arnaud B, Cornily JC, *et al*. Influence of omeprazole on the antiplatelet action of clopidogrel associated with aspirin: the randomized, double-blind OCLA (Omeprazole CLopidogrel Aspirin) Study. J Am Coll Cardiol 2008;51:256–60.

25 Laine L, Hennekens C. Proton pump inhibitor and clopidogrel interaction: fact or fiction? Am J Gastroenterol 2010;105:34–41.

26 Ho PM, Maddox TM, Wang L, *et al*. Risk of adverse outcomes associated with concomitant use of clopidogrel and proton pump inhibitors following acute coronary syndrome. JAMA 2009;301:937–44.

27 Ray WA, Murray KT, Griffin MR, *et al*. Outcomes with concurrent use of clopidogrel and proton-pump inhibitors: a cohort study. Ann Intern Med 2010;152:337–45.

28 www.fda.gov/Drugs/DrugSafety/PostmarketDrugSafetyInformationforPatientsand Providers/DrugSafetyInformationforHeathcareProfessionals/ucm190784.htm

29 Bhatt DL, Scheiman J, Abraham NS, *et al*. American College of Cardiology Foundation, American College of Gastroenterology, American Heart Association. ACCF/ACG/AHA 2008 expert consensus document on reducing the gastrointestinal risks of antiplatelet therapy and NSAID use. Am J Gastroenterol 2008; 103:2890–907.

30 O'Donoghue ML, Braunwald E, Antman EM, *et al*. Pharmacodynamic effect and clinical efficacy efficacy of clopidogrel and prasugrel with or without a proton-pump inhibitor: an analysis of two randomized trials. Lancet 2009;374:989–97.

31 Bhatt DL, Cryer BL, Contant CF, *et al*., COGENT Investigators. Clopidogrel with or without omeprazole in coronary artery disease. N Engl J Med 2010;363:1909–17.

32 www.fda.gov/Drugs/DrugSafety/ucm231161.htm.

33 Juurlink DN, Gomes T, Marndarni MM, *et al*. The safety of proton pump inhibitors and clopidogrel in patients after stroke. Stroke 2011;42:128–32.

34 Abraham NS, Hlatky MA, Antman EM, *et al*. ACCF/ACG/AHA 2010 expert consensus document on the concomitant use of proton pump inhibitors and thienopyridines: a focused update of the ACCF/ACG/AHA 2008 expert consensus document on reducing the gastrointestinal risks of antiplatelet therapy and NSAID use. Am J Gastroenterol 2010;105:2533–49.

35 Banerjee S, Weideman RA, Weideman MW, *et al.* Effect of concomitant use of clopidogrel and proton pump inhibitors after percutaneous coronary intervention. Am J Cardiol 2011;107(6):871–8.

36 Chan FKL, Ching JYL, Hung LCT, *et al.* Clopidogrel versus aspirin and esomeprazole to prevent recurrent ulcer bleeding. N Engl J Med 2005;352:238–44.

37 Ma L, Elliott SN, Cirino G, Buret A, Ignarro LJ, Wallace JL. Platelets modulate gastric ulcer healing: role of endostatin and vascular endothelial growth factor release. Proc Natl Acad Sci USA 2001;98:6470–5.

38 Hus PI, Lai KH, Liu CP. Esomeprazole with clopidogrel reduces peptic ulcer recurrence compared with clopidogrel alone, in patients with atherosclerosis. Gastroenterology 2011;140:791–8.

39 Wandall JH. Effects of omeprazole on neutrophil chemotaxis, super oxide production, degranualation and translocation of cytochrome b-245. Gut 1992;33:617–21.

40 Laheij RJ, Sturkenboom MD, Hassing RJ, *et al.* Risk of community-acquired pneumonia and use of gastric acid-suppressive drugs. JAMA 2004;292:1955–60.

41 Gulmez SE, Holm A, Frederiksen H, *et al.* Use of proton pump inhibitors and the risk of community-acquired pneumonia: a population-based case-control study. Arch Intern Med 2007;167:950–5.

42 Herzig SJ, Howell MD, Ngo LH, Marcantonio ER. Acid-suppressive medication use and the risk for hospital-acquired pneumonia. JAMA 2009;301:2120–8.

43 Johnstone J, Nerenberg K Loeb M. Meta-analysis: proton pump inhibitor use and the risk of community-acquired pneumonia. Aliment Pharmacol Ther 2010;31:1165–77.

44 Sarkar M, Hennessy S, Yang YX. Proton-pump inhibitor use and the risk for community-acquired pneumonia. Ann Intern Med 2008;149:391–8.

45 Dublin A, Walker RL, Kackson ML, *et al.* Use of proton pump inhibitors and H2 blockers and risk of pneumonia in older adults: a population-based case-control study. Pharmacoepidemiol Drug Saf 2010;19:792–802.

46 DuPont HL. Travellers' diarrhoea: contemporary approaches to therapy and prevention. Drugs 2006;66:303–14.

47 Cobelens FG, Leentvaar-Kuijpers A, Kleijnen J, *et al.* Incidence and risk factors of diarrhoea in Dutch travellers: consequences for priorities in pre-travel health advice. Trop Med Int Health 1998;3:896–903.

48 Leonard J, Marshall JK, Moayyedi P. Systematic review of the risk of enteric infection in patients taking acid suppression. Am J Gastroenterol 2007;102:2047–56.

49 Dial MS. Proton pump inhibitor use and enteric infections. Am J Gastroenterol 2009;104(Suppl 2):S10–S16.

50 Howell MD, Novack V, Grgurich P, *et al.* Iatrogenic gastric acid suppression and the risk of nosocomial Clostridium difficile infection. Arch Intern Med 2010;170:784–90.

51 Lombardo L, Foti M, Ruggia O, Chiecchio A. Increased incidence of small intestinal bacterial overgrowth during proton pump inhibitor therapy. Clin Gastroenterol Hepatol 2010;8(6):504–8.

52 Bajaj JS, Zadvornova Y, Heuman DM, *et al.* Association of proton pump inhibitor therapy with spontaneous bacterial peritonitis in cirrhotic patients with ascites. Am J Gastroenterol 2009;104:1130–4.

53 Campbell MS, Obstein K, Reddy KR, Yang YX. Association between proton pump inhibitor use and spontaneous bacterial peritonitis. Dig Dis Sci 2008;53:394–8.

54 Sierra F, Suarez M, Rey M, *et al.* Systematic review: proton pump inhibitor associated acute interstitial nephritis. Aliment Pharmacol Ther 2007;26:545–53.

CHAPTER 6

Gastroesophageal Reflux Disease Treatment: Side-Effects and Complications of Fundoplication

Joel E. Richter

Division of Digestive Diseases and Nutrition, and Joy M. Culverhouse Center for Esophageal Diseases, University of South Florida, Tampa, FL, US

Key points

- Even skilled surgeons will have complications after anti-reflux surgery. All patients should be warned about these complications.
- After laparoscopic anti-reflux surgery, mortality is rare (<1%), immediate postoperative morbidity is uncommon (5–20%), and conversion rates to an open operation should be less than 2.5%.
- Common late postoperative complications include gas-bloat syndrome (1–85%), dysphagia (10–50%), diarrhea (18–33%), and recurrent heartburn (10–62%).
- Most of these symptoms improve over the initial 3–6 months after surgery. Dietary modifications, prokinetic drugs, esophageal dilations (bougies or pneumatic balloons), and anti-diarrheal agents may be helpful. Many patients go back on antacid therapy but only 25% have documented recurrent acid reflux.
- Failures after anti-reflux surgery usually occur within the first 2 years of the initial operation. The most common patterns are herniation of the fundoplication into the chest, slipped fundoplication, tight fundoplication, paraesophageal hernia, and malposition of the fundoplication.
- Reoperation rates range from 0–15% for laparoscopic Nissen fundoplication and 4–10% for laparoscopic Toupet fundoplication. Redo fundoplications must be performed by experienced surgeons.

Potential pitfalls

- Anti-reflux surgery is never an emergency procedure. All patients should be carefully evaluated prior to surgery.
- At a minimum, preoperative testing should include upper endoscopy, esophageal manometry and pH testing (the latter primarily patients with non-erosive gastro-esophageal reflux disease). Don't take short cuts.
- Even skilled surgeons will have complications after anti-reflux surgery. All patients should have a frank discussion with their gastroenterologist and surgeon about postoperative dysphagia, gas-bloat, diarrhea, and the durability of the operation with return of heartburn.
- Treat these common complications with conservative therapy and never rush into redo anti-reflux surgery. Most problems will improve over 3–6 months.
- A redo operation requires a very experienced surgeon. The keys to success must not be violated. These include careful review of the patient's prior work-up and repeat studies as necessary, recognition of esophageal shortening, and complete takedown of the original fundoplication.

Introduction

In the past 15 years, there has been an increase in the number of anti-reflux operations being performed. The reasons for this increase include the development and proliferation of laparoscopic techniques, the increase in the fraction of the population that is overweight, and possibly the increased willingness of the population to undergo an operation to avoid a lifetime of medications or lifestyle changes. The operation is now widely available in community hospitals, the length of stay ranges between 1 and 4 days, some operations are even done as day surgery, and most patients return to normal activity within 2 weeks [1,2]. Patients over 65 years of age can expect an excellent outcome after laparoscopic surgery in at least 90% of cases, similar to younger patients [3]. Based on the US Nationwide Inpatient Sample, there were 9173 adult anti-reflux operations in 1993, which increased nearly 3.5-fold, reaching a peak at 32,980 in 2000 [4]. For poorly understood reasons, the most recent available data for 2006 show a 40% decline to 19,688 operations [5].

This review will focus on the surgical and medical complications primarily reported after laparoscopic anti-reflux surgery (Box 6.1). The available reports on this subject are numerous so I have relied on summary data available from the Society of American Gastrointestinal and Endoscopic Surgeons (SAGES) [1] and the Agency for Healthcare Research and Quality Effective Health Care Program [6]. The chapter will summarize mortality and morbidity data for laparoscopic anti-reflux operations, review the common perioperative and postoperative complications, and discuss the common reasons for fundoplication failure.

Box 6.1 Prevalence of medical and surgical complications of anti-reflux surgery

- Mortality (<30 days): 1% or less
- Perioperative and immediate postoperative morbidity: 8–17%
- Open conversion rate: 0–24%
- Early postoperative complications:
  - bowel perforation: 0–4%
  - bleeding and splenic injury: <1%
  - pneumothorax: 0–10%
  - severe postoperative nausea and vomiting: 2–5%
- Late postoperative complications:
  - gas-bloat syndrome: 1–85%
  - dysphagia:
    early: 10–50%
    late: 3–24%
  - diarrhea: 18–33%
  - recurrent heartburn: 10–62%
- Need for revisional surgery:
  - laparoscopic Nissen fundoplication: 0–15%
  - laparoscopic Toupet fundoplication: 4–10%

General mortality, morbidity and conversion rate to open operation

By all measures, laparoscopic anti-reflux surgery is safe when performed by experienced surgeons. Postoperative 30-day mortality has rarely been reported and is usually <1% [1]. Using the US Nationwide Inpatient Sample (20% stratified sample of US non-federal hospitals recording 5–8 million hospital stays for about 1000 hospitals each year), we reported that the inpatient mortality after anti-reflux surgery decreased from 0.82% in 1993 to 0.26% in 2000, but it increased to 0.54% by 2006 [5]. The latter increase in mortality was associated with the patients being older, having a longer length of hospital stay and more complications. A review of the Department of Veterans Affairs administrative databases from 1990 to 2001 identified 3145 patients undergoing anti-reflux surgery [7]. Of this group, 28 patients died for a mortality rate of 0.8%. The major causes of death were gastrointestinal hemorrhage, necrosis of the stomach, perforation of the esophagus and colon, cardiac arrest, respiratory complications, and pulmonary embolism.

The perioperative and immediate postoperative morbidity rate of laparoscopic anti-reflux surgery varies widely related to experience, technique, and degree of follow-up. One review suggested a rate up to 17% [8]. Our National Inpatient Sample database found that 8.3% of adults hospitalized for anti-reflux surgery had at least one complication in 1993. This rate decreased to 4.7% in 2000 but increased to 6.1% in 2006 [5]. In these reviews and reports, the most important complications include perforation, hemorrhage, splenic injury, pneumothorax, and wrap herniation from intractable nausea and vomiting.

The rate of open conversion during laparoscopic anti-reflux surgery ranges from 0% to 24%; however, most series from high-volume centers report conversion rates less than 2.4% [1]. The intraoperative conversion rate seems to parallel the surgeons' experience and the operative volume in the hospital [9]. The reasons for conversion may be loosely divided into three categories: complications, surgeon comfort, and equipment failure. Surgeon comfort is a broad category that encompasses such problems as adhesions from previous operations, difficult exposure secondary to a large liver, or failure to progress. In addition, the category boundaries are indistinct because surgeon comfort plays a variable role in the decision to convert after most complications or equipment failures. The distribution among categories in one review representing 135 open conversions was 34.1% complications, 59.3% surgeon comfort, and 6.7% equipment failure [10].

Acute perioperative and immediate postoperative complications

Poor functional outcome after anti-reflux surgery often can be traced to inadequate patient selection or technical problems encountered during the operation. In other cases, a different set of complications become manifest clearly during the operation or immediately postoperatively and may lead to significant morbidity if not immediately recognized and treated [11].

Bowel perforation

Bowel perforation, especially of the esophagus and stomach, may be life-threatening and lead to longer hospital stay. The perforation rate varies according to technique and exposure, ranging from 0% to 4% [1], with the highest incidence being reported with redo fundoplications [12]. The injury may occur during placement of the camera port with a trocar, from excessive retraction on the stomach, passage of the esophageal bougie or during lysis of adhesions [11]. Because it is not possible to palpate a bougie or nasogastric tube during a laparoscopic procedure, correction of the esophagogastric angulation by appropriate traction of the stomach is critical to avoid damage. The importance of experience in passing the tube or dilator is also central [8]; this should be done by an experienced anesthesiologist or surgeon. The frequency of perforation during laparoscopic operation is no higher than in the conventional open approach of laparotomy [8]. The greatest threat to the patient is unrecognized damage to the esophagus or stomach, which can be at least partly prevented by frequent leakage testing during the operation. If the perforation is recognized and repaired during the index operation, the patient's subsequent course is usually uneventful and the functional results excellent [13].

Bleeding and splenic injury

Usually the bleeding encountered during anti-reflux surgery is minor and easily controlled. Most commonly, bleeding occurs during division of the short gastric vessels which is necessary to mobilize the fundus of the stomach [11]. This technique generally includes dissecting and cutting the short gastric vessels arising from the spleen. Bleeding and tears of the splenic capsule were common after open laparotomy and fundoplication, requiring splenectomy in 5–11% of cases; however, the rate has decreased to less than 1% after laparoscopic procedures [14]. This decrease in morbidity is due to better exposure induced by the pneumoperitoneum and laparoscopic technological developments that facilitate division of the short gastric vessels with less trauma to the spleen. Not unexpectedly, patients in whom accidental splenectomy has to be carried out have an increased rate of infection complications as well as a slight but definite increased postoperative mortality rate [15].

Pneumothorax

During mediastinal dissection, it is not uncommon to create a tear of one or both pleura. Rates of pneumothorax during laparoscopic anti-reflux surgery in most series range from 0% to 1.5%, but may be as high as 10%, especially in repairing paraesophageal hernias [1].

Postoperative nausea and vomiting

This can be a major problem after laparoscopic anti-reflux surgery, causing both discomfort and harm to the newly created fundoplication. Up to 60% of patients have problems with severe postoperative nausea, with as many as 5% experiencing vomiting in the recovery unit or hospital room after laparoscopic fundoplication [16]. Aggressive prophylactic treatment with intravenous antiemetics such as ondansetron has been recommended [17]. Patients who retch or vomit in the early postoperative period are at risk for disruption of the crural closure and/or intrathoracic herniation of the fundoplication. Patients with early postoperative vomiting should undergo immediate barium esophagram to access the integrity of the fundoplication. If a disruption is identified, the patient should be taken back to surgery as early as possible. If reoperation is performed within 4–10 days, the procedure is usually relatively simple but if delayed until adhesions develop, the anatomy may be difficult to discern and manage [17].

Late postoperative complications

Gas-bloat syndrome

The gas-bloat syndrome comprises an ill-defined and variable group of complaints assumed to result from the inability to vent gas from the stomach into the esophagus after fundoplication. The predominant complaint is bloating but other symptoms include abdominal distension, early satiety, nausea, upper abdominal pain, flatulence, inability to belch, and inability to vomit. The cause of the syndrome is unclear but proposed mechanisms include:

- inability of the surgically altered gastroesophageal junction to relax in response to gastric distension
- aerophagia, a frequent habit among patients with severe gastroesophageal reflux disease (GERD), which becomes problematic after fundoplication when the air cannot be vented
- impairment of meal-induced receptive relaxation and accommodation of the stomach with rapid gastric emptying
- surgical injury to the vagus nerve, which delays gastric emptying and interferes with transient relaxation that is part of the normal belch reflux [18].

The reported frequency of gas-bloat syndrome has ranged widely from 1% to 85%, depending on the definition of the disorder as well as underlying population and type of fundoplication [6]. For example, an early VAH trial of medication and surgical therapies for GERD found by questionnaire that 81% of the surgical patients had at least one symptom of the gas-bloat syndrome, but the comparable medically treated patients also had a 60% rate of gas-bloat symptoms [19]. These symptoms seem to be worse with a total compared to a partial fundoplication [8]. Symptoms tend to be worse immediately after surgery, with most improving or resolving over the first year.

Recommended therapies, albeit without convincing evidence of effectiveness, include dietary modifications to avoid gas-producing foods, eating slower to avoid aerophagia, cessation of smoking, gas-reducing agents such as simethicone, and prokinetic drugs. Debilitating cases need further evaluation for small bowel obstruction secondary to adhesions from the original surgery and delayed gastric emptying. Up to 40% of patients with GERD may have some element of delayed gastric emptying [20] but anti-reflux surgery usually accelerates the emptying of both solids and liquids [21].

Inadvertent vagotomy, especially common with redo fundoplications, can delay gastric emptying of solids by interfering with antral motility and pyloric relaxation. Severe cases may require surgical revision which could include conversion to a partial fundoplication, allowing easier gas venting, and pyloromyotomy when delayed gastric emptying is documented.

Dysphagia

Approximately 50% or more of patients experience solid foods passing slowly through the esophagus immediately after fundoplication, presumably as a consequence of postsurgical edema and inflammation [6]. Marked dysphagia for liquids is rare and should suggest an important anatomical dysfunction. These patients are initially treated with dietary modification (soft diets, plenty of fluids) and reassurance, with the dysphagia usually resolving spontaneously within 2–3 months. However, 3–24% of patients experience dysphagia that persists beyond 3 months requiring more than dietary management [22]. This group of patients usually have a fundoplication which is too tight for their functional esophageal pump, but other problems include previously unrecognized achalasia, healed peptic stricture, paraesophageal hernia, slipped fundoplication into the chest with a recurrent hernia or distal migration of the wrap onto the stomach creating a two-compartment stomach. Preoperative manometry is mandatory to exclude achalasia but esophageal function testing otherwise is poor in defining those patients likely to be troubled with postoperative dysphagia. Therefore, "tailoring" the type of fundoplication to the esophageal pump has lost favor with the exception of a partial fundoplication in patients with aperistalsis [23]. Patients with dysphagia prior to surgery are more likely to have dysphagia after surgery, regardless of the type of fundoplication [24].

Patients with persistent dysphagia will need further investigation to determine whether the fundoplication is too tight or long versus an anatomical disruption. These tests include barium esophagram with a 13 mm tablet, esophageal manometry, and/or endoscopy. If the fundoplication is intact, bougie and/or through-the-scope balloon dilation will relieve symptoms in one-half to two-thirds of cases, usually with one series of dilations up to 18 mm (54 Fr) [22,25]. This can be done within a month of the fundoplication and does not produce new reflux symptoms [22]. More recently, pneumatic dilation (30–40 mm balloons) has been advocated, if the patients fail to respond to bougie dilation and the nadir lower esophageal sphincter (LES) pressure on manometry is ≥10 mmHg [26]. About two-thirds of patients not responding to bougie dilation with tight fundoplications will respond to pneumatic dilation. The remainder will need revision surgery converting the complete fundoplication to a partial wrap. On the other hand, patients with slipped fundoplications or paraesophageal hernias usually will require reoperation as less than 30% respond to bougie dilation alone [22].

Diarrhea

Diarrhea is a frequent complication of fundoplication, often not discussed prior to surgery. In a study of 84 patients responding to a telephone survey after anti-reflux surgery, 15 (18%) described the new onset of diarrhea [27]. The diarrhea usually developed within 6 weeks of the operation, was low volume and worse after meals. Sometimes it can be explosive and associated with fecal incontinence. In this study, only two of 15 patients (13%) had complete resolution of their diarrhea after 2 years. Other reports describe rates as high as 33%, but these studies do not describe whether the diarrhea was present before surgery [28].

The cause of postfundoplication diarrhea is not known. Proposed mechanisms include rapid gastric emptying from the fundoplication overloading the small intestine's ability to handle the osmotic bolus, vagal injury with subsequent small bowel bacterial overgrowth, and exacerbation of underlying irritable bowel syndrome [27]. Anti-motility agents including codeine, antibiotics for small bowel bacterial overgrowth and cholestyramine may ease the diarrhea, but the management is empirical.

Recurrent heartburn

Much interest and research have recently been focused on the durability of anti-reflux surgery. This was spurred by the 10-year follow-up of a large randomized VAH trial of medical versus surgical therapy [29]. Among the medically treated patients, 92% were still on medications while surprisingly, 62% of those undergoing surgical fundoplication were back on reflux medications (50% proton pump inhibitors (PPIs), 50% H2 receptor antagonists (H2RAs)). Furthermore, 16% of the surgical patients had at least one additional operation. In a large Veterans Affairs (VA) administrative database review of 3145 patients undergoing surgery from 1990 to 2001 with at least 4.5 years of follow-up, antacid prescriptions were dispensed regularly, including H2RAs (23.8%), PPIs (34.3%), and prokinetic drugs (9.2%). Overall, 49.8% of patients received at least three prescriptions for one of these drugs [30]. Other centers of excellence studies suggest postoperative use of acid-reducing medications rates of less than 20% [1].

Does the fact that the patient is back on PPIs prove that surgery has failed? This can only be accurately assessed with postoperative pH testing in symptomatic patients. Two studies have adequately addressed this issue with similar findings. Lord *et al.* [31] identified 37 patients (43%) who were taking acid suppression medications after fundoplication. However, only 24% (9 of 37) had abnormal 24-h pH testing. Recurrent heartburn and regurgitation were the only symptoms associated with abnormal pH results. Likewise, Wijnhoven *et al.* [32] identified, by postal survey, 312 patients (37%) who primarily were taking PPIs after an average of 6 years after fundoplication. Postoperative pH studies were abnormal in 16/61 patients (26%) on medication and in 5/78 patients (6%) not taking medication. Although small studies, these results suggest that many patients may inappropriately be back on medications for non-specific peptic symptoms such as dyspepsia or extraesophageal symptoms or have other reasons for antacid therapy such as peptic ulcer disease. An empirical trial of PPIs is reasonable with recurrent "reflux" symptoms post fundoplication, but the requirement for progressively higher doses of PPIs or possible revision surgery requires documentation that the patient actually has recurrent pathological acid reflux.

Redo anti-reflux surgery

Although long-term results with anti-reflux surgery are generally good, especially if performed by experienced surgeons, failures are unavoidable. Most failures occur within the first 2 years of the initial operation [1]. In large reviews, the most common symptoms are recurrent heartburn and/or dysphagia, with pain and bloating being less common [10,33].

Figure 6.1 illustrates several of the primary patterns of fundoplication failure [34]. Herniation of the fundoplication into the chest (type 1A) is the most common failure, reported in 30–80% of cases [10,33,34]. These failures usually result from disruption of the crural repair or failure to perform the initial wrap over a tension-free segment of intraabdominal esophagus. To avoid these failures, there must be at least 2–3 cm of tension-free intraabdominal esophagus below the hiatus and the gastroesophageal junction must be clearly identified. A slipped Nissen fundoplication occurs when part of the stomach lies both above and below the wrap (type 1B). This defect, accounting for 15–30% of failures [10,33,34], may arise from the stomach slipping through the fundoplication or incorrect positioning of the wrap around the stomach at the time of the original operation [33] Type II failures present as a posterior paraesophageal hernia and accounted for 23% of redo operations in one series [34]. The mechanism is thought to include inadequate hiatal closure or a redundant wrap with some excess portion of the wrap serving as a lead point in the formation of the hernia. This can be prevented by the "shoe-shine" maneuver, insuring the wrap is not twisted or redundant and is positioned appropriately on the distal esophagus. Type III failure occurs as a consequence of malposition of the wrap at the initial operation, accounting for about 10% of failures.

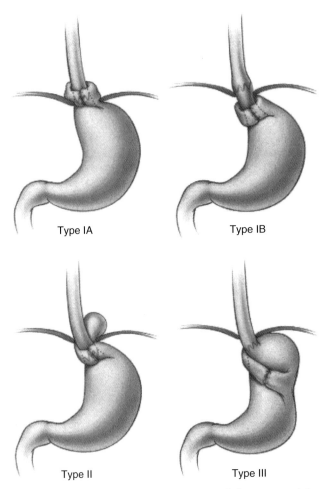

Figure 6.1 Common patterns of primary fundoplication failures. Type I failures occur with displacement of the gastroesophageal junction into the chest through the esophageal hiatus. Type 1A has herniation of the wrap and GE junction both into the chest. Type 1B presents with recurrence of the hiatal hernia, but the wrap remains below the diaphragm. Type II failures are defined as failures secondary to paraesophageal hernia. Type III failures occur as a consequence of malposition of the wrap at the time of initial surgery, usually on the cardia of the stomach. Reproduced from Hatch *et al.* [34], with permission from Elsevier.

A tight fundoplication represents an anatomically appropriately placed wrap which generates too much resistance for the esophageal pump. The primary complaint is dysphagia rather than heartburn. Studies suggest this may account for 8–16% of redo operations [10,33]. Careful preoperative manometry to recognize a weak esophageal pump, performance of the fundoplication over a large bougie (52–56 Fr) or a floppy Nissen fundoplication or partial wrap may minimize this problem [35]. Other factors associated with recurrent symptoms include too loose a fundoplication, vagal injury and pseudoachalasia [35]. Interestingly, complete fundoplication disruptions are much less common (3–14%) in the laparoscopic era than with open operations (greater than 30%) [33].

The keys to success of a redo fundoplication are careful review of the patient's prior work-up and repeat studies as necessary, recognition of esophageal shortening, and complete takedown of the original fundoplication [35]. Although controversial, it is hypothesized that long-standing reflux leads to circumferential esophageal scarring and, in more severe cases, varying degrees of longitudinal scarring and esophageal shortening. A short esophagus should be suspected in the presence of a moderate or large non-reducible hiatal hernia, difficult-to-manage peptic stricture or long-segment Barrett's esophagus [36]. Adequate laparoscopic mobilization of the mediastinal esophagus is critical in constructing a tension-free intraabdominal fundoplication. If esophageal shortening is identified and adequate intraabdominal esophageal length cannot be obtained, a Collis gastroplasty will be required.

The most important principle during reoperation is to restore normal anatomy before recreating the fundoplication [35]. This requires the wrap be completely taken down, the fundus restored to its normal location, and the degree of esophageal shortening determined. The restoration can be tedious and it is very tempting to convert the Nissen fundoplication to what appears to the surgeon to be a posterior wrap. Taking this shortcut only increases the likelihood that the patient will not benefit from the reoperation. Dysphagia is often the result of an improperly constructed wrap, and to relieve this symptom the fundoplication must be completely dismantled.

Redo fundoplications must be done by experienced surgeons [1]. In these settings, laparoscopic approaches to reoperative anti-reflux surgery offer similar results to open surgery, but conversion rates are higher than with the initial operation [1]. Reoperation rates range from 0% to 15% for laparoscopic Nissen fundoplication and 4–10% for laparoscopic Toupet fundoplication [6]. Compared to primary repair, redo surgery requires longer operation times, has higher complication rates (20–45%) and the mortality rates are higher, from 0% to 17% [1,6]. Finally, the likelihood of success for controlling GERD decreases with subsequent reoperations, approaching at least 10% per each revisional surgery and being no better than 50% or less in patients undergoing three or more reoperations [37]. For these latter unusual cases, serious consideration should be given to an esophagectomy.

CASE STUDY

A 42-year-old man was referred to his local gastroenterologists for surgical evaluation due to long-standing heartburn and regurgitation. His heartburn was improved by a b.i.d. proton pump inhibitor, but the regurgitation was still a daily problem after meals and interfered with sleep. Endoscopy showed a 3 cm hiatal hernia with Los Angeles Grade B esophagitis despite his PPI regimen. Esophageal manometry found a low LES pressure (5 mmHg) with peristalsis present but in the low normal range (25–40 mmHg). He underwent a "loose" Nissen fundoplication performed laparoscopically by an experienced surgeon over a 54 Fr bougie.

For the first 6 weeks postoperatively, he was on a soft diet. Initially, postprandial bloating and increased flatus were an issue. These resolved, but the patient began to experience substernal chest pain and dysphagia if he ate too rapidly or the food was of firm texture (i.e. meats, hard breads and sandwiches). He was pleased his heartburn and regurgitation were relieved, but these new symptoms interfered with his general activities, especially his many evening business dinners. His gastroenterologist performed an endoscopy, finding the fundoplication to be intact, and there was no resistance to passage of the endoscope. Repeated bougie dilations to 20 mm (60 Fr) gave transient relief for about 2 weeks but then the dysphagia recurred, requiring modification of his diet.

A discussion began considering the possibility of surgically revising the fundoplication to a partial wrap. Preoperative testing included a barium swallow showing the wrap was intact below the diaphragm, intermittent peristalsis was observed and a 13 mm tablet passed over 3–5 min after drinking more barium. Esophageal manometry found an increase in LES pressure to 35 mmHg with incomplete relaxation. Peristalsis was present after 70% of wet swallows with the amplitude increased on average to 45 mmHg. A diagnosis of a "tight" Nissen fundoplication was made. Prior to revising the fundoplication, the gastroenterologist and surgeon suggested one last attempt at aggressive dilation with a 30 mm pneumatic balloon. This was performed under fluoroscopic guidance. The patient tolerated the procedure and has been symptom free for the last 6 months.

References

1 Stefanidis D, Hope WW, Kohn GP, *et al.* Guidelines for surgical treatment of gastro-esophageal reflux disease. Surg Endosc 2010;24:2647–69.

2 Jensen CD, Gilliam AD, Horgan LF, *et al.* Day-care laparoscopic Nissen fundoplication. Surg Endosc 2009;23:1745–9.

3 Pizza F, Rossetti G, Limongelli P, *et al.* Influence of age on outcome of total laparoscopic fundoplication for gastroesophageal reflux disease. World J Gastroenterol 2007;13:740–7.

4 Finks JF, Wei Y, Birkmeyer JD. The rise and fall of antireflux surgery in the United States. Surg Endosc 2006;20:1698–701.

5 Wang YR, Dempsey DT, Richter JE. Trends and perioperative outcomes of inpatient antireflux surgery in the United States, 1993–2006. Dis Esophagus 2011;24(4):215–23.

6 Agency for Healthcare Research and Quality – the Effective Healthcare Program. *Comparative effectiveness of management strategies for gastroesophageal reflux disease – an update to the 2005 report.* Washington, DC: Agency for Healthcare Research and Quality, 2011.

7 Dominitz JA, Dire CA, Billingsley KG, Todd-Steinberg JA. Complications of antireflux medication use after antireflux surgery. Clin Gastroenterol Hepatol 2006;4:299–305.

8 Lundell L. Complications of anti-reflux surgery. Best Pract Res Clin Gastroenterol 2004;18(5):935–45.

9 Zacharoulis D, O'Boyle CJ, Sedman PC, et al. Laparoscopic fundoplication: a 10-year learning curve. Surg Endosc 2006;20:1662–70.

10 Carlson MA, Frantzides CT. Complications and results of primary minimally invasive antireflux procedures: a review of 10,735 reported cases. J Am Coll Surg 2001;193:428–39.

11 Bizekis C, Kent M, Luketich J. Complications after surgery for gastroesophageal reflux disease. Thorac Surg Clin 2006;16:99–108.

12 Neuhauser B, Hinder RA. Laparoscopic reoperation after failed antireflux surgery. Semin Laparosc Surg 2001;8:281–6.

13 Rantanen TK, Salo JA, Sipponen JT. Fatal and life-threatening complications in antireflux surgery: analysis of 5,502 operations. Br J Surg 1999;86:1573–7.

14 Flum DR, Koepsell T, Heagerty P, Pellegrini C. The nationwide frequency of major adverse outcome in antireflux surgery and the role of surgeon experience, 1992–1997. J Am Coll Surg 2002;195:611–18.

15 Rogers DM, Herrington JL, Morton C. Incidental splenectomy associated Nissen fundoplication. Ann Surg 1980;191:153–6.

16 Bradshaw WA, Gregory BC, Finley C, et al. Frequency of postoperative nausea and vomiting in patients undergoing laparoscopic foregut surgery. Surg Endosc 2002;16:777–80.

17 Meyers BF, Soper NJ. Complications of surgery for gastroesophageal reflux. In: Patterson GA, Cooper JD, Deslauriers J, Lerut AEMR, Luketic JD, Rice TW (eds) *Person's thoracic and esophageal surgery*, 3rd edn. Philadelphia: Churchill Livingstone, 2008: pp. 376–86.

18 Spechler SJ. The management of patients who have "failed" antireflux surgery. Am J Gastroenterol 2004;99:552–61.

19 Spechler SJ. Comparison of medical and surgical therapy for complicated GERD in veterans. Department of Veterans Affairs Gastroesophageal Reflux Study Group. N Engl J Med 1992;326:786–92.

20 McCallum RW, Berkowitz DM, Lerner E. Gastric emptying in patients with gastro-esophageal reflux disease. Gastroenterology 1981;80:285–91.

21 Bias JE, Samson M, Boudesteijn CG, et al. Impact of delayed gastric emptying on the outcome of antireflux surgery. Ann Surg 2001;234:139–46.

22 Wo JM, Trus TL, Richardson WS, et al. Evaluation and management of post fundoplication dysphagia. Am J Gastroenterol 1996;91:2318–22.

23 Fibbe C, Layer P, Keller J, et al. Esophageal motility in reflux disease before and after fundoplication: a prospective randomized, clinical and manometric study. Gastroenterology 2001;121:5–14.

24 Watson DL. Laparoscopic treatment of gastroesophageal reflux disease. Best Pract Res Clin Gastroenterol 2004;18:19–35.

25 Malki-Chowla N, Gorecki P, Bammer T, et al. Dilation after fundoplication: timing, frequency, indications and outcome. Gastrointest Endosc 2002;55:219–23.

26 Hui JM, Hunt DR, Carle DJ, et al. Esophageal pneumatic dilation for post fundoplication dysphagia: safety, efficacy and predictors of outcome. Am J Med 2002;97:2986–91.

27 Klaus A, Hinder RA, deVault KR, Achem SR. Bowel dysfunction after laparoscopic antireflux surgery: incidence, severity and clinical course. Am J Med 2003; 114:6–9.

28 Swanstrom L, Wayne R. Spectrum of gastrointestinal symptoms after laparoscopic fundoplication. Am J Surg 1994;167:538–41.

29 Spechler SJ, Lee E, Ahnen D, *et al.* Long-term outcome of medical and surgical therapies for gastroesophageal reflux disease: follow-up of a randomized controlled trial. JAMA 2001;285:2331–8.

30 Domintz JA, Dire C, Billingsley KG, Todd-Steinberg JA. Complications and antireflux medication use after antireflux surgery. Clin Gastroenterol Hepatol 2006; 4:299–305.

31 Lord RVN, Kaminski A, Oberg S, *et al.* Absence of gastroesophageal reflux disease in a majority of patients taking acid suppression medications after Nissen fundoplication. J Gastrointest Surg 2002;6:3–10.

32 Wijnhoven BPL, Lally CJ, Kelly JJ, *et al.* Use of antireflux medication after antireflux surgery. J Gastrointest Surg 2008;12:510–17.

33 Hunter JG, Smith CS, Branum GD, *et al.* Laparoscopic fundoplication failure: patterns of failure and response to fundoplication revision. Ann Surg 1999;23:595–606.

34 Hatch KF, Daily MF, Christiansen BJ, Glasgow RE. Failed fundoplications. Am J Surg 2004;188:786–91.

35 Bizekis C, Kent M, Luketich J. Complications after surgery for gastroesophageal reflux disease. Thorac Surg Clin 2006;16:99–108.

36 Gastal OL, Hagen JA, Peters JH, *et al.* Short esophagus: analysis of predictors and clinical implications. Arch Surg 1999;134:633–6.

37 Smith CD, McClusky DA, Rajad MA, *et al.* When fundoplications fails: redo? Ann Surg 2005;241:861–71.

PART 2

Gastroesophageal Reflux Disease: Management of Specific Clinical Presentations

CHAPTER 7

Evaluation and Management of Refractory Gastroesophageal Reflux Disease

John E. Pandolfino and Sabine Roman
Division of Gastroenterology, Northwestern University, Chicago, IL, USA

Key points
- Four phenotypes of proton pump inhibitor non-responders are described:
  - phenotype 1: persistent acid reflux
  - phenotype 2: non-acid reflux
  - phenotype 3: functional overlap with gastroesophageal reflux disease
  - phenotype 4: functional heartburn.
- Choice of physiological testing is based on pretest probability for baseline gastroesophageal reflux disease.
- Treatment strategy should be based on proton pump inhibitor non-responder phenotype.

Potential pitfalls
- Proton pump inhibitor non-responder phenotypes are defined in patients compliant to optimized proton pump inhibitor therapy.
- Physiological testing should be performed off therapy when the pretest probability for baseline gastroesophageal reflux disease is low.

Introduction

Proton pump inhibitor (PPI) therapy for gastroesophageal reflux disease (GERD) is highly effective; however, there are a substantial number of patients who do not respond to this therapy and seek further medical care. While success rates in healing esophagitis may reach 80–90%, a large number of patients (up to 30%) remain symptomatic or unsatisfied despite continued PPI therapy [1,2]. Additionally, patients with non-erosive reflux

---

Practical Manual of Gastroesophageal Reflux Disease, First Edition.
Edited by Marcelo F. Vela, Joel E. Richter and John E. Pandolfino.

disease (NERD) tend to have even lower response rates to PPI therapy, with symptom resolution rates ranging from 30% to 70% [3]. Given the large baseline prevalence of GERD, with approximately 7,000,000 ambulatory care visits per year constituting 17.5% of all digestive system diagnoses, PPI non-responders now represent a substantial utilization of healthcare resources in gastroenterology clinics [4].

Proton pump inhibitor non-responders are an extremely challenging population to manage for many reasons. First, there is a lack of consensus regarding the definition of a PPI non-responder or refractory GERD; this is largely due to the heterogeneity of the patient group, including individual response to medication, type of symptoms, and the mechanism behind continued symptom generation. For example, some patients have a partial response to medication that may be associated with a reduction of heartburn or resolution of the primary symptom with continued secondary symptoms. Others will have no change in their symptoms despite aggressive acid suppressive therapy. Furthermore, patients are heterogeneous in terms of the mechanism behind the generation of symptoms in this patient population. Some patients will exhibit no evidence of abnormal reflux or symptom reflux correlation, while others will have refractory symptoms with continued acid or non-acid reflux-related symptoms. Thus, all PPI non-responders are not the same and many do not have refractory GERD.

The following review will focus on evaluating patients with reflux symptoms that are not responding to PPI therapy (PPI non-responders). The first section will focus on defining the phenotypes of PPI non-responders in the context of clinical presentation and objective physiological evidence of abnormal reflux. The second section will focus on a management algorithm to assess and evaluate mechanisms behind the lack of response to PPI therapy. Finally, the third section will focus on alternative strategies to manage patients not responding to PPI therapy beyond acid suppression.

Definition of refractory gastroesophageal reflux disease and proton pump inhibitor non-responders

How to define proton pump inhibitor non-responders?

As PPIs are extremely effective at healing virtually all esophagitis grades and virtually all patients referred for refractory GERD symptoms are taking or have taken PPI therapy, most patients will have a negative endoscopy. Patients who continue to have erosive esophagitis despite PPI therapy are a true refractory GERD subtype that typically does not require a sophisticated work-up and therapy can be focused on escalating anti-reflux therapy based on endoscopic findings. Although there can be alternative explanations apart from acid reflux that may cause esophagitis, such as pill esophagitis and various infections, endoscopy is very specific for defining peptic injury and further physiological evaluation may only be required to determine why the PPI is not working. However, the more important group of patients that we are currently evaluating in gastroenterology clinics are the endoscopy-negative patients with continued symptoms. Therefore, the real management issue in current practice is focused on dealing with refractory symptoms in patients who are on optimized PPI therapy. A more accurate definition of this clinical dilemma should focus on the lack of response to therapy and thus, PPI non-responder is a much more appropriate definition. The mechanism behind PPI non-response may be related to non-reflux pathophysiology or to refractory gastro-esophageal reflux and therefore, the latter is actually a subcategory of PPI non-response causes.

Two additional important issues must be addressed before defining patients as PPI non-responders: the response to PPI therapy in terms of partial or complete non-response, and what dose constitutes an appropriate trial before someone is considered a failure. In terms of response to therapy, some patients may have a partial response with their primary symptom being partially reduced or completely reduced with continued secondary symptoms. In contrast, some patients may have absolutely no response to therapy and their symptoms will show no improvement with escalation of therapy or no worsening symptoms with discontinuation of therapy. These clinical issues are extremely important in defining the pretest probability of whether or not these patients actually have abnormal reflux at baseline. Given the success of PPI therapy in reducing acid reflux-related symptoms, it would be unusual for patients with GERD to have absolutely no response to PPI therapy. Patients who do not respond at all and can undergo discontinuation of PPI therapy without an escalation of symptoms likely have an alternative diagnosis that is not acid or reflux mediated. Therefore, this first question focused on response to therapy does provide an extremely useful starting point to assess pre-test probability that gastroesophageal reflux is causing the current subjective complication.

Even before one assesses the level of response, one would also have to document compliance to medical therapy at an appropriate dose sufficient to treat most grades of reflux severity. In evaluating the dose of proton pump inhibitor therapy that would reasonably be seen as a failure, one would likely utilize a dose that is higher than the current FDA-approved doses for the various available PPIs. Based on current treatment guidelines [5] and physiological testing data available on patients on single-dose therapy and double-dose therapy [6], a reasonable approach would be to consider patients who fail twice the FDA-approved dose in either a single-dose or split (b.i.d.)-dose regimen as a failure. Most guidelines advocate for physiological reflux testing after patients have attempted an escalation of PPI therapy to double dose [5,7]. In addition, studies assessing abnormal acid exposure on PPI therapy in patients with continued symptoms suggest that up to 30% of symptomatic patients on single-dose PPI therapy will have abnormal acid exposure. In contrast, less than 10% of symptomatic patients on double-dose PPI therapy will have abnormal acid exposure. Given that the primary mechanism of PPI therapy is to reduce overall acid reflux and reflux burden, it would appear that the yield of reducing acid burden by increasing the PPI dose to double the FDA-approved dose is significant and would warrant this degree of escalation as the threshold for someone to be considered a PPI failure.

Thus, in addition to defining phenotypes of PPI non-responders, defining level of response to therapy on adequate treatment is an important component of the evaluation and management of these refractory patients.

Conceptual phenotypes of proton pump inhibitor non-responders

Once patients are documented to have a poor or inadequate response to optimized PPI therapy (double-dose PPI), the next most important steps are to document whether or not the patients actually have abnormal gastroesophageal reflux and to document whether or not their symptoms experienced on medication are associated with reflux. By focusing on these two specific issues, one can define four specific phenotypes of PPI non-responders. This will require further physiological testing that will focus on ambulatory reflux monitoring and will be discussed in the section describing the appropriate utilization of ambulatory reflux monitoring.

The four specific phenotypes of PPI non-responders are described below and illustrated in Table 7.1.

• Phenotype 1: persistent acid reflux
• Phenotype 2: non-acid reflux
• Phenotype 3: functional overlap with GERD
• Phenotype 4: functional heartburn

As mentioned above, the first distinction in the phenotypes is focused on determining whether or not the patient has baseline abnormal gastroesophageal reflux. Phenotypes 1–3 are patients who have abnormal gastroesophageal reflux off PPI therapy, but continue to have symptoms that are either partially treated or secondary complaints that may (phenotypes 1 and 2) or may not (phenotype 3) be related to reflux. Phenotypes 1 and 2 have continued symptoms that are related to reflux and these subtypes are truly refractory GERD. Phenotype 1 will have evidence of abnormal acid exposure on ambulatory pH reflux testing and/or a positive

Table 7.1 Phenotypes of PPI non-responders based on physiological testing.

	Phenotype 1	Phenotype 2	Phenotype 3	Phenotype 4
	Persistent acid reflux	Non-acid reflux	Functional overlap with GERD	Functional heartburn
Acid esophageal exposure **off** PPI*	+	+	+	–
Acid esophageal exposure **on** PPI*	+	–	–	–
Excessive number of reflux events with impedance **on** PPI	+/–	+/–	+	–
Positive reflux-symptom association with impedance **on** PPI	+/–	+	–	–

*Prolonged wireless pH monitoring both off and on PPI may be used to evaluate esophageal acid exposure in a single examination [19].
GERD, gastroesophageal reflux disease; PPI, proton pump inhibitor.

symptom-reflux correlation in the context of overt abnormal acid exposure or normal acid exposure associated with an acid hypersensitivity. Similarly, phenotype 2 will also have a positive symptom reflux correlation; however, the correlation is predominantly with weakly acidic reflux events. Phenotype 2 will have no overt abnormality in distal esophageal acid exposure and is likely hypersensitive to volume, other components of the gastric refluxate or refluxate with a pH above 4. These particular phenotypes will likely respond to an escalation of anti-reflux therapy focused on reducing acid burden and the overall number of reflux events.

It is important to distinguish phenotypes 3 and 4 from phenotypes 1 and 2 because they should exhibit a lack of response to more aggressive anti-reflux therapy. However, phenotype 3 patients do have baseline reflux disease and many require PPI therapy to maintain control of other symptoms that are related to abnormal reflux. This particular group of patients will exhibit pathological acid reflux off PPI therapy and normalization on PPI therapy with a negative symptom correlation with all types of reflux events. Ambulatory reflux testing on PPI therapy incorporating impedance may reveal an increased number of overall reflux events suggesting underlying baseline GERD. Thus, these patients will be unable to discontinue PPI therapy and will require an evaluation for alternative causes and therapy beyond reflux suppression. In contrast, phenotype 4 patients will have no evidence of abnormal reflux or a symptom-reflux correlation at baseline or on PPI therapy. This group of patients can be labeled as functional heartburn once an endoscopy has ruled out alternative causes and manometry has not revealed an underlying esophageal motor disorder. These patients should have their PPI therapy discontinued and will likely require therapy focused beyond acid suppression and reflux inhibition.

Evidence to support this phenotypic classification can be found in recent studies assessing large series of referral patients for combined pH impedance testing both off and on PPI therapy. Savarino *et al.* noted in a series of 200 patients with non-erosive reflux disease that 27% had normal esophageal acid exposure and negative symptom association probability on 24-h pH impedance monitoring performed off PPI (phenotype 4) [8]. Eleven percent of the patients presented with a positive association between symptoms and non-acid reflux events only in the absence of PPI therapy. Mainie *et al.* also observed different phenotypes of PPI non-responders in a series of 168 patients who underwent 24-h pH impedance monitoring on PPI for refractory GERD symptoms [9]. Eleven percent of subjects had a persistent pathological esophageal acid exposure despite PPI twice daily (phenotype 1), 31% had a positive association between symptoms and

---

CASE STUDY

A 28-year-old woman complained of heartburn, chest pain and gurgling in the throat for the past 10 years. She tried different PPIs (dexlansoprazole, omeprazole, esomeprazole) without any improvement of her symptoms. The symptoms were worse after a meal and with stress. She had no significant previous health history. Her Body Mass Index (BMI) was 21.4 kg/m². No hiatal hernia was seen on esophagogastroduodenscopy. Two small tongues of pink mucosa extending 1 cm maximally from the squamocolumnar junction were observed. The corresponding biopsies showed esophageal squamous and gastric mucosa with chronic carditis.
A 24-h pH impedance monitoring was performed on PPI therapy (esomeprazole 40 mg b.i.d.). The esophageal acid exposure was normal at 0.6%. The number of reflux episodes was also normal (23 episodes, three acid and 20 non-acid). During the recording, the patient reported 17 episodes of heartburn. The symptom index and the symptom association probability were both equal to 0%.

What do you propose for the management of this patient?
As the pH impedance on PPI was normal without any positive correlation between symptom and reflux event, the current symptoms presented by the patient were not linked to persistent pathological GERD on PPI. An alternative therapy triggering visceral hypersensitivity should be proposed.
  Should PPI therapy be discontinued in this patient? In the absence of GERD documentation off medicine, it is not possible to differentiate a phenotype 4 (functional heartburn) from a phenotype 3 (functional overlap with GERD). An evaluation off PPI (pH or pH impedance monitoring) would be helpful to diagnose a "baseline" GERD. If the patient presented a pathological acid esophageal exposure, PPIs should be maintained. Otherwise they should be stopped.

non-acid reflux (phenotype 2), and 58% had no evidence of pathological reflux and/or positive association on PPI (phenotypes 3 and 4). As data on esophageal pH monitoring off PPI were not available for these patients, it is not possible to differentiate phenotypes 3 and 4.

Diagnostic algorithm for managing proton pump inhibitor non-responders

The evaluation of patients who are not responding to PPI therapy begins by first documenting that the patient is compliant with medical management. This is an important component of the work-up of the refractory patient as a large population-based study suggests that over 50% of patients on PPI therapy are not compliant with medication [10,11]. In addition to daily compliance, less than 50% of patients take their PPI optimally (timing, frequency, and dose) [12]. Most of the current guidelines support empiric treatment with single FDA-approved dose PPI therapy for a 4–8-week period for a patient presenting with typical GERD symptoms [13]. If the patient fails single-dose therapy, it is reasonable to escalate therapy to double dose as there is little risk to this practice and a small group of patients may respond.

One caveat to empiric treatment focuses on the presence or absence of warning signs. Although there is controversy regarding the predictive value of warning symptoms [14], an upfront endoscopy is reasonable if there is evidence of dysphagia, odynophagia, gastrointestinal (GI) bleeding, unintentional weight loss, early satiety or age at presentation greater than 55 to rule out significant complications and malignancy. In the absence of warning signs, patients are typically not referred for endoscopy unless they have failed a course of optimized PPI therapy. The timing of endoscopy in the algorithm and the dose of PPI that is considered a failure which warrants endoscopic evaluation are unclear. However, we would recommend a trial of double-dose therapy.

A diagnostic algorithm is presented in Figure 7.1. The test choice is firstly determined by the pretest probability for baseline GERD. This algorithm allows the differentiation of the different phenotypes of PPI non-responders.

As mentioned above, patients who fail initial single-dose FDA-approved PPI therapy will have their acid suppression therapy increased to at least double the FDA-approved dose [5]. The data to support the yield of an escalation of PPI therapy to double dose in patients not responding to single dose are marginal and likely in the range of 10–20% [15]. Thus, the majority of patients who are escalated to double dose still have continued symptoms and do warrant further evaluation with ambulatory reflux testing.

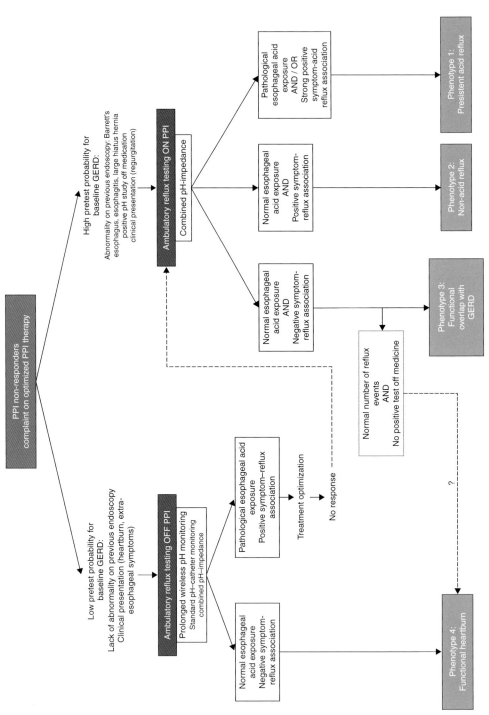

Figure 7.1 Diagnosis algorithm to identify the four phenotypes of PPI non-responders. Modified from Pandolfino and Vela [16], with permission from Elsevier.

The approach to ambulatory reflux monitoring is outlined in Figure 7.1 and mirrors the American Society for Gastrointestinal Endoscopy (ASGE) guidelines published in 2009 [16]. Decisions regarding the type of device utilized for the evaluation of PPI non-responders are beyond the scope of this particular chapter and are covered in Chapter 3. However, a few important concepts should be reviewed regarding whether or not to study patients off or on medical therapy.

The decision to study patients off and on medication should focus on the pretest probability that the patient has baseline pathological acid reflux and also on the specific question that needs to be answered. If the pretest probability is low based on the clinical presentation and lack of overt abnormalities on endoscopy (esophagitis, Barrett's esophagus, large hiatus hernia), the first and most important question in the evaluation of refractory symptoms should be whether or not the patient actually has baseline abnormal reflux/pathological acid exposure. Thus, these patients should have ambulatory pH monitoring off medication to document whether or not abnormal reflux/pathological acid exposure is present at baseline (Plate 7.1). This can be accomplished with a standard pH catheter, combined pH impedance catheter or wireless pH capsule. Data suggesting that the wireless capsule pH monitoring system is superior in diagnosing abnormal reflux are limited; however, there are studies that suggest that extending the duration of pH monitoring from 24 h to 48–96 h may improve the yield of documenting abnormal reflux. For example, among 38 patients with negative 24-h pH catheter-based results, prolonged (48–96 h) wireless pH monitoring revealed a pathological acid esophageal exposure in 37% and 47% using average and worst day analysis respectively [17]. Overall, GERD was diagnosed in 61% (average analysis) and 76% (worst day) based on either pathological acid exposure or positive symptom association.

If the pretest probability for baseline GERD is high secondary to a documented abnormality found previously on endoscopy (large hernia, esophagitis, Barrett's esophagus), a positive pH study off medication or strong clinical scenario where the patient is likely to have baseline GERD, the patient should undergo ambulatory reflux testing on PPI therapy using combined pH impedance (Plate 7.2). In this instance, the question of whether or not baseline GERD exists is less important and the focus of the evaluation is on defining the mechanism behind the refractory symptoms. Moreover, it has been shown that 93% of patients with symptoms refractory to twice-daily dosage of PPI and abnormal pH impedance monitoring on PPI have abnormal acid esophageal exposure off PPI [18]. Thus, this technology can define the remaining phenotypes (2–4) and direct appropriate management. In the absence of evaluation off PPI, the distinction between phenotypes 3 and 4 may be difficult. If the total number of reflux events is normal, the patient likely fits a phenotype consistent with functional heartburn. However, the threshold number of reflux events to distinguish phenotype 3 from 4 is not clear when patients are studied on PPI therapy. An alternative to answer the question of whether to test on or off medication is prolonged wireless pH monitoring both off and on PPI (BOOP testing) in a single examination (2 days off PPI followed by 2 days on PPI) [19]. This test is sufficient to identify patients with phenotypes 1 and 4 but does not allow one to differentiate phenotype 2 from phenotype 3.

Treatment of proton pump inhibitor non-responders

Unfortunately, the treatment strategies and management options for PPI non-responders are poorly defined and draw from open label studies or small clinical trials. In addition, most trials assessing refractory GERD have not clearly defined the relevant phenotypes and thus, it has been difficult to assess the overall benefit of specific therapies. Given this fact, this section will focus on the available therapies and also discuss which phenotype would be most likely to respond to the various therapies.

Acid suppression

Although the majority of this chapter has focused on the evaluation and management of refractory symptoms in endoscopy-negative patients, one important aspect of true refractory GERD is patients with refractory esophagitis, peptic strictures, and continued symptoms in Barrett's esophagus. These patients may require higher doses of PPI therapy or other adjunct treatment focused on reducing the overall reflux burden. These patients tend to have the most severe abnormalities in the anti-reflux barrier (hiatus hernia, hypotensive lower esophageal sphincter (LES)) and esophageal clearance (weak peristalsis, hiatus hernia). Improving acid suppression can be accomplished by either increasing the dose of PPI therapy or adding an H2 blocker at night [20]. The data supporting the efficacy of these particular treatments are limited, but this strategy represents a reasonable approach with limited risk and a valid endpoint to follow on endoscopy. Occasionally, ambulatory pH monitoring without impedance can be performed to assess the effectiveness of PPI therapy by studying patients on medication. However, this is an exception and once again, it is probably better to study these patients with combined pH impedance on PPI therapy.

The data supporting the efficacy of increasing PPI therapy to double dose or adding an H2 blocker at night in endoscopy-negative patients with refractory symptoms are limited. The therapeutic benefit of increasing PPI dose was reported in a study by Fass [15]. In patients with persistent heartburn on PPI once-daily treatment, two therapeutic strategies were compared: increasing PPI dosage to twice daily (lansoprazole 30 mg b.i.d) versus switching to another PPI (esomeprazole 40 mg). These two strategies were equivalent in terms of heartburn symptom control. However, these results would not necessarily be similar with other PPIs as esomeprazole may have a better bioavailability than the other PPIs. Finally, Becker *et al.* showed that increasing PPI dosage was more effective in patients with pathological findings in pH impedance monitoring on standard PPI therapy (persistent abnormal acid exposure and/or increased number of reflux events) than in patients without any pathological findings on pH impedance (91% symptom relief versus 43%, $P < 0.001$) [21]. This study emphasizes the benefit of acid suppression intensification in patients with phenotypes 1 and 2.

Another strategy to augment acid suppression has been focused on adding an H2 blocker at night to help control the histamine-generated nocturnal acid breakthrough common with PPI therapy [22]. This strategy was shown to obliterate nocturnal acid breakthrough on pH studies but a clinical correlation with symptom improvement is still unproven. Furthermore, there have been potential issues with tachyphylaxis as evidenced by a study by Fackler *et al.* that revealed a blunting of the H2 blocker effect after 4 weeks [23]. However, the addition of an H2 blocker at night is reasonable as the medication is safe and could potentially be effective in a small proportion of patients with significant nocturnal symptoms, especially if the medication is used intermittently when symptoms are exacerbated.

Treatment beyond acid suppression

A number of therapies have been proposed to treat refractory symptoms in PPI non-responders that go beyond acid suppression and focus on reflux inhibition and reducing visceral hypersensitivity.

Reflux inhibition

Targeting transient lower esophageal sphincter relaxations (TLESRs) provides an opportunity to develop reflux inhibitors. Baclofen, a gamma-aminobutyric acid B (GABA$_B$) receptor agonist, is a potential add-on treatment for patients with persistent symptomatic reflux events despite PPI. It decreases the number of postprandial acid and non-acid reflux events [24]. The dose of 20 mg three times daily has been proposed in refractory GERD [25]. However, no controlled trial of baclofen in PPI non-responders is available. Moreover, because the drug crosses the blood–brain barrier, neurological side-effects including somnolence, dizziness, and drowsiness are important limiting factors in the use of baclofen in clinical practice. Novel GABA$_B$ agonists are currently in clinical development for the treatment of refractory GERD. Arbaclofen placarbil, a pro-drug of the pharmacologically active *R*-isomer of baclofen, decreased the number of postprandial reflux events and associated symptoms [26]. The safety profile could be better compared to baclofen. Lesogabaran, a new GABA$_B$ agonist, was developed to overcome the side-effects of baclofen. It decreased the number of postprandial TLESRs, but its effect is modest [27].

As metoclopramide may improve gastric emptying and basal lower esophageal sphincter pressure [28], it represents a reasonable treatment option in GERD. However, side-effects and lack of efficacy limit recommendation of this drug in GERD management [13]. Current strategies would only advocate using this medication in patients with poor gastric emptying and for patients who have shown a dramatic benefit from the medicine. Short trials to determine if the medication is associated with improvement in symptoms should be performed with close follow-up and a careful discussion of potential adverse events. If no improvement on metoclopramide occurs, it should be discontinued given the significant neurological side-effects.

Visceral hypersensitivity

There is growing evidence to suggest that altered hypersensitivity and central sensitization may be important components of the visceral pain perception pathway. This concept was first acknowledged when balloon distension studies were noted to reproduce heartburn and chest pain in a higher proportion of patients with non-cardiac chest pain compared to healthy volunteers. Subsequently, studies in non-cardiac chest pain and functional heartburn have shown a reduced perception threshold to balloon distension and acid perfusion [29–31]. Most models of hyperalgesia suggest that both hypersensitivity of peripheral nociceptors and aberrant central modification of pain may be responsible for this phenomenon. Previous injury in the esophagus related to reflux of gastric contents may elicit inflammation and release cytokines that could potentially induce greater afferent firing and central delivery of pain mediators. This response could be implicated in the hyperalgesia that may be associated with weakly acidic events in a subgroup of PPI non-responders. Additionally, chronic neuropathic injury may also cause spontaneous neuropathic pain which may elicit symptoms independent of the stimulus and thus could potentially explain why functional heartburn patients have no evidence of symptom reflux correlation.

Given the importance of sensitivity in visceral pain perception, PPI non-responders may be better suited for interventions focused on reducing esophageal hypersensitivity or central perception. Furthermore, even those patients with a clear reflux symptom relationship may require *both* acid suppression and an adjunct therapy focused on esophageal hypersensitivity [32,33].

Low-dose antidepressants

Low-dose antidepressants have been shown to reduce symptoms in patients with non-cardiac chest pain. Currently, this class of medication is commonly used as adjunct therapy for patients with refractory GERD symptoms despite lack of efficacy data and a significant side-effect profile [7]. Although experimental physiological data suggest that these agents may alter symptom perception thresholds to artificial stimuli such as balloon distension and catheter-delivered acid infusion [30], it is unclear how effective these agents are in reducing symptoms.

Acupuncture

Alternative approaches to treating visceral pain may be useful in PPI non-responders. In a series of 30 patients who presented refractory heartburn on standard dose PPI, acupuncture in combination with single-dose PPI therapy has been shown to be more effective than double-dose PPI [34]. This promising result has to be confirmed in larger series.

Hypnotherapy

Response to PPI may be dependent on the level of psychological distress [35]. Moreover, patients with poor correlation between symptoms and reflux events display a higher level of anxiety than patients with a good correlation between symptoms and reflux [36]. Hypnotherapy is effective in pathology associated with high levels of anxiety. In patients with non-cardiac chest pain, hypnotherapy improved pain relief and was associated with a decrease in medication use [37]. Therefore, this alternative approach may be useful to improve PPI response not only in patients with refractory symptoms associated with reflux events but also in patients with functional heartburn.

The role of surgery in refractory gastroesophageal reflux disease

Few data are available on the efficacy of fundoplication in refractory GERD. Broeders *et al.* recently showed that patients with PPI-refractory non-erosive reflux disease and erosive reflux disease benefit equally from Nissen fundoplication [38]. It is important to note that all the patients included in this study presented with pathological esophageal acid exposure on ambulatory 24-h pH testing performed off PPI and thus, phenotype 4 was ruled out. In a series of 19 patients who underwent fundoplication for refractory GERD with a positive symptom index on pH impedance monitoring, Mainie *et al.* noted a significant improvement of GERD symptoms in 17 patients 14 months after fundoplication [39]. However, response to surgery has not been tested in large controlled trials and careful selection before treatment is a requirement. Before referring the patient to the surgeon for refractory GERD, an objective evaluation is always required to rule in pathological acid exposure and rule out alternative causes, such as achalasia and eosinophilic esophagitis [13]. Only patients with proven pathological GERD and persistent positive association between reflux events and symptoms despite PPI therapy should be eventually considered for surgery.

Conclusion

Proton pump inhibitor non-responders represent a large group of patients being seen in both primary care and gastroenterology clinics. Among patients compliant on optimized PPI therapy, four different phenotypes can be identified using ambulatory reflux testing: persistent acid reflux (phenotype 1), non-acid reflux (phenotype 2), functional overlap with GERD (phenotype 3), and functional heartburn (phenotype 4). The choice of which ambulatory reflux test (catheter, wireless or combined with impedance) and whether to study the patient off or on medication should be based on the pretest probability for baseline GERD. When the probability is low, pH monitoring off medication allows one to identify patients with functional heartburn. When the pretest probability is high, combined pH impedance on PPI should be the preferred method as the main question now focuses on why the medicine is not working. The treatment of refractory GERD also remains challenging and identification of PPI non-responder phenotypes may provide the pathophysiological basis to help guide therapy. Improving reflux control may be proposed in patients with phenotypes 1 and 2, whereas treatment strategies targeting visceral hypersensitivity may be more relevant in phenotypes 3 and 4. Further studies are required to evaluate this treatment strategy.

References

1 El-Serag H, Becher A, Jones R. Systematic review: persistent reflux symptoms on proton pump inhibitor therapy in primary care and community studies. Aliment Pharmacol Ther 2010;32(6):720–37.

2 Castell DO, Kahrilas PJ, Richter JE, et al. Esomeprazole (40 mg) compared with lansoprazole (30 mg) in the treatment of erosive esophagitis. Am J Gastroenterol 2002;97(3):575–83.

3 Lind T, Havelund T, Carlsson R, et al. Heartburn without oesophagitis: efficacy of omeprazole therapy and features determining therapeutic response. Scand J Gastroenterol 1997;32(10):974–9.

4 Everhart JE, Ruhl CE. Burden of digestive diseases in the United States part I: overall and upper gastrointestinal diseases. Gastroenterology 2009;136(2):376–86.

5 Tytgat GN, McColl K, Tack J, *et al.* New algorithm for the treatment of gastro-oesophageal reflux disease. Aliment Pharmacol Ther 2008;27(3):249–56.

6 Charbel S, Khandwala F, Vaezi MF. The role of esophageal pH monitoring in symptomatic patients on PPI therapy. Am J Gastroenterol 2005;100(2):283–9.

7 Fass R, Shapiro M, Dekel R, Sewell J. Systematic review: proton-pump inhibitor failure in gastro-oesophageal reflux disease – where next? Aliment Pharmacol Ther 2005;22(2):79–94.

8 Savarino E, Pohl D, Zentilin P, *et al.* Functional heartburn has more in common with functional dyspepsia than with non-erosive reflux disease. Gut 2009;58(9):1185–91.

9 Mainie I, Tutuian R, Shay S, *et al.* Acid and non-acid reflux in patients with persistent symptoms despite acid suppressive therapy: a multicentre study using combined ambulatory impedance-pH monitoring. Gut 2006;55(10):1398–402.

10 El-Serag HB, Fitzgerald S, Richardson P. The extent and determinants of prescribing and adherence with acid-reducing medications: a national claims database study. Am J Gastroenterol 2009;104(9):2161–7.

11 Hungin AP, Rubin G, O'Flanagan H. Factors influencing compliance in long-term proton pump inhibitor therapy in general practice. Br J Gen Pract 1999;49(443):463–4.

12 Gunaratnam NT, Jessup TP, Inadomi J, Lascewski DP. Sub-optimal proton pump inhibitor dosing is prevalent in patients with poorly controlled gastro-oesophageal reflux disease. Aliment Pharmacol Ther 2006;23(10):1473–7.

13 Kahrilas PJ, Shaheen NJ, Vaezi MF, *et al.* American Gastroenterological Association Medical Position Statement on the management of gastroesophageal reflux disease. Gastroenterology 2008;135(4):1383–91.

14 Vakil N. Review article: test and treat or treat and test in reflux disease? Aliment Pharmacol Ther 2003;17(Suppl 2):57–9.

15 Fass R, Sontag SJ, Traxler B, Sostek M. Treatment of patients with persistent heartburn symptoms: a double-blind, randomized trial. Clin Gastroenterol Hepatol 2006;4(1):50–6.

16 Pandolfino JE, Vela MF. Esophageal-reflux monitoring. Gastrointest Endosc 2009;69(4):917–30.

17 Sweis R, Fox M, Anggiansah A, Wong T. Prolonged, wireless pH-studies have a high diagnostic yield in patients with reflux symptoms and negative 24-h catheter-based pH-studies. Neurogastroenterol Motil 2011;23(5):419–26.

18 Pritchett JM, Aslam M, Slaughter JC, Ness RM, Garrett CG, Vaezi MF. Efficacy of esophageal impedance/pH monitoring in patients with refractory gastroesophageal reflux disease, on and off therapy. Clin Gastroenterol Hepatol 2009;7(7):743–8.

19 Garrean CP, Zhang Q, Gonsalves N, Hirano I. Acid reflux detection and symptom-reflux association using 4-day wireless pH recording combining 48-hour periods off and on PPI therapy. Am J Gastroenterol 2008;103(7):1631–7.

20 Rackoff A, Agrawal A, Hila A, Mainie I, Tutuian R, Castell DO. Histamine-2 receptor antagonists at night improve gastroesophageal reflux disease symptoms for patients on proton pump inhibitor therapy. Dis Esophagus 2005;18(6):370–3.

21 Becker V, Bajbouj M, Waller K, Schmid RM, Meining A. Clinical trial: persistent gastro-oesophageal reflux symptoms despite standard therapy with proton pump inhibitors – a follow-up study of intraluminal-impedance guided therapy. Aliment Pharmacol Ther 2007;26(10):1355–60.

22 Hatlebakk JG, Katz PO, Kuo B, Castell DO. Nocturnal gastric acidity and acid breakthrough on different regimens of omeprazole 40 mg daily. Aliment Pharmacol Ther 1998;12(12):1235–40.

23 Fackler WK, Ours TM, Vaezi MF, Richter JE. Long-term effect of H2RA therapy on nocturnal gastric acid breakthrough. Gastroenterology 2002;122(3):625–32.

24 Vela MF, Tutuian R, Katz PO, Castell DO. Baclofen decreases acid and non-acid postprandial gastro-oesophageal reflux measured by combined multichannel intraluminal impedance and pH. Aliment Pharmacol Ther 2003;17(2):243–51.

25 Koek GH, Sifrim D, Lerut T, Janssens J, Tack J. Effect of the GABA(B) agonist baclofen in patients with symptoms and duodeno-gastro-oesophageal reflux refractory to proton pump inhibitors. Gut 2003;52(10):1397–402.

26 Gerson LB, Huff FJ, Hila A, et al. Arbaclofen placarbil decreases postprandial reflux in patients with gastroesophageal reflux disease. Am J Gastroenterol 2010;105(6): 1266–75.

27 Boeckxstaens GE, Beaumont H, Mertens V, et al. Effects of lesogaberan on reflux and lower esophageal sphincter function in patients with gastroesophageal reflux disease. Gastroenterology 2010;139(2):409–17.

28 Durazo FA, Valenzuela JE. Effect of single and repeated doses of metoclopramide on the mechanisms of gastroesophageal reflux. Am J Gastroenterol 1993;88(10):1657–62.

29 Yang M, Li ZS, Chen DF, et al. Quantitative assessment and characterization of visceral hyperalgesia evoked by esophageal balloon distention and acid perfusion in patients with functional heartburn, nonerosive reflux disease, and erosive esophagitis. Clin J Pain 2010;26(4):326–31.

30 Broekaert D, Fischler B, Sifrim D, Janssens J, Tack J. Influence of citalopram, a selective serotonin reuptake inhibitor, on oesophageal hypersensitivity: a double-blind, placebo-controlled study. Aliment Pharmacol Ther 2006;23(3):365–70.

31 Nasr I, Attaluri A, Hashmi S, Gregersen H, Rao SS. Investigation of esophageal sensation and biomechanical properties in functional chest pain. Neurogastroenterol Motil 2010;22(5):520–6.

32 Shi G, Bruley des Varannes S, Scarpignato C, Le Rhun M, Galmiche JP. Reflux related symptoms in patients with normal oesophageal exposure to acid. Gut 1995;37 (4):457–64.

33 Fass R, Tougas G. Functional heartburn: the stimulus, the pain, and the brain. Gut 2002;51(6):885–92.

34 Dickman R, Schiff E, Holland A, et al. Clinical trial: acupuncture vs. doubling the proton pump inhibitor dose in refractory heartburn. Aliment Pharmacol Ther 2007;26(10):1333–44.

35 Nojkov B, Rubenstein JH, Adlis SA, et al. The influence of co-morbid IBS and psychological distress on outcomes and quality of life following PPI therapy in patients with gastro-oesophageal reflux disease. Aliment Pharmacol Ther 2008;27(6):473–82.

36 Rubenstein JH, Nojkov B, Korsnes S, et al. Oesophageal hypersensitivity is associated with features of psychiatric disorders and the irritable bowel syndrome. Aliment Pharmacol Ther 2007;26(3):443–52.

37 Jones H, Cooper P, Miller V, Brooks N, Whorwell PJ. Treatment of non-cardiac chest pain: a controlled trial of hypnotherapy. Gut 2006;55(10):1403–8.

38 Broeders JA, Draaisma WA, Bredenoord AJ, Smout AJ, Broeders IA, Gooszen HG. Long-term outcome of Nissen fundoplication in non-erosive and erosive gastro-oesophageal reflux disease. Br J Surg 2010;97(6):845–52.

39 Mainie I, Tutuian R, Agrawal A, Adams D, Castell DO. Combined multichannel intraluminal impedance-pH monitoring to select patients with persistent gastro-oesophageal reflux for laparoscopic Nissen fundoplication. Br J Surg 2006;93(12): 1483–7.

CHAPTER 8

Functional Heartburn

Stanislas Bruley des Varannes,[1] Frank Zerbib,[2] and Jean-Paul Galmiche[1]

[1]Institut des Maladies de l'Appareil Digestif, Centre Hospitalier Universitaire de Nantes, Nantes, France
[2]Département de Gastroentérologie, CHU de Bordeaux and Centre Hospitalier Saint André de Bordeaux, Bordeaux, France

Key points

- The diagnostic criteria of functional heartburn according to the ROME III definition (presence for at least 3 months, with onset at least 6 months before diagnosis, of burning retrosternal discomfort or pain; and absence of evidence that gastroesophageal acid reflux is the cause of the symptom; and absence of histopathology-based esophageal motility disorders).
- Functional heartburn is frequently associated with other functional disorders and psychological co-morbidities.
- In endoscopy-negative patients with heartburn unresponsive to a proton pump inhibitor trial, the diagnosis of functional heartburn should be considered and gastroesophageal reflux disease excluded by the appropriate investigations, esophageal pH monitoring or, better still, pH impedance monitoring performed off medication.
- Although no treatment has been proven to be effective by well-conducted randomized controlled trials, pain modulators and behavioral therapies may be of benefit to some patients.

Potential pitfalls

- Continue proton pump inhibitor despite treatment failure in a patient with refractory functional heartburn.
- Miss or underestimate the role of other functional gastrointestinal disorders (e.g. dyspepsia) in the pathogenesis of symptom complaints.
- Perform anti-reflux surgery in a patient with functional heartburn.

Practical Manual of Gastroesophageal Reflux Disease, First Edition.
Edited by Marcelo F. Vela, Joel E. Richter and John E. Pandolfino.
© 2013 John Wiley & Sons, Ltd. Published 2013 by John Wiley & Sons, Ltd.

Introduction

Heartburn occurring at least once a month is reported by 10–20% of the general population in the US [1], but very few sufferers actually seek medical help. Heartburn seems to be more prevalent in the US and Europe than in Asia, although the incidence is probably rising in this part of the world [2]. Typical heartburn has been considered traditionally to be a specific symptom for gastroesopheal reflux disease (GERD), thus allowing diagnosis without the need for any further, invasive investigation [3]. However, with the development of more accurate diagnostic tools such as pH monitoring and, more recently, pH impedance monitoring [4], it has become increasingly evident that the perception of heartburn is not always associated with a reflux event, either acid or non-acid (i.e. weakly acidic or weakly alkaline [5]). Of note, the majority of acid reflux episodes occurring either physiologically or in GERD are not perceived and remain asymptomatic. Conversely, slight decreases in esophageal pH which do not reach the (arbitrary) threshold of pH 4 may be perceived as painful sensations (heartburn or chest pain) in some individuals. Finally, physiological studies have clearly established that mechanical stimuli such as esophageal balloon distension can also elicit the perception of heartburn [6], rendering the saying "no acid, no heartburn" in fact wrong, even if acid plays a major role in the pathogenesis of symptoms for the large majority of GERD patients.

Considering the complexity and diversity of esophageal functional disorders and GERD phenotypes, several attempts have been made to better characterize GERD with and without esophageal injury (non-erosive reflux disease or NERD) and to reclassify the group(s) of patients with typical heartburn but no evidence of the presence of GERD, either at endoscopy or after pH monitoring.

Functional heartburn (FH) is a term that has been introduced by the ROME group of experts to fully recognize this entity and to encourage further research [7–9]. As a result of the progress accomplished in the characterization of functional esophageal disorders, the definition of FH itself has evolved in the time between the implementation of the ROME II and ROME III systems [7,9]. Notably, the so-called acid-sensitive esophagus (characterized by a statistically significant relationship between acid reflux and symptom events, despite a normal acid exposure of the esophagus [10,11]), initially included in the FH group by the ROME II criteria, has been requalified in ROME III as part of the GERD spectrum. In Rome III, only patients with normal acid exposure and no correlation between reflux episodes qualify as having functional heartburn [12].

Irrespective of the academic aspects of this debate, it is clinically relevant to point out that the simple presence of heartburn, even if typical, does not correlate exactly with a homogeneous group of patients suffering from the

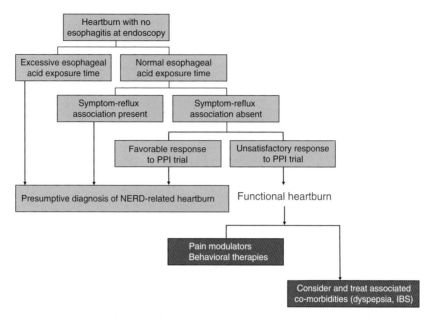

Figure 8.1 Classification of patients with heartburn and no evidence of esophagitis at endoscopy, using pH and response to a therapeutic trial of PPIs; the group classified as functional heartburn (FH) corresponds to the ROME III definition of FH. Adapted from Galmiche *et al.* [8], with permission from Elsevier. IBS, irritable bowel syndrome; NERD, non-erosive reflux disease; PPI, proton pump inhibitor.

same disease. This heterogeneity likely contributes to the explanation of why 30–40% of patients with typical heartburn are completely or partially refractory to acid suppression with a proton pump inhibitor [13]. In this chapter we have adopted the ROME III definition of FH (Figure 8.1), but it should be acknowledged that a large part of the referenced literature is not based on similar definitions of FH, making comparisons between studies in some cases difficult [8,14–17].

Definition and diagnostic criteria

According to the ROME III definition, "retrosternal burning in the absence of GERD that meets other essential criteria for the functional esophageal disorders typifies the diagnosis of FH". The diagnostic criteria are the following.
• Presence for at least 3 months, with onset at least 6 months before diagnosis, of burning retrosternal discomfort or pain; and
• Absence of evidence that gastroesophageal acid reflux is the cause of symptom; and
• Absence of histopathology-based esophageal motility disorders.

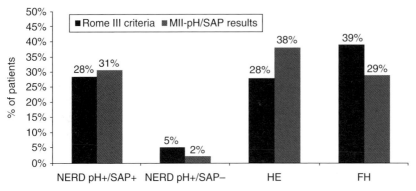

Figure 8.2 Contribution of pH impedance monitoring with Symptom Association Probability (SAP) analysis in identifying various subgroups of endoscopy-negative patients suffering from typical reflux symptoms. Comparison with the strategy consisting of pH-metry plus PPI response (used for the definition of FH according to Rome III criteria). pH impedance monitoring reduced the percentage of patients classified as FH. FH, functional heartburn; HE, hypersensitive esophagus; NERD, non-erosive reflux disease. Reproduced from Savarino *et al.* [24] with permission from Elsevier.

The minimal frequency of heartburn that is required to consider the patient's condition as an illness is not well defined. However, two or more days per week of mild heartburn is sufficient in GERD to influence quality of life and the same threshold can be applied in FH [2].

Overall, one of the weaknesses inherent in the definition of a functional disorder in general, and FH in particular, is that the diagnosis is largely influenced by the different constraints in the ability to fully recognize the presence or importance of GERD. This is illustrated by the decision to exclude patients with normal esophageal acid exposure, yet acid-related symptom events on ambulatory pH monitoring (hypersensitive esophagus), from the FH entity. The reason is that this group resembles other GERD patients in terms of presentation, manometric findings, impact on quality of life, natural history, and response to anti-reflux therapy in general, even if increased acid suppression may be required to relieve heartburn [11,18,19]. The same reasoning applies to patients with symptoms which respond well to a trial of proton pump inhibitor (PPI). Indeed, although a favorable response to a brief therapeutic trial using high doses of a PPI is not specific for GERD [20–22], the lack of response probably has a high negative predictive value for GERD. As anticipated by the authors of the Rome III definition of FH, studies using pH impedance monitoring [4,23,24] have clearly established that when more accurate investigations are used to detect acid and non-acid reflux and to assess the temporal relationship of reflux events and symptoms, the proportion of patients with a residual diagnosis of FH decreases (Figure 8.2).

Epidemiological studies using stringent definitions of FH are scarce. The female predominance and the younger age of patients with FH, as

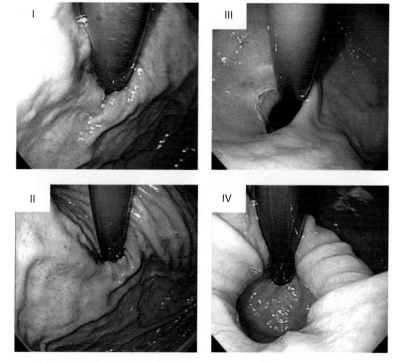

Plate 1.1 Endoscopic grading of the gastroesophageal flap valve. Grade I: a prominent ridge of tissue is present along the lesser curvature that is closely approximated to the endoscope. Grade II: the ridge is present but less well defined than in grade I, it opens rarely with respiration and closes promptly. Grade III: the ridge is barely present and there is often failure to close around the endoscope. It is nearly always accompanied by a hiatal hernia. Grade IV: there is no muscular ridge at all. The lumen of the esophagus gapes open, allowing the squamous epithelium to be viewed from below. A hiatal hernia is always present. Classification described by Hill LD *et al.* Gastrointest Endosc 1996;44:541–7. Reproduced from Kim GH *et al.* J Gastroenterol 2006;41:654–61 with permission from Springer.

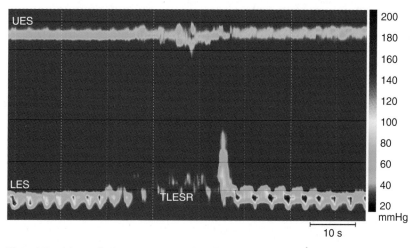

Plate 1.2 High-resolution manometry plot of a TLESR characterized by an abrupt fall in pressure at the position of the LES, a prominent after-contraction and esophageal shortening.

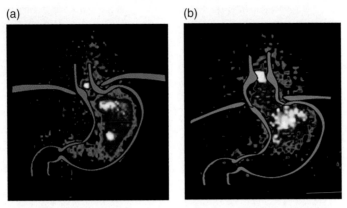

Plate 1.3 Scintigraphic image of the postprandial acid pocket with respect to the crural diaphragm. (a) Normal subdiaphragmatic position of the acid pocket in a patient without hiatal hernia. (b) Supradiaphragmatic position of the pocket in a patient with a large hiatal hernia.

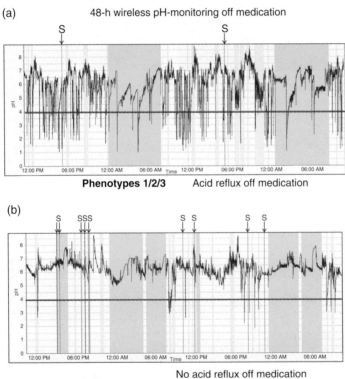

Plate 7.1 48-h wireless pH monitoring off medication is depicted for two patients with typical GERD symptoms (heartburn and chest pain). Esophageal pH was recorded 6 cm above the squamocolumnar junction. The horizontal red line corresponds to pH 4. Acid reflux is defined as a pH drop <4. Meal periods are represented in yellow and supine position in green. Symptom occurrence (S) is indicated by black arrows. (a) The patient presented with an esophageal pH <4 during 11.2% of total time on day 1 and during 7.9% on day 2. He had pathological acid reflux off medication and could present as phenotype 1, 2 or 3. (b) The patient presented with an esophageal pH <4 during 0.8% of total time on both day 1 and day 2. The symptoms were not correlated with acid reflux (symptom index 0%) and thus, he would fulfil criteria for phenotype 4.

(a)

pH-impedance monitoring on medication

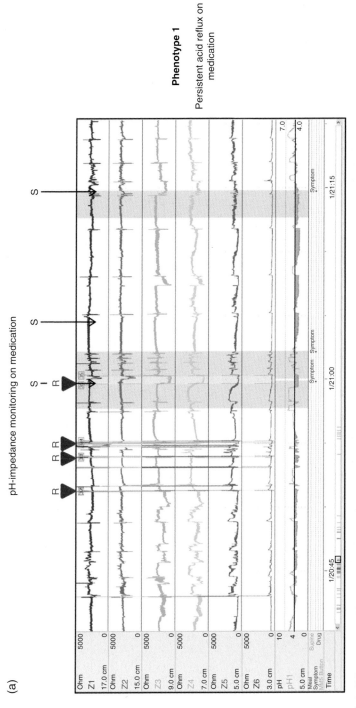

Phenotype 1

Persistent acid reflux on
medication

Plate 7.2 Representative 40-min pH impedance monitoring on medication given for three patients with typical GERD symptoms on medication. The pH was recorded 5 cm above the proximal border of the lower esophageal sphincter (LES) determined by high-resolution esophageal manometry. The impedance was recorded 3, 5, 7, 9, 15 and 17 cm above the LES. The horizontal black line represents pH 4. All occurrences of pH <4 are shaded in salmon on the pH tracing. Reflux events (R) defined by an abrupt 50% drop of impedance baseline are indicated by red head arrow and shaded in light purple on the impedance tracings. Symptom occurrence (S) is indicated by black arrow and the 2-min period preceding symptom occurrence is shaded in orange on impedance and pH tracings. (a) The patient presented with persistent pathological acid exposure despite esomeprazole 40 mg b.i.d (esophageal pH <4 during 8.9% of total time). This pattern corresponds to phenotype 1.

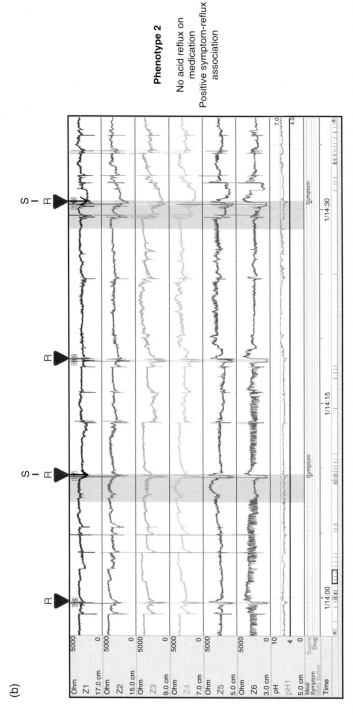

Plate 7.2 (Cont'd) (b) The patient had no pathological esophageal acid exposure (esophageal pH <4 during 1.3% of total time) on dexlansoprazole 60 mg but 40 weakly acidic reflux events per 24 h and a positive symptom association (symptom index 64% and symptom association probability 100%). Therefore he presented as a phenotype 2.

Phenotype 2

No acid reflux on medication

Positive symptom-reflux association

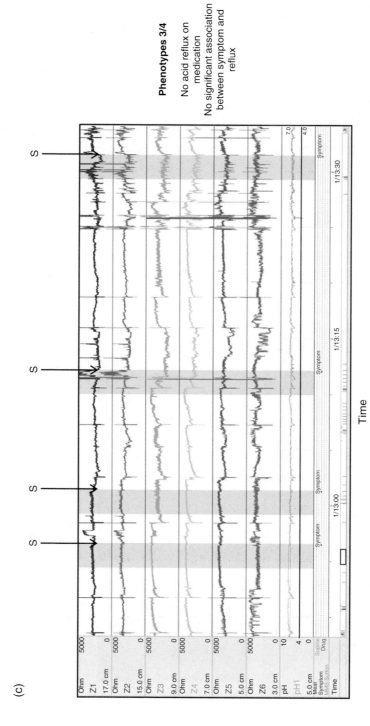

Plate 7.2 (Cont'd) (c) The patient presented with GERD symptoms despite esomeprazole 40 mg b.i.d. The pH impedance on medication revealed a normal esophageal acid exposure (0.6%), 25 reflux events per 24 h and a negative symptom association (symptom index 0%). This patient could potentially be a phenotype 3 or 4. Studies to determine an appropriate number of reflux events on PPI therapy that clearly distinguish phenotypes 3 and 4 are still lacking.

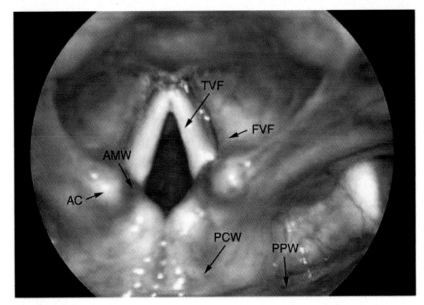

Plate 10.1 Normal laryngeal tissue. AC, arytenoid complex; AMW, arytenoid medial wall; FVF, false vocal fold; PCW, posterior cricoid wall; PPW, phosterior pharyngeal wall; TVF, true vocal fold. Adapted from Vaezi *et al.* [1] with permission from Elsevier.

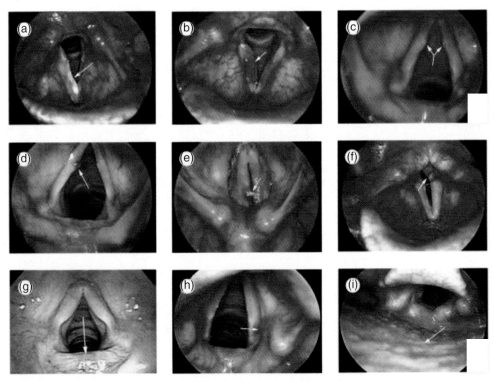

Plate 10.2 Abnormal larynx. (a) Leukoplakia. (b) Reinke's edema. (c) Bilateral true vocal cord nodules. (d) True vocal fold hemorrhagic polyp. (e) True vocal fold erythema. (f) Vocal fold granuloma. (g) Interarytenoid bar. (h) Arytenoid medial wall erythema. (i) Posterior pharyngeal wall cobblestoning. Adapted from Vaezi *et al.* [1] with permission from Elsevier.

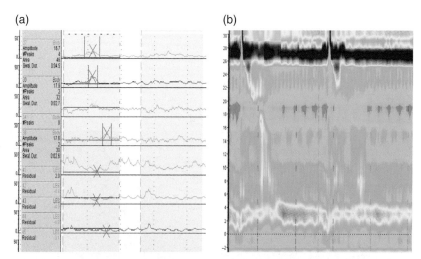

Plate 14.1 Manometric appearance of ineffective esophageal manometry (IEM). (a) Waveform images showing hypotensive contractions. (b) High-resolution manometry topographic plot exhibiting low-pressure peristaltic contractions.

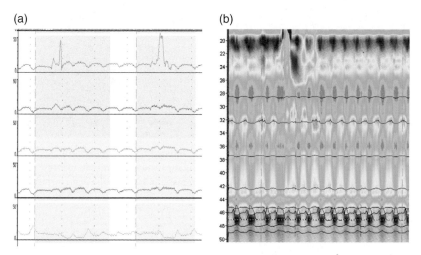

Plate 14.2 Manometric appearance of scleroderma. (a) Waveform images showing no smooth muscle contractions. (b) High-resolution manometry topographic plot exhibiting prominent pharyngeal contraction and weak distal esophageal pressure.

(a) (b)

(c) (d)

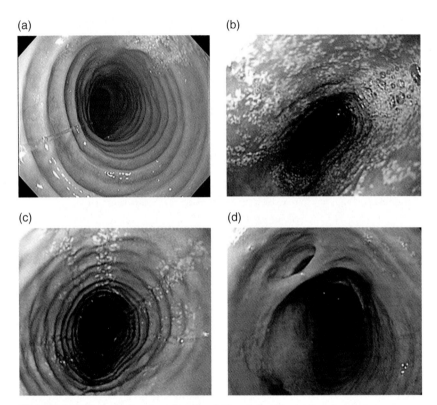

Plate 15.1 Endoscopic features of eosinophilic esophagitis. (a) Esophgeal rings.
(b) Esophageal exudates. (c) Esophgeal rings, exudates and longitudinal furrows.
(d) An esophageal pseudodiverticulum likely the result of healing of a deep intramural
esophageal tear.

opposed to NERD, are not really evident once patients with acid-sensitive esophagus have been excluded from the definition of FH [17]. Interestingly, and irrespective of the clinical setting (i.e. primary care or specialty practice), FH frequently occurs in association with symptoms usually considered to be components of dyspeptic syndrome, such as postprandial fullness, bloating, nausea, and early satiety [25–27]. Irritable bowel syndrome (IBS) symptoms also seem to be more prevalent in FH than in GERD patients [28,29].

In summary, the prevalence of FH depends on the defining and diagnostic criteria. Studies using both endoscopy and ambulatory pH monitoring to objectively establish evidence of GERD indicate that FH is likely to represent less than 10% of heartburn patients presenting to gastroenterologists [30]. The proportion is probably higher in primary care settings, when all patients with GERD symptoms which are non-responsive to PPI given empirically are considered. Conversely, in tertiary centers,

---

CASE STUDY

A 40-year-old female patient is referred for refractory heartburn. She has a history of appendectomy and irritable bowel syndrome. She has been complaining of heartburn for the previous 2 years. She describes a burning sensation behind the breastbone, occurring almost daily, mainly during the daytime. The symptoms appear to be more severe in the postprandial period, during which she also complains of epigastric bloating, nausea, and fullness. She has a long history of constipation and lower abdominal pain related to IBS. She has not lost weight over time (Body Mass Index (BMI) 23 kg/m²). There is no evidence of a psychiatric disorder such as depression or anxiety. She has been prescribed several PPIs at single and double dose without any significant improvement of heartburn. Compliance with PPI therapy, and also dosing times, appear to be adequate. An endoscopic work-up has been performed. There were no mucosal breaks at endoscopy and no eosinophilic infiltration of esophageal mucosa on the esophageal biopsies. Colonoscopy findings were also normal.

The patient is referred for refractory heartburn and advice regarding anti-reflux surgery. High-resolution esophageal manometry is performed, demonstrating no significant abnormality of esophageal motility. Lower esophageal sphincter pressure is within the normal range (23 mmHg). Wireless, 48-h pH monitoring is performed off therapy Both the number of acid reflux episodes and esophageal acid exposure are within normal limits during this 48-h period. Symptom association analysis does not demonstrate any correlation between heartburn episodes reported by the patient and the reflux events.

The final diagnosis is functional heartburn associated with functional dyspepsia and irritable bowel syndrome. Treatment with pain modulators is proposed to the patient who initially refuses it. Two months later, she finally accepts and is prescribed amitriptyline. The initial dose is 10 mg at bedtime, increased by 10 mg increments weekly. As the patient experiences side-effects (dry mouth, somnolence), the dose cannot be increased above 40 mg daily. After a period of 3 months, there is a significant improvement in both the frequency and severity of heartburn symptoms. There is no significant effect on functional dyspepsia and IBS symptoms.

when pH impedance monitoring is performed with statistical symptom analysis for acid and non-acid reflux episodes (including Symptom Associated Probability (SAP) [31] or Symptom Index (SI) determination), the proportion of remaining patients with a final diagnosis of FH is certainly smaller.

Pathogenesis of heartburn in functional heartburn

One difficulty in adequately analyzing the available data on the pathogenesis of FH is that the literature, at least with regard to the earliest reports, is clouded by the inclusion of subjects with undetected GERD in patient groups with presumed FH. This is actually the case for the excellent review published in 2002 by Fass and Tougas [32] on the role of peripheral and central factors in the pathogenesis of esophageal symptoms in NERD. Nevertheless, the conceptual model proposed by these authors remains valid as a representative overview of the mechanisms involved in esophageal perception in general (Figure 8.3). From a more mechanistic point of view, noxious esophageal stimuli are known to activate nociceptive receptors such as the TRPV1 (vanilloid) receptor, the transient receptor potential acid-sensing ion channel (ASIC), and the PX 2 family of ligand-gated ion channels responsive to adenosine triphosphate (ATP) (for a review see [33]). Activation of these receptors generates signals that are transmitted to the central nervous system (CNS) via either vagal or spinal nerves (Figure 8.4). Whether the same pathways are involved in NERD and FH remains unknown; if differences are present, they may contribute to explain the differences encountered in therapeutic response to acid suppression. It is also worth considering that, apart from pathways activated by topical chemical stimuli such as bile or acid, even in minute amounts, vagal afferents may also play a role in the perception of esophageal distension.

Regarding FH in particular, the prevailing view is to consider disturbed visceral perception as a major factor involved in its pathogenesis [32]. Hypersensitivity includes allodynia (defined by the perception of stimuli which are not normally perceived, for example slight changes in intraluminal esophageal pH) and hyperalgesia (pain greater than normally expected for a given stimulus). Both phenomena may be involved in FH. Moreover, "esophageal hypersensitivity" can include peripheral, central and possibly psychological factors which may act independently or, more likely, in concert.

Among other factors which are potentially involved in the pathogenesis of esophageal symptoms, hormonal pathways may also play a role. Indeed, the most frequent trigger of heartburn is eating a meal, suggesting that

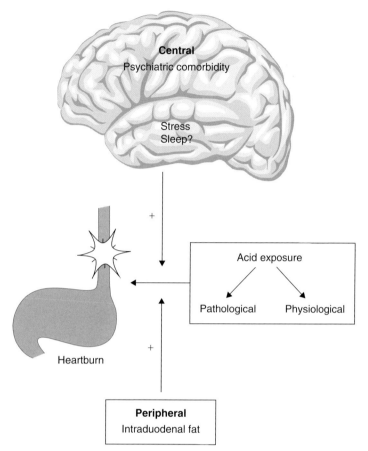

Figure 8.3 Proposed conceptual model for symptom generation in patients with non-erosive reflux disease. This model suggests that central (through brain–gut interactions) and peripheral mechanisms are essential for intraoesophageal stimuli (either physiological or pathological) to reach the conscious level and thus be perceived. Reproduced from Fass and Tougas [32] with permission from BMJ Publishing Group.

some food components, especially fats, may induce or exacerbate symptoms through a hormonal pathway. For example, Meyer *et al.* [34] showed that infusion of fat into the duodenum of reflux patients reduced the latency of occurrence of heartburn in response to esophageal acid infusion and increased symptom severity. Although the interpretation of this phenomenon remains largely speculative, a role for cholecystokinin has been proposed but other neurotransmitters also, e.g. calcitonin gene-related peptide or substance P, may influence esophageal perception by either peripheral (on vagal afferences) or central action.

The role of corticocerebral processing of esophageal signals has been investigated recently in a few studies using the recording of cortical

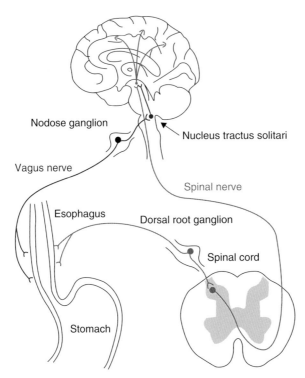

Figure 8.4 Sensory pathway from esophagus to brain. Esophageal nociceptive stimuli are conveyed to the brain via two major sensory pathways – a sympathetic pathway and a vagal pathway. Reproduced from Miwa *et al.* [33] with permission from the Korean Society of Neurogastroenterology and Motility.

potentials evoked by esophageal balloon distension or acid perfusion [35] and by newer imaging technologies such as positron emission tomography (PET) and functional magnetic resonance imaging [36,37]. These studies have all indicated strongly that the central processing of esophageal signals, after either noxious or physiological (normally non-painful) stimuli, may be different between healthy subjects and patients with GERD or FH. FH patients (Rome III definition) seem to be more sensitive to mechanical or chemical stimuli than NERD patients. Moreover, a phenomenon of acid chemoreceptor sensitization may significantly influence the response of pressure-sensitive receptors, suggesting cooperative interaction between these two receptor types in the process of esophageal hyperalgesia [38].

Irrespective of the esophageal stimulus considered, the conventional theory of the pathogenesis of heartburn implies a penetration of the noxious component either through mucosal breaks (in reflux esophagitis) or because of an increased permeability of the epithelial esophageal barrier. These alterations of the esophageal barrier are themselves the consequence

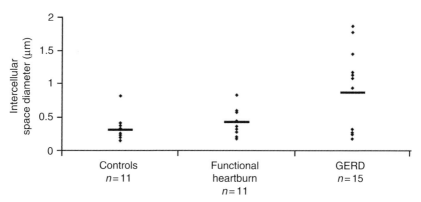

Figure 8.5 Scatter plot of mean intercellular space diameter (ISD) in μm for the three study groups. GERD, gastroesophageal reflux disease. Reproduced from Vela *et al.* [39] with permission from Blackwell Publishing.

of chronic exposure of the mucosa to a noxious agent (usually acid in GERD) refluxing from the stomach.

In recent decades, the consistent observation by several authors of an increased intercellular space between epithelial cells in both erosive esophagitis and NERD has lent support to this penetration theory. Indeed, this morphological change (called dilated intercellular space or DIS) is postulated to allow the noxious component of the refluxate to reach the nerve endings which run below the epithelial layer. However, the role of DIS in FH has recently been challenged by an important study by Vela *et al.* [39]. These authors used pH impedance monitoring (for acid and non-acid reflux detection) and electron microscopy (to measure intercellular space) in patients with heartburn refractory to PPI therapy. Patients were carefully phenotyped according to the ROME III criteria and then compared with healthy controls. While the mean intercellular distance was increased in GERD patients compared with controls, there was no significant difference between FH and controls (Figure 8.5). Moreover, only 9% of the FH patients had an intercellular distance greater than the normal range (compared with 60% of those with GERD).

These results, although requiring further confirmation using larger patient cohorts, are the first to support the use of a morphological marker capable of distinguishing FH from GERD. They also indicate that the perception of heartburn may arise even if the integrity of the mucosa is maintained. In these cases, sustained esophageal contractions can represent another mechanism in the pathogenesis of heartburn, as well as an explanation for the lack of temporal relationship between symptom events and reflux episodes during pH monitoring. Conversely, esophageal acid infusion has been shown to induce such sustained esophageal contractions [40].

Therefore different mechanisms are probably associated which may interact between each other and facilitate pain perception [41].

Role of psychological factors

It is now well established that acute experimental stress enhances the perception of esophageal acid in GERD patients. Indeed, Bradley *et al.* [42] showed in 1993 that reflux patients who are chronically anxious and exposed to prolonged stress may perceive low-intensity acid stimuli as painful symptoms. Of interest, in this controlled study the stress tasks did not significantly influence acid reflux parameters. More recently, the effect of life stress on symptoms of heartburn was studied by Naliboff *et al.* [43] in a cohort of patients followed prospectively for 4 months. The presence of severe, sustained life stress during the previous 6 months significantly predicted increased heartburn symptoms during the subsequent 4 months. Anxiety was strongly associated with impaired quality of life, and depression with heartburn medication use.

In another study, whereas psychological profiles did not differentiate subjects with normal esophageal acid exposure and no esophagitis from those having elevated acid exposure times, patients with FH had greater anxiety and somatization scores and poorer social support levels than those with reflux-provoked symptoms [44]. Shapiro *et al.* [45] conducted a study comparing the physiological and clinical characteristics of a group of 22 NERD patients (with abnormal pH test) with those of 30 FH patients (ROME II definition). There were no statistical differences in demographic parameters, frequency of hiatal hernia and *H. pylori* infection rates between the two groups. In contrast, FH patients had increased reports of chest pain, somatization and altered autonomic function (assessed by heart rate variability and skin conductance). In addition to stress and anxiety, sleep disorders may also enhance the perception of low-intensity esophageal stimuli [46]. Finally, some studies have suggested that a lower social status may be associated with FH [44].

Clinical evaluation

Clarification of the nature of the symptom is an essential first step [7]. Heartburn is characterized by pain or discomfort of burning quality that originates high in the epigastrium with intermittent cephalad retrosternal radiation. There are no evidence-based data to determine the specific symptom features of FH, including diurnal characteristics, exacerbating factors and ameliorating maneuvers. The benefit of structured questionnaires to better identify and categorize patients suffering from heartburn in a primary care setting remains controversial. Functional heartburn usually occurs during the day and, like the heartburn of GERD, may be elicited or exacerbated by certain foods and by lying down or bending over. However, it is difficult to extrapolate from data representing the whole "heartburn spectrum" to those of FH.

By definition, the diagnosis of FH requires specific investigations, at least endoscopy and pH monitoring and, if available, pH impedance monitoring in order first to exclude GERD as the cause of heartburn. In clinical practice, patients in whom FH is suspected are usually referred to a tertiary center after a long history of troublesome heartburn that has been partially or completely unresponsive to a PPI trial, usually consisting of a double-dose regimen administered for several months.

Concerning pH monitoring (or pH impedance monitoring), it is insufficient to limit the assessment to the measure of acid exposure. A careful analysis of the temporal relationships between the occurrence of symptoms and reflux events (both acid and non-acid) is of the utmost importance and the results must be expressed using SAP or SI values [31]. In routine practice, it is likely that many investigators do not perform such statistical analyses, with the risk of missing acid- or non-acid-sensitive esophagus. Extending the duration of pH monitoring by using the Bravo® capsule technology [47] increases the diagnostic yield of the investigation and allows the detection of a greater number of patients for whom a final GERD diagnosis can be made. Interestingly, patients with FH may be more likely to report retrosternal discomfort during wireless pH monitoring [48]. Although there is some controversy about whether pH (or pH impedance) monitoring should be performed "on" or "off" PPI therapy in patients with GERD refractory to PPI, the diagnosis of FH *always* requires the discontinuation of PPI therapy for at least 7 days before the procedure is performed.

Finally, other esophageal (e.g. achalasia, eosinophilic esophagitis) and non-esophageal (e.g. coronary artery disease) sources should be considered and appropriately evaluated when atypical or unusual symptom characteristics (e.g. exercise exacerbations) associated with heartburn are present. Similarly, it is important to carefully consider the associated burden related to other symptoms such as dyspepsia or IBS, because these functional manifestations may contribute to the impairment of quality of life. Understanding the main expectations of the patient, taking into consideration his/her socioeconomic status, is also an important part of a good clinical evaluation.

Treatment

By definition, the diagnosis of functional heartburn is considered when a patient with heartburn fails to improve on PPI therapy. Recent reviews on the management of refractory GERD have been published [49,50] and different algorithms have been proposed. As some patients with FH may be sensitive to small amounts of acid or acidic fluid with a pH >4, a trial of more vigorous acid suppression therapy is usually considered first. The addition of a prokinetic to acid suppression is not supported by evidence and a recent, randomized, placebo-controlled trial conducted in NERD patients failed to show any significant benefit of mosapride citrate (5 mg t.i.d.) plus omeprazole (10 mg o.d.) versus omeprazole alone [51].

The role of diet is frequently advocated by patients with functional gastrointestinal disorders but there is no clear evidence for a benefit of excluding specific foods (e.g. acidic or spicy foods). On the contrary, there are some arguments suggesting that the chronic ingestion of chili, which contains capsaicin, may improve functional dyspepsia and reflux symptoms by desensitization of TRPV 1 receptors [52]. Similarly, as fat and cholesterol could increase esophageal sensitivity to acid [53], heavy meals are usually avoided spontaneously by the patients themselves. Changing the composition of the refluxate may, at least in theory, represent an alternative approach; for example, in patients who are sensitive to bile salts, it might be possible to change the bile composition by the administration of ursodeoxycholic acid [54]. In fact, in clinical practice it is important to reassure the patient concerning the harmless effects of many foods and to convince him/her to avoid overly restrictive dietary regimens. Although the role of obesity in FH has not really been investigated, it is common sense to attempt to reduce excess weight.

Because the pathophysiology of FH may be quite similar to that of non-cardiac chest pain, and involve heightened visceral sensation, the use of low-dose tricyclic antidepressants, and possibly selective serotonin reuptake inhibitors, is reasonable. Similarly, psychological approaches such as behavioral modification, acupuncture [50], hypnotherapy or relaxation therapy [55] may be beneficial. However, to date no published controlled trials have demonstrated efficacy of any of these interventions in FH patients.

Several molecules may, potentially, influence visceral perception and this may be exploited in functional esophageal disorders in general, and in FH in particular. For example, the effect of tegaserod, a 5-HT4 agonist, was tested in a placebo-controlled, cross-over trial conducted in patients with overlapping symptoms of FH and functional dyspepsia (ROME II definition). The severities of heartburn, regurgitation, early fullness, and bloating were significantly lower after tegaserod compared with a placebo [56]. In the same study, mechanical sensitivity was assessed using the barostat technique and tegaserod was shown to increase the pressure threshold for gastric pain. However, the study conclusions are limited by the small sample of patients included and the cross-over design of the trial. Moreover, tegaserod is not available in many countries, especially in Europe and

North America, making applications of these findings very limited. Among other molecules, antagonists of the TRPV 1 receptor (AZD1386) have recently been developed and proof-of-concept studies have been published [57]. In healthy human subjects, AZD1386 increased esophageal and skin heat pain thresholds and was well tolerated. Thus this new class of drug may have a potential in NERD and also FH but it is too early to extrapolate from pharmacodynamic effects to the clinic.

Anti-reflux surgery in patients with FH has not been fully evaluated, but surgical management is unlikely to provide relief for these patients with frequently overlapping symptoms of dyspepsia and IBS, and in whom testing for pathological reflux is negative. Although the predictive value of preoperative esophageal acid exposure on postsurgical outcome remains controversial, some studies have indicated worse results in patients with a normal pH test [58]. Moreover, it is now well established that a proportion of patients with recurrent heartburn after anti-reflux surgery have normal esophageal pH values. Thompson *et al.* [59] reported that in such patients heartburn is frequently associated with psychiatric co-morbidities such as depression, suggesting that FH rather than GERD recurrence may be responsible for the persisting heartburn. The same prudent limitation should be applied to endoscopic anti-reflux procedures, although some of these procedures, such as a radiofrequency energy delivery (Stretta procedure), may affect esophageal sensitivity independently of their effect on cardial continence [60,61]. That said, endoscopic therapies cannot be recommended for FH at the present time.

In summary, once PPI failure has been confirmed and GERD excluded by appropriate tests, the treatment of FH remains largely empirical and an individual approach is therefore recommended. The clinician should provide reassurance and refrain from performing too many invasive tests or therapeutic procedures. Although the long-term natural history of FH is poorly known, some studies, as well as clinical experience, suggest a considerable "turnover" of functional gastrointestinal disorders with the appearance and disappearance of different categories of functional disorders in the same patient. In this context, Boyd *et al.* [62] reported a decrease in the prevalence of FH over time in a cohort of patients with associated eating disorders. Such findings may have important implications in favor of a very conservative and non-invasive approach in FH patients.

References

1 Locke GR, Talley NJ, Fett SL, *et al.* Prevalence and clinical spectrum of gastroesophageal reflux: a population-based study in Olmsted Country, Minnesota. Gastroenterology 1997;112:1448–56.

2 Dent J, Armstrong D, Delanye B, *et al.* Symptom evaluation in reflux disease: workshop, background, process, terminology, recommendations and discussion outputs. Gut 2004;53:iv1–iiv24.

3 Carlsson R, Dent J, Bolling–Sternevalde E, *et al.* The usefulness of a structured questionnaire in the assessment of symptomatic gastroesophageal reflux disease. Scand J Gastroenterol 1998;33:1023–9.

4 Zerbib F, Roman S, Ropert A, *et al.* Esophageal pH-impedance monitoring and symptom analysis in GERD. A study in patients off and on therapy. Am J Gastroenterol 2006;101:1956–63.

5 Sifrim D, Castell D, Dent J, *et al.* Gastro-oesophageal reflux monitoring: review and consensus report on detection and definitions of acid, non-acid, and gas reflux. Gut 2004;53:1024–31.

6 Karamanolis G, Stevens W, Vos R, *et al.* Oesophageal tone and sensation in the transition zone between proximal striated and distal smooth muscle oesophagus. Neurogastroenterol Motil 2008;20:291–7.

7 Clouse RE, Richter JE, Heading RC, *et al.* Functional esophageal disorders. In: Drossman DA, Corazziari E, Talley NJ, Thompson WG, Whitehead WE (eds) *Rome II. The functional gastrointestinal disorders*, 2nd edn. McLean, VA: Degnon Associates, 2000: pp. 247–98.

8 Galmiche JP, Clouse RA, Balint A, *et al.* Functional esophageal disorders. Gastroenterology 2006;130:1459–65.

9 Galmiche JP, Clouse RE, Balint A, *et al.* Functional esophageal disorders. In: Drossman DA, Corazziari E, Spiller R, *et al.* (eds) *Rome III .The functional gastrointestinal disorders*, 3rd edn. McLean, VA: Degnon Associates, 2006: pp. 369–418.

10 Shi G, Bruley des Varannes S, Scarpignato C, *et al.* Reflux related symptoms in patients with normal oesophageal exposure to acid. Gut 1995;37:457–64.

11 Trimble KC, Douglas S, Pryde A, *et al.* Clinical characteristics and natural history of symptomatic but not excess gastroesophageal reflux. Dig Dis 1995;40:1098–104.

12 Fass R, Ofman JJ. Gastroesophageal reflux disease – should we adopt a new conceptual framework? Am J Gastroenterol 2002;97:1901–9.

13 Fass R, Shapiro M, Dekel R, *et al.* Systematic review: proton-pump inhibitor failure in gastro-oesophageal reflux disease – where next? Aliment Pharmacol Ther 2005;22:79–94.

14 Frazzoni M, de Michell E, Zentilin P, Pathophysiological characteristics of patients with non-erosive reflux disease differ from those of patients with functional heartburn. Aliment Pharmacol Ther 2004;20:81–8.

15 Fry LC, Monkemuller K, Malfertheiner P. Functional heartburn, non-erosive reflux disease, and reflux esophagitis are all distinct conditions – a debate: con. Curr Treat Options Gastroenterol 2007;10:305–11.

16 Hershcovici T, Zimmerman J. Functional heartburn vs non-erosive reflux disease: similarities and differences. Aliment Pharmacol Ther 2008;27:1103–9.

17 Fass R. Functional heartburn: what it is and how to treat it. Gastrointest Endosc Clin North Am 2009;19:23–33.

18 Sacher-Huvelin S, Gournay J, Amouretti M, *et al.* Acid sensitive esophagus: natural history and quality of life of patients with acid hypersensitive esophagus syndrome. Comparison with classical gastro-esophageal reflux disease. Gastroenterol Clin Biol 2000;24:911–16.

19 Watson RGP, Tham TCK, Johnston BT, *et al.* Double blind cross-over placebo controlled study of omeprazole in the treatment of patients with reflux symptoms and physiological levels of acid reflux – the "sensitive" esophagus. Gut 1997;40:587–90.

20 Numans ME, Lau J, de Wit NJ, *et al.* Short-term treatment with proton-pump inhibitors as a test for gastroesophageal reflux disease: a meta-analysis of diagnostic test characteristics. Ann Intern Med 2004;140:518–27.

21 Bruley des Varannes S, Sacher-Huvelin S, Vavasseur F, *et al.* Rabeprazole test for the diagnosis of gastro-esophageal reflux disease: results of a study in a primary care setting. World J Gastroenterol 2006;28:2569–73.

22 Meineche-Schmidt V, Christensen E, Bytzer P. Randomised clinical trial: identification of responders to short-term treatment with esomeprazole for dyspepsia in primary care – a randomised, placebo-controlled study. Aliment Pharmacol Ther 2011;33:41–9.

23 Savarino E, Zentilin P, Tutuian R, *et al.* The role of nonacid reflux in NERD: lessons learned from impedance pH monitoring in 150 patients off therapy. Am J Gastroenterol 2008;103:2685–93.

24 Savarino E, Marabotto E, Zentilinn P, *et al.* The added value of impedance-pH monitoring to Rome III criteria in distinguishing functional heartburn from non-erosive reflux disease. Dig Liver Dis 2011;43(7):542–7.

25 Savarino E, Pohl D, Zentilin P, *et al.* Functional heartburn has more in common with functional dyspepsia that with non-erosive reflux disease. Gut 2009;58:1185–91.

26 Hershcovici T, Fass R. GERD: are functional heartburn and functional dyspepsia one disorder? Nat Rev Gastroenterol Hepatol 2010;7:71–2.

27 Xiao YL, Peng S, Tao J. Prevalence and symptom pattern of pathologic esophageal acid reflux in patients with functional dyspepsia based on the Rome III criteria. Am J Gastroenterol 2010;105:2626–31.

28 Lee KJ, Kwon HC, Cheong JY, *et al.* Demographic, clinical and psychological characteristics of the heartburn groups classified using the Rome III criteria and factors associated with the responsiveness to proton pump inhibitors in the gastroesophageal reflux disease group. Digestion 2009;79:131–6.

29 Kaji M, Fujiwara Y, Shiba M. Prevalence of overlaps between GERD, FD and IBS and impact on health-related quality of life. J Gastroenterol Hepatol 2010;25:1151–6.

30 Martinez SD, Malagon IB, Garewal HS, *et al.* Non-erosive reflux disease (NERD) – acid reflux and symptom patterns. Aliment Pharmacol Ther 2003;17:537–45.

31 Weusten BLAM, Roelofs JMM, Akkermans LM, *et al.* The symptom-association probability: an improved method for symptom analysis of 24-hour esophageal pH data. Gastroenterology 1994;107:1741–5.

32 Fass R, Tougas G. Functional heartburn: the stimulus, the pain, and the brain. Gut 2002;51:885–92.

33 Miwa H, Kondo T, Oshima T, *et al.* Esophageal sensation and esophageal hypersensitivity – overview from bench to bedside. J Neurogastroenterol Motil 2010;16:353–62.

34 Meyer JH, Lembo A, Elashoff JD, *et al.* Duodenal fat intensifies the perception of heartburn. Gut 2001;40:624–8.

35 Yang M, Li ZS, Xu XR. Characterization of cortical potentials evoked by oesophageal balloon distention and acid perfusion in patients with functional heartburn. Neurogastroenterol Motil 2006;18:292–9.

36 Kern MK, Birn RM, Jaradeh S, *et al.* Identification and characterization of cerebral cortical response to esophageal mucosal acid exposure and distention. Gastroenterology 1998;115:1353–62.

37 Kern M, Hofmann C, Hyde J, *et al.* Characterization of the cerebral cortical representation of heartburn in GERD patients. Am J Physiol Gastrointest Liver Physiol 2004;286:G174–81.

38 Yang M, Li ZS, Chen DF, *et al.* Quantitative assessment and characterization of visceral hyperalgesia evoked by esophageal balloon distention and acid perfusion in

patients with functional heartburn, nonerosive reflux disease, and erosive esophagitis. Clin J Pain 2010;26:326–31.

39 Vela MF, Craft BMM, Sharma N, *et al*. Refractory heartburn: comparison of intercellular space diameter in documented GERD vs functional heartburn. Am J Gastroenterol 2011;106:844–50.

40 Pehlivanov N, Liu J, Mittal RK. Sustained esophageal contraction: a motor correlate of heartburn symptom. Am J Physiol Gastrointest Liver Physiol 2001;281:G743–G751.

41 Barlow WJ, Orlando RC. The pathogenesis of heartburn in nonerosive reflux disease: a unifying hypothesis. Gastroenterology 2005;128:771–8.

42 Bradley LA, Richter JE, Pulliam TJ, *et al*. The relationship between stress and symptoms of gastroesophageal reflux: the influence of psychological factors. Am J Gastroenterol 1993;88:11–19.

43 Naliboff BD, Mayer M, Fass R, *et al*. The effect of life stress on symptoms of heartburn. Psychosom Med 2004;66:426–34.

44 Johnston BT, Lewis SA, Collins JS, *et al*. Acid perception in gastro-oesophageal reflux disease is dependent on psychosocial factors. Scand J Gastroenterol 1995;30:1–5.

45 Shapiro M, Green C, Bautista JM. Functional heartburn patients demonstrate traits of functional bowel disorder but lack a uniform increase of chemoreceptor sensitivity to acid. Am J Gastroenterol 2006;10:1084–91.

46 Schey R, Dickman R, Parthasarathy S, *et al*. Sleep deprivation is hyperalgesis in patients with gastroesophageal reflux disease. Gastroenterology 2007;133:1787–95.

47 Prakash C, Clouse RE. Value of extended recording time with a wireless esophageal pH system in patients with gastroesophageal reflux disease. Clin Gastroenterol Hepatol 2005;3:329–34.

48 Lee YC, Wang HP, Chiu HM, *et al*. Patients with functional heartburn are more likely to report retrosternal discomfort during wireless pH monitoring. Gastrointest Endosc 2005;62:834–41.

49 Fass R, Sifrim D. Management of heartburn not responding to proton pump inhibitors. Gut 2009;58:295–309.

50 Hershcovici T, Fass R. An algorithm for diagnosis and treatment of refractory GERD. Best Pract Res Clin Gastroenterol 2010;24:923–36.

51 Miwa H, Inoue K, Ashida K. Randomised clinical trial: efficacy of the addition of a prokinetic, mosapride citrate, to omeprazole in the treatment of patients with nonerosive reflux disease – a double-blind, placebo-controlled study. Aliment Pharmacol Ther 2011;33:323–32.

52 Gonlachanvit S. Are rice and spicy diet good for functional gastrointestinal disorders? J Neurogastroenterol Motil 2010;16:131–8.

53 Shapiro M, Green C, Bautista JM, *et al*. Assessment of dietary nutrients that influence perception of intra-oesophageal acid reflux events in patients with gastro-oesophageal reflux disease. Aliment Pharmacol Ther 2007;25:93–101.

54 Siddiqui A, Rodriguez-Stanley S, Zubaidi S. Esophageal visceral sensitivity to bile salts in patients with functional heartburn and in healthy control subjects. Dig Dis Sci 2005;50:81–5.

55 McDonald-Haile J, Bradley LA, Bailey MA, *et al*. Relaxation training reduces symptom reports and acid exposure in patients with gastroesophageal reflux disease. Gastroenterology 1994;107:61–9.

56 Miner PB Jr, Rodriguez-Stanley S, Proskin HM, *et al*. Tegaserod in patients with mechanical sensitivity and overlapping symptoms of functional heartburn and functional dyspepsia. Curr Med Res Opin 2008;24:2159–72.

57 Krarup AL, Ny L, Astrand M. Randomised clinical trial: the efficacy of a transient receptor potential vanilloid 1 antagonist AZD1386 in human oesophageal pain. Aliment Pharmacol Ther 2011;33:1113–22.

58 Khajanchee YS, Hong D, Hansen PD, *et al*. Outcomes of antireflux surgery in patients with normal preoperative 24-hour pH test results. Am J Surg 2004;187:599–603.

59 Thompson SK, Cai W, Jamieson GG. Recurrent symptoms after fundoplication with a negative pH study – recurrent reflux or functional heartburn? J Gastrointest Surg 2009;13:54–60.

60 Galmiche JP, Bruley des Varannes S. Endoluminal therapies for gastro-oesophageal reflux disease. Lancet 2003;361:1119–21.

61 Arts J, Tack J, Galmiche JP. Endoscopic antireflux procedures. Gut 2004;53:1207–14.

62 Boyd C, Abraham S, Kellow J. Appearance and disappearance of functional gastrointestinal disorders in patients with eating disorders. Neurogastroenterol Motil 2010;22:1279–83.

CHAPTER 9

The Role of Acid Reflux in Non-Cardiac Chest Pain

Cristina Almansa and Sami R. Achem

Division of Gastroenterology, Mayo Clinic Florida, Jacksonville, FL, USA

Key points box

- Non-cardiac chest pain is a common clinical problem.
- The esophagus is the main source of non-cardiac chest pain.
- Gastroesophageal reflux disease is a frequent cause of non-cardiac chest pain.
- Gastroesophageal reflux disease can co-exist with other causes of chest pain.
- A diagnosis of gastroesophageal reflux disease-related non-cardiac chest pain should not be established unless a cardiac source of the symptoms has been reasonably excluded.
- An empirical treatment with a proton pump inhibitor is a helpful tool to identify gastroesophageal reflux disease-related non-cardiac chest pain.
- Ambulatory reflux monitoring is recommended if there is lack of response to proton pump inhibitor therapy.
- There is insufficient evidence to recommend anti-reflux surgery as an alternative to proton pump inhibitor therapy in patients with non-cardiac chest pain.

Potential pitfalls

- Do not assume the patient's chest pain is esophageal until objective cardiac studies and/or a cardiology consultation are done.
- A negative endoscopy does not exclude gastroesophageal reflux disease but it is often done to exclude structural disease.
- Symptom association studies may be useful but have limitations; therefore, a negative Symptom Association Index does not rule out gastroesophageal reflux disease as the cause of chest pain, especially in patients with sporadic symptoms.
- Esophageal motility testing is frequently normal in non-cardiac chest pain but should be done in patients with persistent chest pain, to exclude certain esophageal motility disorders such as achalasia.
- While some esophageal spastic disorders as nutcracker and esophageal spasm have been frequently invoked as causes of non-cardiac chest pain, such relationship might be biased by their frequent association with gastroesophageal reflux disease.

Practical Manual of Gastroesophageal Reflux Disease, First Edition.
Edited by Marcelo F. Vela, Joel E. Richter and John E. Pandolfino.
© 2013 John Wiley & Sons, Ltd. Published 2013 by John Wiley & Sons, Ltd.

Introduction

Non-cardiac chest pain (NCCP) is defined as recurrent episodes of chest pain resembling angina after cardiac origin has been excluded. NCCP is a common clinical problem. Population studies estimated a prevalence ranging from 12% in European countries like Sweden and Spain to 33% in Australia [1–3]. In the United States, approximately 23% of the population have NCCP [4]; thus, more than 70 million Americans suffer from this condition. A prospective multicenter study of patients presenting to the emergency department at 10 US hospitals found that as many as 55% of those with chest pain had no evidence of cardiac disease [5]. For patients undergoing cardiac catheterization for chest pain, as many as 14–30% have normal or insignificant coronary artery disease [6]. Despite the widespread prevalence of the problem, an Australian study suggests that only a small proportion of patients with episodes of recurrent chest pain consult a physician [7]. However, the economic impact of this condition is still high. In 2007, in the US almost 6 million patients visited the emergency department for chest pain at an estimated cost of at least $19 billion (average cost per visit of $3205 according to Medicare) [8,9]. NCCP is also an important cause of work absenteeism and impaired productivity. A survey performed in patients attending an emergency department in Australia found that 29% of subjects with NCCP (*n*=126) missed work or school in the previous year with an average number of 23 missed days (range 1–240). In addition, up to two-thirds of those presenting with NCCP mentioned some kind of interruption to their daily activities (including work) relating to the condition [10].

The purpose of this chapter is to focus on the role of gastroesophageal reflux disease (GERD) as a cause of NCCP.

Reflux in non-cardiac chest pain

The esophagus is the most common source of NCCP [11]. Several factors have been associated with NCCP including esophageal motility disorders, visceral hyperalgesia, autonomic dysregulation, and GERD. GERD is by far the most common cause of NCCP [12]. Evidence supporting the role of GERD comes from different sources: symptom-derived studies, endoscopy and ambulatory pH testing data, and therapeutic trials.

In a population-based study that included 672 subjects in Australia, Eslick *et al.* demonstrated that the frequency of heartburn was the only independent risk factor for NCCP (odds ratio (OR) 1.74%, 95% confidence interval (CI) 1.08–2.79) [7].

A population-based study in Olmsted County, Minnesota (*n*=1511), found that NCCP was significantly more common among subjects with weekly typical GERD symptoms than in those without typical symptoms (37% versus 7.9%, $P < 0.001$) [4]. In another study, the same researchers at the Mayo Clinic explored the prevalence and risk factors for NCCP in the same geographical area ($n = 1524$) [13]. In this later study, 65 (52%) of 124 subjects with frequent NCCP also complained of GERD symptoms. Independent risk factors for NCCP were similar to those found in GERD, including obesity and family history of GERD [13].

Symptom-oriented studies suggest a high prevalence of GERD in NCCP but ambulatory pH testing and endoscopy-based studies have also noted a high association of GERD in this setting. Hewson *et al.* observed that 48 of 100 patients with NCCP exhibited abnormal acid exposure during 24-h pH monitoring [14]. Beedassy *et al.* assessed 104 patients with NCCP and documented a similar proportion (48%) with abnormal acid exposure [15]. A review of the utility of 24-h pH monitoring in patients with NCCP estimated that 22–75% (average 43%) have abnormal acid reflux [16]. In a cohort of 94 patients with NCCP, 50% also had GERD on pH testing and/or endoscopy [17]. Though patients with NCCP have a lower prevalence of GERD endoscopic findings than those with typical GERD symptoms, an endoscopic chart review of 161 patients who underwent upper endoscopy for NCCP found that as many as 18.6% had esophagitis and 21% had Barrett's esophagus (20% short and 1% long segment) [18]. Dickman *et al.* reported a prevalence of 19.4% for esophagitis and 4.4% for Barrett's esophagus in a cohort of 3688 consecutive patients with NCCP undergoing endoscopy [19].

In addition to the aforementioned studies confirming a strong association between GERD and NCCP, a causal relationship between both entities has also been implied on the basis of a temporal correlation between episodes of reflux and chest pain during ambulatory 24-h pH monitoring [14,16] and the reproduction of chest pain following esophageal acid perfusion [20,21]. Hewson *et al.* evaluated 100 consecutive patients with recurrent NCCP and found that 50 (60%) had a temporal symptom correlation or positive Symptom Index (SI) during 24-h pH monitoring [14]. Lam *et al.* reported that 17 of 48 patients (35%) with recurrent NCCP who were symptomatic during ambulatory pH monitoring presented a positive SI correlation [22].

Attempts at reproducing acid-related chest pain have used the acid perfusion test or Bernstein test (a measure of esophageal acid sensitivity). In patients with NCCP, the results of the Bernstein test have been variable, ranging from 6.7% in a study by Katz *et al.* that included 910 patients with NCCP [23] to 100% in a small series of 11 patients with NCCP reported by Behar *et al.* [24]. Richter *et al.* compared the accuracy of the acid perfusion test with 24-h pH monitoring and use of the SI at different cut-off levels (25%, 50% and 75%) in 75 consecutive patients with NCCP. They concluded that the acid perfusion test was highly specific (83% for a SI $\geq$75%, 94% for a SI $\geq$25%) but very insensitive (32% for a SI $\geq$25%, 46% for a SI $\geq$75%) [21]. In view of those findings and for practical reasons, most investigators have now replaced the acid perfusion test with ambulatory pH testing. In addition, impedance pH monitoring enables measurement of non-acid reflux; the clinical importance of this phenomenon in patients with NCCP awaits further study.

In summary, several lines of evidence such as symptom-driven surveys and pH-based studies and, to a lesser extent, endoscopy-related investigations report a strong prevalence of GERD in NCCP. Given the ubiquitous nature of GERD, it is unclear whether GERD is a cause of chest pain or an associated phenomenon. Whether cause and effect exists may be best determined by direct therapeutic trials aimed at acid suppression. The introduction of proton pump inhibitor (PPI) agents during the late 1980s provided an additional tool to explore the relationship between GERD and NCCP. PPIs are effective acid inhibitor compounds. Today, the most widely used approach in clinical practice to demonstrate a causal relationship between GERD and NCCP is the clinical response to anti-reflux therapy [25,26]. This approach and its success will be reviewed in a subsequent section.

Mechanisms of pain

Nociceptors

Esophageal pain can be the consequence of stimulation of esophageal nociceptors by acid [27]. Experimental studies have shown that esophageal mucosa exposure to acid and pepsin damages the intercellular junction complex, increasing paracellular permeability and the development of dilated intercellular spaces. This results in enhanced permeability of the esophageal mucosa to noxious stimuli such as acid. The enhanced permeability allows contact with the chemical-sensitive nociceptors, leading to irritation of these cells [28]. It has also been suggested that the volume of the acid refluxate may cause esophageal wall distension, triggering local intramural reflexes that generate abnormal contractility [27,29]. Following stimulation of chemo- and mechanoreceptors, sensory information is passed on to nociceptors which transmit their signals through C-fibers (unmyelinated) or A-delta fibers (myelinated). Functional differences between both types of fibers might explain different painful perceptions among individuals exposed to the same stimulus; myelinated fibers conduct nervous impulses fast and their stimulation causes a well-localized, sudden, sharp pain, while unmyelinated fibers are slower conductors and produce a poorly localized, dull, burning pain [27].

Visceral hypersensitivity

Richter *et al.* demonstrated that patients with NCCP have lower painful thresholds (allodynia) to mechanical stimulation. In their experiment, progressive balloon distension of the distal esophagus up to a maximum of 10 mL induced pain more often in patients with NCCP than in controls (60% versus 20%, $P < 0.005$). In addition, patients with NCCP developed chest pain at lower volumes (≤ 8 mL) compared to controls (≥ 9 mL) [30]. The increased esophageal sensitivity in patients with NCCP may be due to either hypersensitive afferent pathways (peripheral sensitization) or abnormal central processing of visceral sensation [31,32].

Gastroesophgeal reflux disease may also be involved in the pathogenesis of visceral hypersensitivity. Hu *et al.* performed an experimental study using an esophageal barostat. They evaluated the sensory esophageal threshold at baseline and after perfusion of normal saline or hydrochloric acid in a group of healthy male volunteers ($n = 12$). They found that, compared to baseline, acid perfusion significantly reduced the first perception (median value 15 mmHg versus 8 mmHg, $P = 0.05$) and pain threshold (32.5 versus 26.5 mmHg, $P = 0.05$) while saline perfusion was not associated with significant changes in the esophageal sensory thresholds [33]. This study suggests that, at least in a subset of patients, acute acid exposure could sensitize the esophageal mechanoreceptors (peripheral sensitization) contributing to the development of visceral hypersensitivity.

In a seminal study, Sarkar *et al.* demonstrated the presence of secondary allodynia (lower pain thresholds distant to the site of the stimuli) as well as the concurrence of visceral and somatic hypersensitivity, characteristic of central sensitization, in patients with NCCP [34]. Acid infusion (but not saline) in the distal esophagus decreased pain thresholds in non-acid-exposed areas (proximal esophagus and the cutaneous area of pain referral) of both patients with NCCP ($n = 7$) and controls ($n = 19$), though the responses were longer and more pronounced in those with NCCP [34]. The same investigators compared the presence of secondary allodynia in patients with chest pain and co-existing GERD and controls; while healthy controls showed a significant decrease in pain thresholds following acid infusion (but not saline), none of the patients with chest pain and GERD developed secondary allodynia in response to saline or acid. The authors explained this finding by suggesting that once esophageal afferent pathways are sensitized by GERD (resting pain thresholds were lower in patients than controls), exposure to additional amounts of acid might not reduce the pain thresholds further. Following PPI therapy (20 mg b.i.d., 6 weeks), resting pain thresholds increased in patients with NCCP (though were still lower than in healthy controls) and a significant decrease in esophageal pain thresholds (secondary allodynia) was seen after acid infusion, suggesting that in the presence of GERD, esophageal pain hypersensitivity could decrease, at least partially, following acid suppression therapy [35].

Sustained esophageal contractions

Balaban *et al.*, using high-frequency intraluminal endosonography in patients with unexplained NCCP, identified prolonged (mean duration 68 sec), sustained esophageal longitudinal smooth muscle contractions (SECs) preceding 75% of chest pain episodes and a temporal correlation between a drop in pH levels and SECs in 78% of GERD-related chest pain events. SECs of shorter duration (mean duration 29 sec) were also identified in 45% of asymptomatic reflux episodes. The authors concluded that in this subset of patients, the cause of chest pain was most likely the duration of SECs rather than the presence of GERD [36]. The mechanism by which SECs produce chest pain and/or why in some patients the same stimuli produce longer or shorter duration SECs are still unknown.

Gastroesophageal reflux in patients with coronary artery disease

Patients with coronary artery disease may suffer from co-existing GERD. A review of the literature estimated that 51% of patients with coronary artery disease (CAD) and chest pain have GERD, and of those, 54% showed a direct correlation between chest pain episodes and acid events on pH testing [37]. The increased association between GERD and CAD may be explained by the fact that both entities share common risk factors [38,39]. In addition, a 2-year-follow-up study of patients with chest pain and CAD ($n=415$) found that those treated with PPI ($n=94$) developed a significant reduction in the number of chest pain episodes (70%), the use of emergency facilities (55%) and the number of hospitalizations for chest pain (53%) compared to a cohort not treated with PPI ($n=321$) [40]. Budzynski *et al.* performed a double-blind, cross-over, placebo-controlled trial to evaluate the effect of acid reduction therapy (omeprazole 20 mg b.i.d. for 2 weeks) in a cohort of patients with chest pain and CAD ($n=48$). They found that treatment with omeprazole was significantly associated with a decrease in the number of chest pain episodes and their severity, and a reduced use of medication (nitrates). Interestingly, omeprazole also reduced the percentage of subjects showing significant decrease of the ST interval during a treadmill stress test [41].

These observations raise the possibility of a close interaction between heart and esophageal disease. This potential interaction was first described by Froment [42] though the term "linked angina" was coined in 1962 by Smith and Papp [43] to describe a condition in which gastrointestinal factors trigger the development of angina in patients with CAD by increasing cardiac workload. Indeed, Mellow *et al.* showed that esophageal acid perfusion induced myocardial ischemia and chest pain in almost two-thirds of patients with CAD, while producing a significant increase in the rate-pressure product (an index of myocardial workload) and electrocardiogram signs of myocardial ischemia (17% of those with pain) [44]. The presence of a cardioesophageal reflex was also suggested by Chauhan *et al.* who demonstrated that esophageal acid instillation in subjects with syndrome X (typical angina pain, positive exercise test, negative coronary angiography) reproduced the pain in more than half of them (11 out of 20). Interestingly, in this subset of subjects, acid instillation was also followed by a significant decrease in coronary blood flow velocity [45]. A later study comparing the results of esophageal acid infusion in a cohort of patients with syndrome X and another cohort of heart transplant recipients showed that reproduction of chest pain and coronary blood flow reduction were exclusively seen in those with syndrome X (57% versus 0%). The lack of symptoms and vascular changes in those with denervated hearts suggests that this cardioesophageal reflex may be mediated by a neural mechanism, most likely vagal [46].

Diagnosis

The diagnosis of NCCP is challenging. This is frequently due to the lack of specificity of symptoms, the insufficient sensitivity of the current diagnostic tests and the potential co-existence of different sources of pain in the same individual [38,39,47].

Data from a multicenter, prospective study suggested that 2.1% of the patients presenting to the emergency department with acute myocardial infarction and 2.3% of those with unstable angina were mistakenly discharged from the emergency department as suffering from NCCP [5]. A review of malpractice claims against emergency doctors in Massachusetts from 1975 to 1993 indicates that a wrong diagnosis of chest pain was one of the leading cause of claims (10.4%) and accounted for the highest percentage of indemnity and expense ($9,974,847 or 25.47%) [48]. When approaching a patient complaining of chest pain, the physician must ensure that a cardiac cause(s) of pain has been considered and properly excluded by cardiology testing and/or consultation. Other sources of chest pain such as pleural, pulmonary, musculoskeletal and gastrointestinal (i.e. peptic ulcer, gallbladder, pancreatic disease) should also be considered. Review of these other causes of NCCP is beyond the scope of this chapter. Once cardiac and other potential non-cardiac causes of chest pain have been excluded, esophageal sources of chest pain are frequently considered.

As previously described, GERD is one of the most common esophageal causes of NCCP. However, GERD-related NCCP is frequently indistinguishable from other types of chest pain, including angina [47]. The identification of heartburn and/or regurgitation in a patient with NCCP is very specific of GERD [49] but the fact that a patient complaining of chest pain also has a clinical history suggestive of GERD does not imply a causal relationship [47]; therefore additional tests are required to reach a diagnosis of GERD-related NCCP.

Barium tests and endoscopy

Barium studies are rarely indicated in the evaluation of NCCP due to their low diagnostic sensitivity. Yet barium radiology can be useful to detect motility disorders causing chest pain such as achalasia [50], define the anatomy of the upper gastrointestinal (GI) tract and exclude abnormalities such as peptic strictures or distal rings [51].

Endoscopy is frequently performed in the evaluation of patients with NCCP, mostly to exclude structural diseases [51]. The prevalence of endoscopic findings in NCCP has been reported to be lower when compared to those with typical GERD symptoms [18]. A review of a large (n=3688) US multicenter endoscopic database revealed that at least a third of patients with NCCP had esophageal findings on upper endoscopy, mostly acid related [19]. Other studies have also shown a low prevalence of endoscopic findings in patients with NCCP and for those with abnormal results, most were acid related too [52,53]. Esophageal cancer in patients complaining only of chest pain has rarely been observed but when patients complained of dysphagia in addition to chest pain, this rate increases to 7% [54]. In certain patients, mainly young-middle aged Caucasian males with an allergic background, upper endoscopy with multiple esophageal biopsies could be justified to rule out eosinophilic esophagitis as a cause of chest pain [55].

Esophageal motility

Esophageal manometry remains the best tool to detect esophageal motility disorders. However, 70% of NCCP patients have normal esophageal motility during manometry testing [23,56]. Although esophageal motility disorders are noted in up to 30% of patients with NCCP, the relationship between these motor abnormalities and chest pain remains unclear. The single largest series of patients undergoing esophageal motility due to NCCP published to date (n=910) identified nutcracker esophagus as the most common motility disorder related to NCCP (48%), followed by non-specific esophageal motility disorder (36%) and diffuse esophageal spasm (10%) [23]. However, a more recent review of a national motility database including data from 140 patients with NCCP found that nutcracker esophagus and non-specific esophageal motility disorder were less common than expected in patients with NCCP, each of them diagnosed in 10% of those with an abnormal motility, while esophageal spasm was definitively a rare diagnosis, only 2% of those with NCCP and a motility disorder [56]. Furthermore, therapeutic trials aimed at improving abnormal motility in NCCP patients have not consistently resulted in symptomatic improvement [57–59]. Thus, the motility abnormalities represent either a marker of sensorimotor dysfunction or an epiphenomenon due to the frequent co-existence of GERD and spastic motility disorders [60,61]. Esophageal motility therefore is reserved for evaluating patients with recurrent chest pain not responding to a therapeutic trial of PPI and/or in whom a motility diagnosis is suspected as the source of pain.

Proton pump inhibitor trials as a diagnostic test

A PPI trial is defined as an empirical treatment for NCCP with any PPI at double dose during a short period of time, such as 1 week [25,26]. Fass *et al.* reported the diagnostic value of a PPI trial for diagnosing GERD in patients with NCCP [62] (the "omeprazole test" since this was the only PPI available at the time). They found that treatment with omeprazole at doses of 40 mg morning and 20 mg evening during 1 week saved an average of $573 per patient and significantly reduced the number of diagnostic procedures performed due to its high positive predictive value (90%) [62]. Previously, there were some attempts to rule out GERD using a single large dose of omeprazole (80 mg) but these experiences were only reported in abstract form [63,64].

Recently, the results of two metaanalyses have confirmed that in patients with NCCP, a brief empirical PPI trial (any PPI at double dose, during 1 week) is an adequate tool to identify GERD-related NCCP, with an overall sensitivity of 80% and a specificity of 74% [25,26]. It is noteworthy, however, that the studies included in these two metaanalyses were small sized, methodologically heterogeneous, evaluated different types and doses of PPIs, used different outcome measures and did not even agree on the definition of NCCP. A recent uncontrolled study performed in Korea has suggested that, at least in the Chinese population, the optimal minimal duration should be 2 weeks. In this study, Kim *et al.* compared the efficacy of 1-week versus 2-week PPI trial (rabeprazole 20 mg b.i.d.) in 42 patients with frequent chest pain. Participants were classified according the results of pH and endoscopy as GERD-related NCCP ($n=16$) and non-GERD-related NCCP ($n=26$). The comparison of outcomes at 1 week of treatment did not differ significantly between groups (50% of response in GERD-related NCCP versus 23% in non-GERD). At the end of the second week there was a significant improvement in patients with GERD-related NCCP compared to those without GERD (81% versus 27%, $P=0.001$) [65]. Of interest, in patients with typical forms of GERD the benefits of a therapeutic trial have also been demonstrated. A prospective study in 612 patients with typical GERD symptoms showed that empirical treatment with PPI (esomeprazole) is cost-effective and does not affect the patients' quality of life when compared with an endoscopy-oriented strategy (perform upper endoscopy and treat according the endoscopic findings) [66]. Table 9.1 shows a summary of the studies assessing the diagnostic efficacy of a short-course PPI trial in NCCP.

Ambulatory reflux monitoring

Ambulatory pH monitoring is the most useful test for diagnosing GERD and may be particularly helpful in ruling out GERD in those patients who fail to respond to a PPI trial [67]. The study can be done on or off PPI therapy. In patients studied off therapy, it can confirm whether reflux is associated with NCCP. In patients on therapy, it can help verify whether sufficient acid inhibition is accomplished. For studying patients on PPI, impedance pH monitoring is felt to be superior to pH-metry because the yield of pH testing on medication is very low and impedance pH monitoring enables measurement of non-acid reflux as a possible cause of chest pain [68]. If the study confirms acid reflux, this raises the possibility that the patient's adherence to treatment may be suspect or that timing of PPI intake may not be adequate (30 min prior to breakfast and dinner) [69].

In addition, ambulatory pH monitoring may also help to determine whether acid reflux episodes correlate to chest pain. Several scores have been developed to attempt to identify whether symptoms occurring during ambulatory pH testing are related to GERD: the Symptom Index (SI), the Symptom Sensitivity Index (SSI), the Symptom Association Probability (SAP) and the Ghillebert Probability Estimate (GPE) [70–73]. The SI has traditionally been the parameter most widely used in NCCP [74]. Despite efforts to secure a useful SI that can correlate symptoms to GERD, this measure is an insensitive parameter whose accuracy depends largely on the presence of symptoms at the time of the patient's evaluation [17,75]. More importantly, there are scarce data suggesting that SI correlates with treatment (acid suppression) outcomes.

Dekel *et al.* evaluated a group of 94 patients with NCCP that were classified as GERD-positive if presenting either esophageal mucosal lesions on upper endoscopy or abnormal acid exposure on the pH monitoring ($n=47$) and GERD negative if both upper endoscopy and pH testing were normal ($n=47$) [17]. Sixteen patients (34%) in the GERD group and 20 (42%) in the GERD-negative group reported pain during the 24-h pH monitoring. The SI was positive in nine (19%) of the GERD-positive patients and five (10.6%) of the GERD-negative group. Eight out of nine (89%) in the GERD-positive group and two of five (40%) in the GERD-negative group responded to a therapeutic PPI trial [17].

Most recently, Kushnir *et al.* assessed the value of different GERD indices, including the acid exposure time, SI and GPE, alone or in combination, to

Table 9.1 Published studies assessing the accuracy of short-term PPI trials in the diagnosis of non-cardiac chest pain.

Author, year	n	Type of study	PPI	Dose (mg)	Length	Response	Sensitivity	Specificity
Fass et al. 1998 [62]	37	Placebo controlled Cross-over	Omeprazole	40/20	1 wk	>50%	78%	86%
Pandak et al. 2002 [81]	37	Placebo controlled Cross-over	Omeprazole	40 b.i.d.	2 wks	>50%	90%	67%
Bautista et al. 2004 [82]	40	Placebo controlled Cross-over	Lansoprazole	60/30	1 wk	>50%	78%	80%
Dekel et al. 2004 [17]	14	Open label	Omeprazole (n=4) Rabeprazole (n=6) Lansoprazole (n=4)	40/20 20/20 60/30	1 wk	>50%	89%	60%
Dickman et al. 2005 [83]	35	Placebo controlled, cross-over	Rabeprazole	20 b.i.d.	1 wk	≥50%	75%	90%
Kim et al. 2009 [65]	16	Open label	Rabeprazole	20 b.i.d.	1 wk 2 wks	≥50%	67% 83%	67% 62%

Modified from Achem [12], with permission from Elsevier.
PPI, proton pump inhibitor.

predict successful response to anti-reflux therapy [76]. They reviewed the charts of 98 subjects who underwent pH monitoring for NCCP: 79 (80.6%) were symptomatic during the procedure, 53% had an elevated acid exposure time (AET), 26.5% had a positive GPE and 25.5% had a positive SI. All patients were treated initially with PPI (regardless of the results of the pH test) and 24 underwent fundoplication. At follow-up (2.8±0.9 years later), 59.2% of the patients had achieved a sustained response. The best outcomes were obtained in those patients who had all parameters positive at baseline. The combination of a positive SI, a positive GPE and elevated AET showed a specificity and negative predictive value of 98% and 85% respectively, though their sensitivity and positive predictive values were only 24% and 15% respectively [76].

Prakash and Clouse conducted a study to evaluate the potential advantages of using a pH wireless system (Bravo®) that prolongs recording to 48 h over the traditional 24-h monitoring [77]. They performed a chart review of 62 patients with NCCP refractory to PPI who underwent 48-h wireless pH monitoring and evaluated the AET, the SI and the GPE at 24 and 48 h. The results showed that extending the recording time increased the number of subjects reporting symptoms from 55 on day 1 to 59 by the end of the study (7.3% increase), increased the number of patients presenting AET from 16 to 22 (9.7% increase), and the number of subjects with a positive GPE from 12 to 25 (increase of 25%). Twelve additional subjects were diagnosed with GERD-related NCCP combining both the AET and the GPE by the second day of the study. SI scores in those patients with a positive GPE at the end of the study remained relatively stable over the time (nine versus 11). This study suggests that there is a slight advantage of the GPE over the SI and that extending the recording time to 48 h using a wireless pH system may improve the detection of GERD-related NCCP, even in patients with poor response to PPI [77].

Though chest pain has been reported as a potential side-effect caused by the attachment of the Bravo capsule to the esophagus [68], which might overestimate the occurrence of NCCP episodes in these patients, results from a recent study comparing patients' acceptance of Bravo and catheter-based studies suggest that Bravo is overall better tolerated and less likely to be associated with chest pain than the catheter-based technique [78].

Combined multichannel intraluminal impedance pH

The combined multichannel intraluminal impedance pH (MII-pH) allows the detection of both acid and non-acid reflux episodes and therefore increases the likelihood of detecting GERD-related events. The impedance probe detects reflux episodes by measuring changes in the intraluminal resistance caused by the presence of gas or liquid in the esophagus, while the pH probe determines the acidity of the refluxate (acidic pH <4, weakly acidic pH 4–7, non-acidic pH >7) [74]. There is scarce information about the usefulness of MII-pH for detecting GERD-related NCCP. The only series reported to date includes 75 consecutive patients with NCCP [79]; 16 (23%) patients had abnormal acid exposure and 40 (53.3%) "pathological bolus exposure." Pathological bolus exposure was defined as "cases in which reflux time was above 1.4% of the total reflux number on impedance tests". Fifty of 54 patients (92.6%) reported symptomatic improvement following PPI treatment regardless of the presence of GERD [79]; whether this improvement was due to placebo effect or acid hypersensitivity was not clear. In summary, despite its limitations (lack of a control group), this study suggests that the use of MII-pH might increase the diagnostic yield of ambulatory wire pH testing, given its ability to detect patients with weakly acidic and non-acidic GERD. Other reent studies using impedance pH monitoring on medication have shown that in some patients, symptoms that persist despite PPI, including non-cardiac chest pain, may be due to non-acid reflux [80]. Therefore, impedance pH monitoring may be especially useful in patients who are refractory to PPI. However, prospective, controlled studies to confirm these observations are not available at the present time.

In summary, several tests are available for the diagnostic evaluation of patients with NCCP including endoscopy, ambulatory reflux monitoring, and esophageal motility. The available data suggest that the use of an initial short course of a PPI therapeutic trial is a sensitive and specific approach to diagnose GERD-related NCCP. Figure 9.1 summarizes our current suggested approach to NCCP.

Treatment

Medical therapy

Several studies, including the previously mentioned metaanalysis, have confirmed the empiric PPI strategy as a useful tool in the diagnosis and treatment of patients with GERD-related NCCP [17,25,26,57,62,81–85]. For patients responding to this initial approach, it is reasonable to maintain them on a PPI for a longer period of time. The length of therapy in GERD-related NCCP has not been critically evaluated. In 1993, Achem *et al.* showed that high doses of ranitidine (300 mg t.i.d.) or omeprazole 20 mg b.i.d. for 8 weeks induced a significant chest pain improvement in patients with NCCP, GERD and nutcracker esophagus following an open label study [86]. The same authors published the first placebo-controlled trial assessing the efficacy of PPI (omeprazole 20 mg twice daily) for 8 weeks in NCCP. They showed a significant clinical improvement in the omeprazole group versus the placebo [57]. These data suggest that patients with NCCP may be treated effectively for up to 2 months. Whether patients need to be

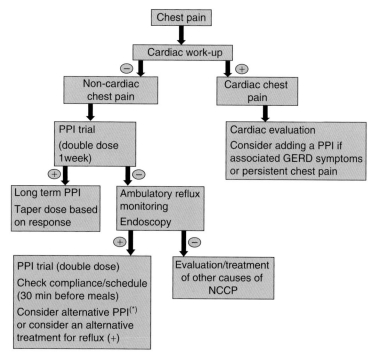

Figure 9.1 Suggested management algorithm. (*) There is no published evidence suggesting that changing the PPI type can improve clinical outcomes. (+) There are no trials supporting the use of alternative treatment modalities for reflux (such as agents acting on transient lower esophageal sphincter relaxation). GERD, gastroesophageal reflux disease; NCCP, non-cardiac chest pain; PPI, proton pump inhibitor.

maintained on a PPI for longer periods or can be gradually tapered is unknown. There is insufficient information to provide guidelines beyond this time. Some experts recommended tapering the dose from twice a day to once daily and subsequently reaching the minimal dose effective to control the symptoms [87].

There are different PPIs available but to date, only omeprazole, lansoprazole, and rabeprazole have been tested in NCCP. Most studies have been done with omeprazole [57, 62, 81, 85], given that this was the first PPI developed, and for some time the only drug of that category that was available. However, more recent trials using other PPIs suggest that these are also effective in relieving GERD-related chest pain [65, 83, 85]. The studies that have evaluated the impact of chronic (>4 weeks) PPI in GERD-related NCCP are summarized in Table 9.2.

Surgery

The outcomes of surgery in patients with GERD-related NCCP have not been systematically studied. The available data suggest that a variable

Table 9.2 Long-term PPI trials (≥4 weeks) in non-cardiac chest pain.

Author, year	n	Type of study	PPI	Dose	Length	Response
Achem et al. 1993* [86]	12	Open label	Ranitidine or omeprazole	300 mg t.i.d., 20 mg/b.i.d.	8 wks	83%
Achem et al. 1997 [57]	36	Placebo controlled	Omeprazole	20 mg/b.i.d.	8 wks	81% omeprazole 6% placebo
Chambers et al. 1998 [84]	23	Open label	Omeprazole	40 mg/d (bedtime)	6 wks	30%
Xia et al. 2003 [85]	68	Placebo controlled parallel group	Lansoprazole	30 mg/d	4 wks	53% lansoprazole 34% placebo

*Patients with non-cardiac chest pain and nutcracker esophagus.
Modified from Achem [12], with permission from Elsevier.
PPI, proton pump inhibitor.

percentage of patients with NCCP, ranging from 41% to 100% [88], may respond to surgery, especially those presenting a positive symptom association on preoperative pH monitoring [89]. However, these data should be interpreted cautiously, given that the information available is based mostly on chart reviews and uncontrolled studies performed in highly specialized centers that evaluated the results of anti-reflux surgery in patients with various extraesophageal manifestations of GERD [58, 90–92]. To date, there are no studies comparing the outcomes of medical versus surgical treatment in patients with NCCP.

Natural history and prognosis

Williams et al. performed a follow-up study, mean 9.8 years (range 1–22 years), to compare the outcomes of patients with NCCP (n=161) and patients with typical GERD (n=1218) [18]. The authors noted that the term "NCCP" or another similar term such as "atypical chest pain" disappeared from the medical records of 96% of the patients within 2 years of the initial evaluation. This was interpreted by the authors as a sign that once evaluated by a cardiologist, the patients' primary care physicians were no longer concerned by the presence of chest pain. When comparing both cohorts of patients, they found significantly higher rates of CAD diagnosis and related events in the NCCP cohort and a significantly increased use of acid suppression drugs in the GERD group. A Kaplan–Meier survival curve did not show any differences in survival between cohorts. This study suggests that patients presenting with NCCP (they did not specify the rate of patients with GERD-related NCCP in the group) and patients with typical GERD symptoms were two separate groups with different characteristics but a similar survival [18].

Eslick and Talley assessed a cohort of patients who presented to the emergency department with chest pain ($n=197$) and surveyed them at baseline, 2 ($n=129$) and 4 years ($n=91$) after the initial consultation. The cohort was divided according to the results of the initial evaluation: those diagnosed with cardiac pain ($n=71$) and those with NCCP ($n=126$). At the 4-year follow-up, 23 of 27 patients with cardiac chest pain and 45 of 64 with NCCP confirmed persistence of the pain. At the end of follow-up, nine of 71 patients with cardiac pain had died, eight of them of myocardial infarction. Eight of the 126 patients in the NCCP cohort were deceased, seven of them of myocardial infarction. A multiple regression logistic model identified only advanced age as an independent predictor of mortality in both groups [93]. Wilhemsen *et al.* also reported increased mortality rate (46%) and cardiovascular mortality (24.5%) in a cohort of 441 patients presenting with NCCP that were followed up longitudinally during a 16-year study in Göteborg, Sweden [94].

It is unclear from these studies whether cardiac disease was missed in the original cohorts or developed subsequently, but the findings underscore the need for periodic reassessment of cardiac disease in patients with persistent unexplained pain during long-term follow-up studies.

Summary and recommendations

Non-cardiac chest pain is a common, expensive and challenging clinical problem. GERD is frequently associated with NCCP and occurs in approximately 43% of the patients. In addition, GERD can co-exist and precipitate chest pain in patients with CAD. After cardiac causes of NCCP have been objectively ruled out, a short therapeutic trial (such as 1–2 weeks) of double-dose PPI is helpful in identifying GERD-related chest pain. Patients with GERD-related NCCP have a high response to PPI therapy. Once symptom improvement has been obtained, treatment is frequently extended up to 8 weeks. Then, patients may be gradually tapered off PPI therapy to achieve the lowest required dose (or no therapy) to sustain symptom control. For patients failing such a trial, further testing such as ambulatory reflux monitoring, endoscopy and motility testing (mostly to exclude achalasia) may be needed.

CASE STUDY

A 48-year-old business woman came to the emergency department (ED) complaining of severe squeezing, non-pleuritic, substernal chest pain radiating to the left arm associated with nausea. The pain lasted about 50 min and resolved spontaneously by the time she reached the ED. She admitted to a prior history of brief recurrent episodes of chest pain related to meals and stress. She had a history of hypertension, hyperlipidemia and the onset of menopause 6 years earlier. Her physical exam showed an anxious patient with a heart rate of 108 beats per minute, but was otherwise unremarkable.

In the ED she had a normal chest x-ray, electrocardiogram, cardiac enzymes, PO_2 saturation (99%), complete blood count, liver chemistries, amylase, and lipase. A stress echo cardiogram showed questionable septum motion abnormalities. A cardiology consultant recommended a coronary angiogram which was negative for obstructive vessel disease. An upper endoscopy was normal. A 24-h pH study showed abnormal acid contact time and several episodes of chest pain correlating with pH <4. The patient was treated with omeprazole 20 mg twice daily and remained symptom free at the 6-month follow-up visit.

References

1 Eslick GD. Epidemiology. In: Fass R, Eslick GD (eds) *Non cardiac chest pain, a growing medical problem*. San Diego, CA: Plural Publishing, 2007: pp.1–12.

2 Rey E, Moreno Elola-Elaso C, Rodriguez Artalejo F, *et al*. Prevalence of atypical symptoms and their association with typical symptoms of gastroesophageal reflux in Spain. Eur J Gastroenterol 2006;18(9):969–75.

3 Agreus L, Svardsudd K, Nyren O, *et al*. The epidemiology of abdominal symptoms: prevalence and demographic characteristics in a Swedish adult population. Scand J Gastroenterol 1994;29:102–9.

4 Locke GR 3rd, Talley NJ, Fett SL, *et al*. Prevalence and clinical spectrum of gastro-esophageal reflux: a population-based study in Olmstead County, Minnesota. Gastroenterology 1997;112(5):1448–56.

5 Pope JH, Aufderheide TP, Ruthazer R, *et al*. Missed diagnoses of acute cardiac ischemia in the emergency department. N Engl J Med 2000;342(16):1163–70.

6 Phan A, Shufelt C, Bairey Mertz CN. Persistent chest pain and no obstructive coronary disease. JAMA 2009;301(14):1468–74.

7 Eslick GD, Jones MP, Talley NJ. Non-cardiac chest pain: prevalence, risk factors, impact and consulting – a population–based study. Aliment Pharmacol Ther 2003;17:1115–24.

8 Niska R, Bhuiya F, Xu J. National Hospital Ambulatory Medical Care Survey: 2007 emergency department summary. National Health Stat Rep 2010;26:1–32.

9 www.healthcaretrendsnewsletter.com/2010/01/ten–most–frequent–outpatient–diagnoses–and–average–cost/

10 Eslick GD, Talley NJ. Non-cardiac chest pain: predictors of health care seeking, the types of health care professional consulted, work absenteeism and interruption of daily activities. Aliment Pharmacol Ther 2004;20(8):909–15.

11 Lam HG, Dekker W, Kan G, *et al*. Acute noncardiac chest pain in a coronary care unit. Evaluation by 24-hour pressure and pH recording of the esophagus. Gastroenterology 1992;102(2):453–60.

12 Achem SR. Noncardiac chest pain – treatment approaches. Gastroenterol Clin North Am 2008;37:859–78.

13 Wise JL, Locke GR, Zinsmeister AR, *et al.* Risk factors for non-cardiac chest pain in the community. Aliment Pharmacol Ther 2005;22:1023–31.

14 Hewson EG, Sinclair JW, Dalton CB, *et al.* Twenty-four-hour esophageal pH monitoring: the most useful test for evaluating noncardiac chest pain. Am J Med 1991;90(5):576–83.

15 Beedassy A, Katz PO, Gruber A, *et al.* Prior sensitization of esophageal mucosa by acid reflux predisposes to a reflux-induced chest pain. J Clin Gastroenterol 2000; 31(2):121–4.

16 Lacima G, Grande L, Pera M, *et al.* Utility of ambulatory 24-hour esophageal pH and motility monitoring in noncardiac chest pain: report of 90 patients and review of the literature. Dig Dis Sci 2003;48:952–61.

17 Dekel R, Martinez-Hawthorne SD, Guillen J, *et al.* Evaluation of symptom index in identifying gastroesophageal reflux disease-related noncardiac chest pain. J Clin Gastroenterol 2004;38(1):24–9.

18 Williams JF, Sontag SJ, Schnell T, *et al.* Non-cardiac chest pain: the long term natural history and comparison with gastroesophageal reflux disease. Am J Gastroenterol 2009;104:2145–52.

19 Dickman R, Mattek N, Holub J, *et al.* Prevalence of upper gastrointestinal tract findings in patients with noncardiac chest pain versus those with gastroesophageal reflux disease (GERD)-related symptoms: results from a national endoscopic database. Am J Gastroenterol 2007;102:1173–9.

20 Smith JL, Opekun AR, Larkai E, *et al.* Sensitivity of the esophageal mucosa to pH in gastroesophageal reflux disease. Gastroenterology.1989;96(3):683–9.

21 Richter JE, Hewson EG, Sinclair JW, *et al.* Acid perfusion test and 24-hour esophageal pH monitoring with symptom index. Comparison of tests for esophageal acid sensitivity. Dig Dis Sci 1991;36(5):565–71.

22 Lam HG, Breumelhof R, van Berge Henegouwen GP, *et al.* Temporal relationships between episodes of non-cardiac chest pain and abnormal oesophageal function. Gut 1994;35(6):733–6.

23 Katz PO, Dalton CB, Richter JE, *et al.* Esophageal testing of patients with noncardiac chest pain or dysphagia. Results of three years' experience with 1161 patients. Ann Intern Med 1987;106(4):593–7.

24 Behar J, Biancani P, Sheahan DG. Evaluation of esophageal tests in the diagnosis of reflux esophagitis. Gastroenterology 1976;71(1):9–15.

25 Cremonini F, Wise J, Moayyedi P, *et al.* Diagnostic and therapeutic use of proton pump inhibitors in non-cardiac chest pain: a metaanalysis. Am J Gastroenterol 2005;100(6):1226–32.

26 Wang WH, Huang JQ, Zheng GF, *et al.* Is proton pump inhibitor testing an effective approach to diagnose gastroesophageal reflux disease in patients with noncardiac chest pain? A meta-analysis. Arch Intern Med 2005;165(11):1222–8.

27 Orlando RC. Esophageal perception and noncardiac chest pain. Gastroenterol Clin North Am 2004;33:25–33.

28 Barlow WJ, Orlando RC. The pathogenesis of heartburn in nonerosive reflux disease: a unifying hypothesis. Gastroenterology 2005;128:771–8.

29 Barlow JD, Gregersen H, Thompson G. Identification of the biomechanical factors associated with the perception of distension in the human esophagus. Am J Physiol Gastrointest Liver Physiol 2002;282:G683–9.

30 Richter JE, Barish CF, Castell DO. Abnormal sensory perception in patients with esophageal chest pain. Gastroenterology 1986;91(4):845–52.

31 Hobson AR, Furlong PL, Sarkar S, *et al.* Neurophysiologic assessment of esophageal sensory processing in noncardiac chest pain. Gastroenterology 2006;130:80–8.

32 Hollerbach S, Bulat R, May A, *et al.* Abnormal cerebral processing of oesophageal stimuli in patients with noncardiac chest pain (NCCP). Neurogastroenterol Motil 2000;12(6):555–65.

33 Hu WH, Martin CJ, Talley NJ. Intraesophageal acid perfusion sensitizes the esophagus to mechanical distension: a Barostat study. Am J Gastroenterol 2000;95(9):2189–94.

34 Sarkar S, Aziz Q, Woolf CJ, *et al.* Contribution of central sensitisation to the development of non-cardiac chest pain. Lancet 2000;356:1154–9.

35 Sarkar S, Thompson DG, Woolf CJ, *et al.* Patients with chest pain and occult gastroesophageal reflux demonstrate visceral pain hypersensitivity which may be partially responsive to acid suppression. Am J Gastroenterol 2004;99(10):1998–2006.

36 Balaban DH, Yamamoto Y, Liu J, *et al.* Sustained esophageal contraction: a marker of esophageal chest pain identified by intraluminal ultrasonography. Gastroenterology 1999;116(1):29–37.

37 Liuzzo JP, Ambrose JA. Chest pain from gastroesophageal reflux disease in patients with coronary artery disease. Cardiol Rev 2005;13:167–73.

38 Mehta AJ, Caestecker JS, Camm AJ, *et al.* Gastro-esophageal reflux in patients with coronary artery disease: how common is it and does it matter? Eur J Gastroenterol Hepatol 1996;8:973–8.

39 Schultz T, Mannheimer C, Dellborg M, *et al.* High prevalence of gastroesophageal reflux in patients with clinical unstable angina and known coronary artery disease. Acute Cardiac Care 2008;10:37–42.

40 Liuzzo JP, Ambrose JA, Diggs P. Proton pump inhibitor use by coronary artery disease patients is associated with fewer chest pain episodes, emergency department visits and hospitalizations. Aliment Pharmacol Ther 2005;22:95–100.

41 Budzynski J, Kłopocka M, Pulkowski G, *et al.* The effect of double dose of omeprazole on the course of angina pectoris and treadmill stress test in patients with coronary artery disease – a randomised, double-blind, placebo controlled, crossover trial. Int J Cardiol 2008;127(2):233–9.

42 Froment R. [Intricated coronary angina; clinical and experimental data]. Brux Med 1955;35(49):2429–42.

43 Smith KS, Papp C. Episodic, postural, and linked angina. BMJ 1962;2(5317):1425–30.

44 Mellow M, Simpson AG, Watt L, *et al.* Esophageal acid perfusion in coronary artery disease: induction of myocardial ischemia. Gastroenterology 1983;85:306–12.

45 Chauhan A, Petch MC, Schofield PM. Effect of esophageal acid instillation on coronary blood flow. Lancet 1993;341:1309–10.

46 Chauhan A, Petch MC, Schofield PM. Cardio-esophageal reflex in humans as a mechanism for 'linked angina'. Eur Heart J 1996;17:407–13.

47 Voskuil JH, Cramer MJ, Breumelhof R, *et al.* Prevalence of esophageal disorders in patients with chest pain newly referred to the cardiologist. Chest 1996;109:1210–14.

48 Karcz A, Korn R, Burke MC, *et al.* Malpractice claims against emergency physicians in Massachusetts: 1975–1993. Am J Emerg Med 1996;14(4):341–5.

49 Mousavi S, Tosi J, Eskandarian R, *et al.* Role of clinical presentation in diagnosing reflux-related non-cardiac chest pain. J Gastroenterol Hepatol 2007;22:218–21.

50 Richter JE, Boeckxstaens GE. Management of achalasia: surgery or pneumatic dilation. Gut 2011;60(6):869–76.

51 Lacy BE, Weiser K, Chertoff J, *et al.* The diagnosis of gastroesophageal reflux disease. Am J Med 2010;123(7):583–92.

52 García-Compeán D, González MV, Galindo G, *et al.* Prevalence of gastroesophageal reflux disease in patients with extraesophageal symptoms referred from otolaryngology, allergy, and cardiology practices: a prospective study. Dig Dis 2000;18(3):178–82.

53 Battaglia E, Bassotti G, Buonafede G, *et al.* Noncardiac chest pain of esophageal origin in patients with and without coronary artery disease. Hepatogastroenterology 2005;52(63):792–5.

54 Gibbs JF, Rajput A, Chadha KS, *et al.* The changing profile of esophageal cancer presentation and its implication for diagnosis. JAMA 2007;99(6):620–6.

55 Achem SR, Almansa C, Murli K, *et al.* Esophageal eosinophilic infiltration in patients with non cardiac chest pain. Aliment Pharm Ther 2011;33(11):1194–201.

56 Dekel R, Pearson T, Wendel C, *et al.* Assesment of esophageal motor function in patients with dyspepsia or chest pain – the Clinical Outcomes Research Initiative experience. Aliment Pharmacol Ther 2003;18(11–12):1083–9.

57 Achem SR, Kolts BE, MacMath T, *et al.* Effects of omeprazole versus placebo in treatment of noncardiac chest pain and gastroesophageal reflux. Dig Dis Sci 1997;42(10):2138–45.

58 Achem SR. Noncardiac chest pain – treatment approaches. Gastroenterol Clin North Am 2008;37:859–78.

59 Achem SR. Treatment of non-cardiac chest pain. Dis Mon 2008;54(9):642–70.

60 Gerson LB, Achem SR. Prevalence of pathologic reflux disease in patients with spastic motility disorders. Gastroenterology 2011;140(5)(Suppl 1):S–232.

61 Almansa C, Heckman MG, Devault KR, *et al.* Esophageal spasm: demographic, clinical, radiographic, and manometric features in 108 patients. Dis Esophagus 2012;25(3):214–21.

62 Fass R, Fennerty MB, Ofman JJ, *et al.* The clinical and economic value of a short course of omeprazole in patients with noncardiac chest pain. Gastroenterology 1998;115(1):42–9.

63 Young MA, Sanowski R, Talbert G, *et al.* Omeprazole administration as a test for gastroesophageal reflux. Gastroenterology 1992;102:192.

64 Squillace SJ, Young MF, Sanowski RA. Single dose omeprazole as a test for non cardiac chest pain. Gastroenterology 1993;104:A197.

65 Kim JH, Sinn DH, Son HJ, *et al.* Comparison of one-week and two-week empirical trial with a high-dose rabeprazole in non-cardiac chest pain patients. J Gastroenterol Hepatol 2009;24(9):1504–9.

66 Giannini EG, Zentilin P, Dulbecco P, *et al.* Management strategy for patients with gastroesophageal reflux disease: a comparison between empirical treatment with esomeprazole and endoscopy-oriented treatment. Am J Gastroenterol 2008;103(2):267–75.

67 Faybush EM, Fass R. Gastroesophageal reflux disease in noncardiac chest pain. Gastroenterol Clin North Am 2004;33:41–54.

68 Pandolfino JE, Vela MF. Esophageal-reflux monitoring. Gastrointest Endosc 2009;69(4):917–30.

69 Fass R. Proton pump inhibitor failure – what are the therapeutic options? Am J Gastroenterol 2009;104(Suppl 2):S33–8.

70 Wiener GJ, Richter JE, Copper JB, *et al.* The symptom index: a clinically important parameter of ambulatory 24-hour esophageal pH monitoring. Am J Gastroenterol 1988;83:358–61.

71 Breumelhof R, Smout APJM. The symptom sensitivity index: a valuable additional parameter in 24-h esophageal pH recording. Am J Gastroenterol 1991;86:160–4.

72 Weusten BL, Rolfs JMM, Akkermans LMA, *et al.* The symptom association probability: an improved method for symptom analysis of 24-h esophageal pH data. Gastroenterology 1994;107:1741–5.

73 Ghillebert G, Janssens J, Vantrappen G, *et al*. Ambulatory 24-h intraesophageal pH and pressure recordings vs provocation test in the diagnosis of chest pain of esophageal origin. Gut 1990;31:738–44.

74 Hirano I, Richter J E. ACG practice guidelines; esophageal reflux testing. Am J Gastroenterol 2007;102:668–85.

75 Taghavi SA, Ghasedi M, Saberi-Firoozi M, *et al*. Symptom association probability and symptom sensitivity index: preferable but still suboptimal predictors of response to high dose omeprazole. Gut 2005;54(8):1067–71.

76 Kushnir VM, Sayuk GS, Gyawali CP. Abnormal GERD parameters on ambulatory pH monitoring predicts therapeutic success in noncardiac chest pain. Am J Gastroenterol 2010;105:1032–8.

77 Prakash C, Clouse RE. Wireless pH monitoring in patients with non-cardiac chest pain. Am J Gastroenterol 2006;101:446–52.

78 Sweis R, Fox M, Anggiansah R, *et al*. Patient acceptance and clinical impact of Bravo monitoring in patients with previous failed catheter-based studies. Aliment Pharmacol Ther 2009;29(6):669–76.

79 Kim BJ, Choi SC, Kim JJ, *et al*. Pathological bolus exposure plays a significant role in eliciting non-cardiac chest pain. J Gastroenterol Hepatol 2010;25(12):1855–60.

80 Mainie I, Tutuian R, Shay S, *et al*. Acid and non-acid reflux in patients with persistent symptoms despite acid suppressive therapy: a multicentre study suing combined ambulatory impedance-pH monitoring. Gut 2006;55:1398–402.

81 Pandak WM, Arezo S, Everett S, *et al*. Short course of omeprazole: a better first diagnostic approach to noncardiac chest pain than endoscopy, manometry, or 24-hour esophageal pH monitoring. J Clin Gastroenterol 2002;35(4):307–14.

82 Bautista J, Fullerton H, Briseno M, *et al*. The effect of an empirical trial of high-dose lansoprazole on symptom response of patients with non-cardiac chest pain – a randomized, double-blind, placebo-controlled, crossover trial. Aliment Pharmacol Ther 2004;19(10):1123–30.

83 Dickman R, Emmons S, Cui H, *et al*. The effect of a therapeutic trial of high-dose rabeprazole on symptom response of patients with non-cardiac chest pain: a randomized, double-blind, placebo-controlled, crossover trial. Aliment Pharmacol Ther 2005;22(6):547–55.

84 Chambers J, Cooke R, Anggiansah A, *et al*. Effect of omeprazole in patients with chest pain and normal coronary anatomy: initial experience. Int J Cardiol 1998;65(1):51–5.

85 Xia HH, Lai KC, Lam SK, *et al*. Symptomatic response to lansoprazole predicts abnormal acid reflux in endoscopy-negative patients with non-cardiac chest pain. Aliment Pharmacol Ther 2003;17(3):369–77.

86 Achem SR, Kolts BE, Wears R, *et al*. Chest pain associated with nutcracker esophagus: a preliminary study of the role of gastroesophageal reflux. Am J Gastroenterol 1993;88(2):187–92.

87 Oranu AC, Vaezi MF. Noncardiac chest pain: gastroesophageal reflux disease. Med Clin North Am 2010;94(2):233–42.

88 Patti MG, Molena D, Fisichella PM, *et al*. Gastroesophageal reflux disease (GERD) and chest pain. Results of laparoscopic antireflux surgery. Surg Endosc 2002;16(4):563–6.

89 So JB, Zeitels SM, Rattner DW. Outcomes of atypical symptoms attributed to gastroesophageal reflux treated by laparoscopic fundoplication. Surgery 1998;124(1):28–32.

90 Chen RYM, Thomas RJS. Results of laparoscopic fundoplication where atypical symptoms coexist with oesophageal reflux. Aust NZ J Surg 2000;70:840–2.

91 Farrell TM, Richardson WS, Trus TL, *et al*. Response of atypical symptoms of gastroesophageal reflux to antireflux surgery. Br J Surg 2001;88(12):1649–52.

92 Rakita S, Valladolid D, Thomas A, *et al.* Laparoscopic nissen fundoplication offers high patient satisfaction with relief of extraesophageal symptoms of gastroesophageal reflux disease. Am Surg 2006;72(3):207–12.

93 Eslick GD, Talley NJ. Natural history and predictors of outcome for non-cardiac chest pain: a prospective 4-year cohort study. Neurogastroenterol Motil 2008;20(9):989–97.

94 Wilhelmsen L, Rosengren A, Hagman M, Lappas G. "Nonspecific" chest pain associated with high long-term mortality: results from the primary prevention study in Göteborg, Sweden. Clin Cardiol 1998;21(7):477–82.

CHAPTER 10

Laryngopharyngeal Reflux

Robert T. Kavitt and Michael F. Vaezi

Division of Gastroenterology, Hepatology, and Nutrition, Vanderbilt University Medical Center, Nashville, TN, USA

Key points
- Gastroesophageal reflux disease is increasingly associated with ear, nose, and throat symptoms, including laryngitis.
- Laryngopharyngeal reflux can be assessed with laryngoscopy, esophagogastroduodenoscopy, and the use of ambulatory pH and impedance monitoring.
- Gastroenterology and otolaryngology specialty societies have released various guidelines in recent years addressing diagnostic and therapeutic approaches to this prevalent and often difficult-to-treat condition.
- Many uncertainties remain, including which patient subgroups might benefit from acid suppressive therapy.

Potential pitfalls
- Laryngopharyngeal reflux symptoms may be associated with, but not necessarily always caused by, acid reflux. It is important to distinguish between potential signs and symptoms of laryngopharyngeal reflux and a true causal relationship with acid reflux.
- One must take a cautious approach in the management of laryngopharyngeal reflux patients with an absence of any symptomatic response to aggressive acid suppression.

Introduction

Reflux of gastroduodenal contents into the laryngopharyngeal region may cause inflammation and symptoms resulting in chronic laryngitis, often referred to as laryngopharyngeal reflux (LPR) [1]. Reports suggest that 4–10% of patients presenting to otolaryngologists demonstrate symptoms attributed in part to gastroesophageal reflux disease (GERD) [2]. Such symptoms include hoarseness, sore or burning throat, chronic cough, globus, dysphagia, postnasal drip, apnea, laryngospasm, and even laryngeal neoplasm, among other complaints (Box 10.1). Chronic laryngitis and throat symptoms are reportedly associated with GERD in up to 60% of

---

Practical Manual of Gastroesophageal Reflux Disease, First Edition.
Edited by Marcelo F. Vela, Joel E. Richter and John E. Pandolfino.
© 2013 John Wiley & Sons, Ltd. Published 2013 by John Wiley & Sons, Ltd.

> **Box 10.1 Symptoms associated with gastroesophageal reflux laryngitis**
>
> - Hoarseness
> - Dysphonia
> - Sore or burning throat
> - Excessive throat clearing
> - Chronic cough
> - Globus
> - Apnea
> - Laryngospasm
> - Dysphagia
> - Postnasal drip
> - Neoplasm

patients [2–8]. Additionally, some studies suggest an association of laryngeal cancer with chronic laryngeal exposure to reflux of gastroduodenal contents [9–13]. Thus, LPR is a significant clinical issue.

The first association between GERD and laryngeal disease was suggested by L.A. Coffin in 1903 [14] with subsequent studies suggesting a role of gastroduodenal contents in the development of "contact ulcer" [15,16] with patient response to antacids, dietary changes, and head of bed elevation. However, since these initial studies, the direct association between reflux of gastroduodenal contents and laryngeal signs and symptoms has been difficult to establish. The 2006 Montreal consensus group distinguished GERD symptoms between esophageal and extraesophageal syndromes [17]. Extraesophageal manifestations with established associations include chronic cough, laryngitis, and asthma, based on population-based studies, with odds ratios (OR) of 1.3–3.0 [18–21]. However, the causal relationship of GERD to these non-specific symptoms is not proven. More recently, the American Gastroenterological Association (AGA) guidelines for GERD recommended against treating for acid reflux for patients with laryngitis or asthma who do not have concomitant typical reflux symptoms [18,22]. Thus, the role of "silent" reflux, extraesophageal symptoms without concomitant heartburn or regurgitation, is controversial and divisive between the gastroenterology and otolaryngology communities.

Prevalence

Gastroesophageal reflux disease is a widely prevalent condition with significant impact on quality of life. A Gallup poll of 1000 adults with heartburn at least weekly conducted for the American Gastroenterology Association found that 79% of respondents noted heartburn symptoms at night [23]. Twenty percent reported supraesophageal symptoms 3–6 times each week, and 43% reported these symptoms once or twice per week. In a population survey study, Locke *et al.* [19] showed that heartburn and acid regurgitation are significantly associated with chest pain, dysphagia, dyspepsia, and globus sensation. A subsequent Veterans Affairs (VA)-based case–control study by El-Serag and Sonnenberg suggested that erosive esophagitis and esophageal stricture were associated with various extra-esophageal symptoms such as sinusitis (OR 1.60, 95% confidence interval (CI) 1.51–1.70), pharyngitis (OR 1.48, 95% CI 1.15–1.89), aphonia (OR 1.81, 95% CI 1.18–2.80), and chronic laryngitis (OR 2.01, 95% CI 1.53–2.63), among others [20]. The authors concluded that patients with reflux esoph-agitis are at an increased risk of harboring a large variety of sinus, pharyn-geal, laryngeal, and pulmonary diseases.

Laryngeal disorders have been shown to be twice as likely in patients with esophagitis compared to those without [20]. Twenty-five percent of patients with LPR are found to have histologic evidence of esophagitis [24]. Thus, epidemiological studies suggest an association between reflux disease and extraesophageal symptoms, including LPR.

Mechanisms of gastroesophageal reflux laryngitis

The two predominant pathophysiological mechanisms for LPR are direct and indirect exposure of the larynx to injurious gastric contents. The direct exposure is due to acid, pepsin, and bile acid exposure to the laryngopha-ryngeal mucosa. The indirect mechanism is thought to be a result of reflux-ate interactions with structures distal to the larynx, evoking a vagally mediated response of bronchoconstriction [25].

The potential agents causing laryngitis may include gastric contents (acid and pepsin) and duodenal contents (bile acids and the pancreatic enzyme trypsin). Animal studies in the past have shown the potential of both acid and pepsin to cause laryngeal injury [26]. The role of conjugated and unconjugated bile and trypsin at pH values of 1–7 was investigated by Adhami *et al.* who did not find histological injury to the canine larynx by the above agents alone. However, they showed that the combination of the bile constituents with acid and pepsin in an acidic pH caused the greatest injury [27]. This is difficult to assess in humans, because refluxate into the esophagus is often a mix of gastric and duodenal contents [28]. However, these data indirectly suggest that reflux of duodenal contents into the larynx, although it may be associated with symptoms such as regurgitation, is less likely to cause mucosal damage unless it occurs in an acidic milieu.

Clinical symptoms

Many patients with gastroesophageal reflux-induced chronic laryngitis present with symptoms such as sore throat, globus, chronic cough, hoarseness, dysphagia, apnea or postnasal drip, among other symptoms (see Box 10.1). However, they may not present with classic GERD symptoms of heartburn and regurgitation. A 1991 study found that of 225 patients with otolaryngological disorders having suspected GERD, only 43% reported symptoms of heartburn or acid regurgitation [6]. Additional symptoms which may be seen in reflux-related laryngitis include frequent throat clearing, dry mouth, prolonged voice warm-up time (greater than 20–30 min), halitosis, excess phlegm, coated tongue, throat tickle, regurgitation of food, nocturnal cough, difficulty breathing especially at night, aspiration, laryngospasm, poorly controlled asthma or pneumonia [29,30].

The Reflux Symptom Index (RSI) is a validated nine-item self-administered instrument published in 2002 to help assess the severity of LPR symptoms at the time of diagnosis and after therapy [31]. Symptoms assessed include throat clearing, difficulty swallowing, hoarseness, excess throat mucus or postnasal drip, coughing after eating or lying down, breathing difficulties or choking episodes, troublesome or annoying cough, sensation of something sticking in the throat or a lump in the throat, and symptoms of heartburn, chest pain or indigestion, on a scale from 0 to 5. An RSI score greater than 12 is defined as abnormal. The RSI was once believed to be significantly higher in untreated patients with LPR than controls; however, more recent studies suggest that it may be of lower clinical utility than previously believed [32]. Reliability of this instrument may vary based on patient population and clinical setting. Additionally, given the complexity of the symptoms and the scoring system, it is not widely used in clinical practice.

Evaluation of the larynx

Physical examination

Physical examination of patients with suspected gastroesophageal reflux laryngitis must be thorough, and include an examination of the head and neck, with assessment of ears and hearing, patency of the nares, oral cavity, temporomandibular joints, and larynx. One should also assess for signs of systemic disease (such as hypothyroidism) or neurological impairment that may manifest with symptoms affecting the throat or voice, including Parkinson's disease, multiple sclerosis or other conditions. When a patient reports symptoms of vocal difficulties, laryngeal examination by an otolaryngologist may include an assessment of the speaking and singing voice and strobovideolaryngoscopy [29]. Objective voice analysis can quantify quality of voice, pulmonary function, harmonic spectral characteristics, valvular efficiency of vocal folds, and neuromuscular function on electromyography [33]. Use of flexible transnasal laryngoscopy plays a vital role in excluding more ominous causes for patients' laryngeal symptoms. Hoarseness is a symptom that can be present in patients with LPR but also may be a symptom in vocal fold paresis, polyps, postviral inflammatory reactions, allergies, vocal abuse, dysplasia, and cancer [34]. If hoarseness persists longer than 2 weeks, laryngoscopy is indicated [35]. Once more ominous diagnoses such as laryngeal cancer are ruled out, LPR is often entertained as a potential contributing etiology for patients' throat symptoms due to laryngeal irritation often found at laryngosocopy.

Laryngeal signs

Normal laryngeal tissue has sharply demarcated landmarks with glistening mucosa with minimal or no laryngeal edema (Plate 10.1), unlike abnormal laryngeal findings (Plate 10.2). The epithelium of the larynx is thin and is not adapted to accommodating injury from acid and pepsin [36]. Several laryngeal signs are attributed to GERD, including edema, erythema, pseudosulcus, ventricular obliteration, and postcricoid hyperplasia (Box 10.2) [1].

In a study reporting the results of a survey of otolaryngologists regarding the signs used to diagnose LPR, subjective signs of laryngeal erythema and edema were the findings most commonly employed to diagnose GERD [37,38]. However, these signs are criticized for their lack of specificity for GERD. Several signs of posterior laryngitis thought to be markers for LPR are actually present in a high percentage of asymptomatic healthy

---

Box 10.2 Potential Laryngopharyngeal Signs Associated with Gastroesophageal Reflux Laryngitis

- Edema and hyperemia of larynx
- Hyperemia and lymphoid hyperplasia of posterior pharynx (cobblestoning)
- Contact ulcers
- Laryngeal polyps
- Granuloma
- Interarytenoid changes
- Subglottic stenosis
- Posterior glottic stenosis
- Reinke's edema
- Tumors

Table 10.1 Advantages and disadvantages of methods for detecting esophageal reflux.

Method	Advantages	Disadvantages
Endoscopy	Easy visualization of mucosal damage/erosions	Poor sensitivity/specificity/PPV Requires sedation High cost
Laryngoscopy	No sedation required Direct visualization of the larynx and laryngeal pathology	No specific laryngeal signs for reflux Overdiagnoses GERD
pH monitoring	Easy to perform Relatively non-invasive Prolonged monitoring possible Ambulatory	Catheter based May have up to 30% false-negative rate No pH predictors of treatment response in LPR
Impedance monitoring	Easy to perform Relatively non-invasive Prolonged monitoring possible Ambulatory Measures acidic and non-acidic gas and liquid reflux (combined with pH)	Catheter based False-negative rate unknown but most likely similar to catheter-based pH monitoring Unknown clinical relevance when abnormal on PPI therapy Unknown importance in LPR
ResTech Dx-pH	Faster detection rate and faster time to equilibrium pH than traditional pH catheters	Unknown if clinically useful in patients with LPR

GERD, gastroesophageal reflux disease; LPR, laryngopharyngeal reflux; PPI, proton pump inhibitor; PPV, positive predictive value.

volunteers, raising questions about the specificity of such findings [39]. Forty-three of 50 healthy subjects (86%) may exhibit one or more findings considered pathognomonic of laryngeal complaints due to GERD. This finding suggests that GERD may be overdiagnosed, as the laryngeal signs used in clinical practice are non-specific [40]. The advantages and disadvantages of laryngoscopy and other diagnostic tests in detecting reflux are shown in Table 10.1.

First described in 2001, the Reflux Finding Score (RFS) received considerable attention initially as a validated sign for reflux-induced laryngeal pathology. This instrument is an eight-item clinical severity scale based on laryngoscopic findings including subglottic edema, vocal fold edema, diffuse laryngeal edema, ventricular obliteration, erythema/hyperemia, posterior commissure hypertrophy, granuloma/granulation tissue, and thick endolaryngeal mucus, ranging from 0 to 26 [41,42]. However, similar to the RSI, the RFS is not commonly employed in clinical practice. A recent study found that both the RSI and RFS have poor specificity, with no significant difference between patients and control groups [32].

The variability of detecting laryngeal signs may also be affected by the quality and sensitivity of the detection instrument. Abnormal laryngeal signs are more likely to be suspected with flexible laryngoscopy as opposed to rigid laryngoscopy in the same individual, indicating that flexible laryngoscopy may be more sensitive and less specific for detecting laryngeal irritation [43]. Laryngeal signs appear to be poorly specific for identifying gastroesophageal reflux. One study showed that lesions of the vocal fold may represent more specific signs for LPR, exhibiting 91% specificity and 88% response to treatment with proton pump inhibitors (PPIs) [44]. The non-specificity of laryngoscopy may also be due to poor inter- and intra-observer variability. A randomized prospective analysis by five otolaryngologists blinded to patient information of 120 video segments of rigid fiberoptic laryngoscopy found poor interrater reliability of the laryngoscopic findings associated with LPR (intraclass correlation coefficient of 0.265), and intrarater reliability was extremely variable for the various physical findings (Kendall correlation coefficients ranging from −0.121 to 0.837). Taken together, these studies suggest that accurate assessment of laryngeal involvement with LPR is quite difficult as interpretation of physical findings is subjective and varies among physicians.

Ambulatory pH studies

Ambulatory pH monitoring allows for detection of esophageal or hypopharyngeal acid exposure. Since even healthy individuals have some reflux, the normal values have a range with an accepted upper limit, based on studies in healthy subjects. Up to 50 acid reflux events into the esophagus each day may occur normally [24]. When compared to physical exam findings, dual pH probe monitoring is reported to have superior sensitivity and specificity [6]. A metaanalysis of 16 studies involving a total of 793 subjects who underwent 24-h pH monitoring (529 patients with LPR, 264 controls) showed that the number of pharyngeal reflux events for the control group and for LPR patients differed significantly ($P < 0.0001$). The authors concluded that the "upper probe gives accurate and consistent information in normal subjects and patients with LPR" and that the acid exposure time and number of reflux events are most important in distinguishing normal subjects from patients with LPR [45]. However, there is a great degree of variability in the reported prevalence of pH abnormalities in the literature for patients with LPR (Table 10.2). This heterogeneity may be due to different patient populations and non-standard pH probe placement [46]. Some investigators utilized direct laryngoscopy for probe placement while others utilized esophageal manometry to identify the upper and lower esophageal sphincters [1]. Current recommendations

Table 10.2 Prevalence of abnormal pH monitoring in distal and proximal esophagus and the hypopharynx.

Study, year (reference)	Proportion of patients with LPR	Number of patients with reflux identified during proximal pH monitoring	Number of patients with reflux identified during distal pH monitoring	Number of patients with reflux identified during hypopharyngeal pH monitoring	Prevalence (%)
Ossakow, 1987 [94]	43/63	NR	43	NR	68
Koufman, 1988 [2]	24/32	NR	24	7	75
Wiener, 1989 [95]	12/15	NR	12	3	80
Wilson, 1989 [96]	17/97	17	NR	NR	18
Katz, 1990 [97]	7/10	NR	7	7	70
Woo, 1996 [98]	20/31	20	20	NR	65
Metz, 1997 [99]	6/10	?	6	NR	60
Vaezi, 1997 [100]	21/21	11	21	NR	100
Chen, 1998 [101]	365/735	NR	229	255	50
Havas, 1999 [71]	10/15	NR	6	4	67
Ulualp, 1999 [102]	15/20	15	15	15	75
Smit, 2001 [103]	7/15	7	3	NR	47
Ulualp, 2001 [52]	28/39	28	28	28	72
Noordzij, 2002 [51]	29/42	NR	29	29	69
Park, 2005 [44]	33/78	20	28	NR	42
Cumulative	**637/1223**	**46%**	**42%**	**38%**	**52**

LPR, laryngopharyngeal reflux; NR, not reported; ?, unclear how many patients tested.

suggest that the hypopharyngeal probe be placed 1–2 cm above the upper esophageal sphincter as determined by manometry, while the distal and proximal pH probes be placed 5 and 15 cm above the manometric lower esophageal sphincter [1].

Initial studies of patients with suspected gastroesophageal reflux laryngitis investigated the role of proximal esophageal pH probes. A 1991 study assessed the prevalence of abnormal acid exposure on the proximal esophagus in 15 patients with typical GERD (group 1), 15 patients with laryngeal symptoms without abnormal findings on laryngoscopy (group 2), and 10 patients with both laryngeal symptoms and findings on laryngoscopy (group 3) [47]. Increased proximal esophageal acid exposure was observed in patients in groups 1 and 2, indicating that proximal esophageal acid exposure may differentiate patients with laryngitis from those with typical GERD. Measurement of hypopharyngeal pH exposure was initially used to objectively measure laryngeal extension of reflux.

An earlier study suggested that hypopharyngeal pH assessment may be useful when used in conjunction with findings on laryngoscopy to identify patients whose symptoms may be related to GERD [48]. In this study, 76 patients with respiratory complaints thought to be related to GERD were divided into three groups based on RFS and pharyngeal reflux events. The patients were classified as RFS+ if the RFS was greater than 7, and pharyngeal reflux positive if they had greater than one episode of reflux noted during pH assessment. Controls were found to have a significantly lower RFS and fewer episodes of pharyngeal reflux. None of the controls had more than one episode of pharyngeal reflux during a 24-h period. Twenty-one patients had both an abnormal RFS and pharyngeal reflux, and these patients also had significantly higher heartburn scores and acid exposure in the distal esophagus. The authors concluded that agreement between detection of pharyngeal reflux by pH monitoring and an increased RFS greater than 7 helps establish or refute the diagnosis of GERD as an etiology of laryngeal symptoms. When both are normal, GERD is most likely not playing a role in a patient's extraesophageal symptoms.

However, initial enthusiasm about the diagnostic ability of hypopharyngeal reflux monitoring has now been replaced by skepticism. The positioning of the hypopharyngeal pH probe is operator dependent and varies with regard to placement via direct visualization with laryngoscopy compared to measurement by manometry [49]. Artifacts commonly occur and computer-driven interpretations must be manually reviewed [50]. Several studies have found that positive results of pharyngeal testing do not predict a favorable response to anti-reflux therapy [51,52]. One study showed that the degree of improvement in symptoms among 19 of 27 patients with pharyngeal reflux was similar to the eight patients not exhibiting pharyngeal reflux [52]. Additionally, there are no universally accepted diagnostic criteria for pH monitoring of the hypopharynx. The range of normal pH values is not uniformly defined, and can vary from none to 4 pH drops less than 4 [51,53,54]. Less restrictive pH values, including a drop in pH of 1.0 or 1.5 units instead of 2.0 units, do not differentiate healthy volunteers from patients with suspected ENT complaints [55].

The 2008 American Gastroenterological Association (AGA) technical review on the management of GERD suggested that the role of pH or impedance pH monitoring in diagnosing extraesophageal reflux is controversial and unproven (Table 10.3) [18]. This evidence-based technical review concludes that the value of a negative pH or impedance pH study is of greater clinical utility, and states "In the absence of troublesome esophageal symptoms or endoscopic findings, with a failed 8-week therapeutic trial of twice-daily PPI therapy, and with normal esophageal acid exposure (PPI therapy withheld) on 24-hour monitoring, one has gone as far as currently possible to rule out GERD as a significant contributor to these non-specific syndromes. Such patients should have etiologies other than GERD explored" [18].

This conclusion is in direct contrast to guidelines published by The American Academy of Otolaryngology-Head and Neck Surgery (AAOHNS) Committee on Speech, Voice, and Swallowing Disorders. The authors of the AAOHNS guidelines state that LPR can be diagnosed based on symptoms or laryngeal findings, but ambulatory 24-h double-probe (simultaneous esophageal and pharyngeal) pH assessment is considered the gold standard diagnostic tool (see Table 10.3) [24]. They also suggested that barium esophagraphy or esophagoscopy provide far less sensitive assessments of LPR, but may be advisable for screening of the esophagus for related pathology [6,24,56]. However, in line with the AGA guidelines, the American College of Gastroenterology (ACG) practice guidelines suggested that pH testing may not be the gold standard diagnostic test in this group of patients (see Table 10.3) [49]. The authors refer to data indicating that the overall pretherapy prevalence of an abnormal pH test in a population with chronic laryngeal symptoms is 53%, with the prevalence of excessive distal, proximal, and hypopharyngeal acid exposure being 42%, 44%, and 38%, respectively [46], suggesting that this population may have abnormal acid reflux exposure but not proving causality. In support of the ACG and AGA guidelines, a placebo-controlled study of 145 patients with suspected GERD-related ENT symptoms treated with high-dose esomeprazole or placebo for 16 weeks found that degree of symptomatic or laryngeal involvement was independent of pretherapy pH findings and that neither esophageal nor hypopharyngeal acid reflux predicted a response to PPI use [57].

In patients who remain symptomatic despite aggressive acid suppressive therapy, recent studies suggest that non-acid reflux may play a role in their

Table 10.3 Summary of AGA, AAOHNS, and ACG guidelines regarding pH testing and treatment modalities for patients with suspected LPR.

	American Gastroenterological Association Institute Technical Review on the Management of Gastroesophageal Reflux Disease, 2008 [18]	Laryngopharyngeal Reflux: Position statement of the Committee on Speech, Voice, and Swallowing Disorders of the American Academy of Otolaryngology-Head and Neck Surgery, 2002 [24]	American College of Gastroenterology Practice Guidelines: Esophageal Reflux Testing, 2007 [49]
pH testing	Role of pH or impedance pH monitoring in diagnosing extraesophageal reflux is controversial and unproven "In the absence of troublesome esophageal symptoms or endoscopic findings, with a failed 8-week therapeutic trial of twice-daily PPI therapy, and with normal esophageal acid exposure (PPI therapy withheld) on 24-hour monitoring, one has gone as far as currently possible to rule out GERD as a significant contributor to these nonspecific syndromes. Such patients should have etiologies other than GERD explore"	Diagnosis of LPR can be made based on symptoms and laryngeal findings, but ambulatory 24-h double-probe pH assessment is considered the gold standard diagnostic too IBarium esophagraphy or esophagoscopy provide far less sensitive assessments of LPR, but may be advisable for screening of the esophagus for related pathology	"The accumulating data seriously question the clinical usefulness of esophageal or hypopharyngeal pH monitoring in the initial evaluation of patients with suspected acid-related ENT complaints" "Studies using impedance pH monitoring in patients with extraesophageal symptoms unresponsive to PPI therapy show little evidence of nonacid reflux, except in the chronic cough patient"
Treatment	Empiric therapy with twice-daily PPI for 2 months for patients with concomitant esophageal GERD syndrome and laryngitis remains a pragmatic clinical strategy (USPSTF grade B, quality fair) Do not support use of once- or twice-daily PPIs (or H2RAs) for acute treatment of potential extraesophageal GERD syndromes, including laryngitis and asthma, in absence of esophageal GERD (USPSTF grade D, quality fair)	Treatment for LPR needs to be more aggressive and prolonged than that for GERD, and depends on symptoms and severity of LPR and on response to therapy Mild or intermittent LPR symptoms can be treated with dietary and lifestyle changes and H2 antagonists, while the majority of patients require at least twice-daily PPI (minimum of 6 months)	"The practical and popular approach is an empiric trial with a BID PPI regimen for several months, reserving pH testing for patients with persistent symptoms. However, here again, the results of acid pH testing have limited clinical utility"

Table 10.3 (cont'd)

American Gastroenterological Association Institute Technical Review on the Management of Gastroesophageal Reflux Disease, 2008 [18]	Laryngopharyngeal Reflux: Position statement of the Committee on Speech, Voice, and Swallowing Disorders of the American Academy of Otolaryngology-Head and Neck Surgery, 2002 [24]	American College of Gastroenterology Practice Guidelines: Esophageal Reflux Testing, 2007 [49]
"Step-down therapy should be attempted in all patients with extraesophageal reflux syndromes after empirical twice-daily PPI therapy. Continuing maintenance PPI therapy should be predicated on either the requirements of therapy for concomitant esophageal GERD syndromes or extraesophageal syndrome symptom response. In both cases, maintenance therapy should be with the lowest PPI dose necessary for adequate symptom relief"	Fundoplication has been shown to be effective	

BID, *bis in die*; ENT, ear, nose and throat; GERD, gastroesophageal reflux disease; H2RA, H2 receptor antagonist; LPR, laryngopharyngeal reflux; PPI, proton pump inhibitor; USPSTF, US Preventive Services Task Force.

symptoms [58–61]. The combination of impedance and pH monitoring allows for distinction between acid, weakly acidic, and weakly alkaline reflux [59]. A multicenter trial using impedance pH-metry in healthy adults developed normal values to be utilized for comparison with reflux patients [62]. Studies assessing patients with heartburn and regurgitation in addition to patients with extraesophageal symptoms suggest that 10–40% of patients on twice-daily PPI therapy may have persistent non-acid reflux [60,63]. However, causation between these non-acid reflux events and persistent symptoms is difficult to establish [28]. A recent study found that abnormal impedance in patients on therapy predicts acid reflux in patients off therapy [64]. It also concluded that in patients with refractory reflux, combined impedance/pH monitoring might provide the single best strategy for evaluating reflux symptoms. However, the clinical significance of abnormal impedance findings in this group of patients awaits further study. The most recent uncontrolled surgical study in patients suspected of having LPR found that on or off therapy impedance monitoring does not predict LPR symptom response to fundoplication but the presence of hiatal hernia, significant acid reflux at baseline and presence of regurgitation concomitantly with the LPR symptom were important predictors of symptom response [65].

The Restech Dx-pH Measurement System™ (Respiratory Technology Corp., San Diego, CA) is a new device developed to detect acid reflux in the posterior oropharynx [66]. A nasopharyngeal catheter is utilized to assess pH in liquid or aerosolized droplets. A comparison of this device to the traditional pH catheters has shown faster detection rate and faster time to equilibrium pH. A recent prospective observational study in healthy volunteers developed normative data for this device at pH cut-offs of 4, 5 and 6 for the distal esophagus and oropharynx [66]. Although the initial studies with this device in patients with LPR are encouraging [67], controlled studies are needed to assess the future role of this new device in patients with LPR.

Managing laryngeal complications of reflux disease

Medical management

Given the poor sensitivity and specificity of diagnostic tests, empiric treatment of suspected gastroesophageal reflux laryngitis using PPIs is common [1]. A recent study assessed response to PPIs based on change in 24-h pH studies in 27 patients with LPR with abnormal pH studies at baseline. Of five patients who did not have a measurable pH response to PPI, four reported improvements in their symptoms, highlighting poor prediction of treatment response based on pH results [68]. Most trials have utilized twice-daily PPIs for 3–4 months [1,69]. The primary reason for this unapproved high-dose acid suppression is based on pH monitoring data indicating that the chance of normalizing exposure of the esophagus to acid in patients with chronic cough, laryngeal symptoms or asthma is 99% with a twice-daily PPI [70]. A prospective cohort study (uncontrolled and open label) assessed optimal PPI dose in patients with LPR, and indicated that twice-daily PPI is more effective than daily PPI in achieving clinical symptom response in patients with suspected LPR [44].

Although PPIs are widely used in patients with suspected LPR, high-quality supporting evidence remains minimal at this time as most trials have utilized small sample sizes and are uncontrolled [1,17,18,69]. Placebo-controlled studies assessing lansoprazole, esomeprazole, pantoprazole, and rabeprazole for 2–4 months' duration have observed no significant difference in symptoms experienced by LPR patients on placebo as compared to PPI

(Table 10.4) [57, 71–73]. Similarly, a metaanalysis of randomized controlled trials assessing PPI use for suspected GERD-related chronic laryngitis noted no benefit of PPIs over placebo (Figure 10.1) [74]. On the other hand, in support of the role of acid suppression in LPR, a more recent double-blind, placebo-controlled trial noted a significant improvement in LPR symptoms with 3 months of esomeprazole therapy [75]. One reason for the positive nature of this study is that the RSI was used as one of the outcome measures assessed. Of all symptoms queried, patients experienced the greatest improvement in heartburn symptoms after 3 months (and less marked improvements in hoarseness, throat clearing, coughing after meals, breathing difficulties, and other symptoms addressed). The improvement in heartburn symptoms had the most significant effect on the overall RSI score.

Similarly, an earlier study comparing lansoprazole with placebo in 22 patients with idiopathic chronic laryngitis noted that after 3 months, 50% of patients in the lansoprazole group had noted resolution of symptoms, compared to 10% of patients in the placebo group [76]. Furthermore, another study reported that LPR patients who tested positive for *H. pylori* antigen were more likely to respond to PPI than those seronegative for *H. pylori* [77]. Finally, in a randomized controlled study of patients with chief complaint of postnasal drainage, Vaezi *et al.* found a benefit for treatment with PPIs, suggesting that PPIs may do more than just suppress reflux in this group of individuals [78]. Thus, the search for the subgroup of patients with suspected LPR or extraesophageal reflux symptoms more likely to respond to PPI therapy continues.

The AGA guidelines advise empiric therapy with twice-daily PPI for 2 months for patients with a concomitant esophageal GERD syndrome (i.e. typical symptoms such as heartburn) and laryngitis (US Preventive Services Task Force (USPSTF) grade B recommendation) [18]. Their recommendations do not support the use of PPIs for acute treatment of laryngitis in the absence of esophageal GERD (USPSTF grade D) [18]. However, the AAOHNS position statement indicates that treatment for LPR needs to be more aggressive and prolonged than that for GERD, and depends on the symptoms and severity of LPR and on the response to therapy [24]. The AAOHNS advises that patients with mild or intermittent symptoms of LPR can be treated with dietary and lifestyle changes and with H2 antagonists, while the majority of patients require at least twice-daily PPI therapy [5,6,25,41,79–84]. Some patients require therapy with both a PPI and an H2 antagonist, and the AAOHNS recommends the use of twice-daily PPI for a minimum of 6 months [24,81]. The authors of the AAOHNS statement suggest that fundoplication has been shown to be an effective treatment for LPR [85,86]. However, this point is controversial, as discussed in the next section.

The need for chronic therapy in patients suspected of GERD-related laryngitis comes from uncontrolled observational studies with small sample

Table 10.4 Placebo-controlled trials assessing use of proton-pump inhibitors in laryngopharyngeal reflux.

Study author (country, year published, reference)	PPI studied	Duration, # of subjects	Inclusion criteria	Important exclusion criteria	pH monitoring	GI endoscopy	Outcome measured	Response to therapy
Havas (Australia, 1999 [71])	Lansoprazole 30 mg twice daily	12 weeks, 15 subjects	Posterior pharyngolaryngitis	CNS disorder, COPD, preexisting acid suppression, severe esophagitis	Yes	Yes	50% reduction in global symptom score	35% reduction in symptoms
Noordzij (USA, 2001 [104])	Omeprazole 40 mg twice daily	8 weeks, 30 subjects	LSx for 3 months LPR 4 episodes	Infection Cancer Allergies	Yes	Optional	50% reduction in global symptom score	Comparable symptom score improvement in both groups
El-Serag (USA, 2001 [76])	Lansoprazole 30 mg twice daily	12 weeks, 20 subjects	LSx for >3 weeks LPR on laryngoscopy	Infection, cancer, previous GI surgery	Yes	Yes	Complete symptom resolution	50% with complete resolution vs 10% in placebo group
Eherer (Austria, 2003 [105])	Pantoprazole 40 mg twice daily	12 weeks, 14 subjects	Hoarseness for 2 months (+) pH test		Yes	Optional	50% reduction in global symptom score	Significant improvement in symptoms in both groups
Steward (USA, 2004 [73])	Rabeprazole 20 mg twice daily	8 weeks, 42 subjects	LSx for >4 weeks LPR on laryngoscopy	GI surgery PPI in 1 month	Optional	Optional	50% reduction in global symptom score	53% resolution in treatment group, 50% resolution in placebo group

Study	Medication	Duration, subjects	Inclusion criteria	Exclusion criteria			Endpoint	Results
Wo (USA, 2006 [72])	Pantoprazole 40 mg daily	12 weeks, 39 subjects	LSx for 3 days a week (+) pH test		Yes	Optional	50% reduction in global symptom score	40% with resolution in both groups
Vaezi (USA, 2006 [57])	Esomeprazole 40 mg twice daily	16 weeks, 145 subjects	LSx for 3 months LPR on laryngoscopy	Heartburn >3/wk PPI in 2 wk	Optional	Optional	50% reduction in symptoms	~15% resolution of symptoms in both groups, with 45% of both groups experiencing improvement in symptoms
Reichel (Germany, 2008 [75])	Esomeprazole 20 mg twice daily	12 weeks, 62 subjects	RFS >7 and RSI >13	PPI in 3 months, GI surgery, laryngeal malignancy	No	No	Reduction of total RSI and RFS	Significantly greater improvement in laryngeal appearance and LPR symptoms

CNS, central nervous system; COPD, chronic obstructive pulmonary disease; GI, gastrointestinal; LPR, laryngopharyngeal reflux; LSx, laryngeal symptoms; PPI, proton pump inhibitor; RFS, Reflux Finding Score; RSI, Reflux Symptom Index.

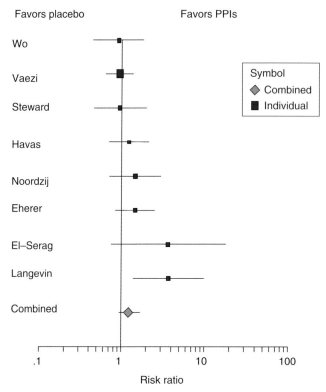

Figure 10.1 Forest plot depicting the risk ratios for studies assessing efficacy of proton pump inhibitor (PPI) in reflux laryngitis and pooled risk ratio by random effects method. Adapted from Qadeer *et al.* [74] with permission from Blackwell Publishing.

sizes. For example, patients with LPR with concomitant GERD symptoms may have esophagitis (12%) and Barrett's esophagus (7%) [87,88]. Studies suggest a possible association between chronic reflux-induced inflammation of the larynx and laryngeal cancer [13,18,34]. However, the main purpose of maintenance use of PPIs in patients with LPR is for control of symptoms and step-down therapy should always follow the initial empiric trial [18]. Long-term PPI is the current practice in many patients, as evidenced by a double-blind placebo-controlled trial finding only 21–48% likelihood of remaining PPI free at 1 year [89]. However, evidence supporting the use of long-term PPI therapy for patients with LPR is primarily anecdotal and future studies are needed to assess appropriate duration and use of PPI in patients with suspected LPR.

Surgical therapy

A number of uncontrolled observational studies have suggested efficacy of anti-reflux surgery in patients with gastroesophageal reflux laryngitis. An earlier study assessed the effect of laparoscopic Hill repair on 145 patients and found that after a mean follow-up of 20 months, reports of sore throat decreased from 43% to 8% of patients. Symptoms of cough decreased from 41% to 8%, and voice loss decreased from 25% to 11% [90]. Similarly, another study evaluated 40 patients who underwent laparoscopic Nissen fundoplication for complaints of reflux laryngitis. After 3 months, 79.3% of patients had decreased inflammation noted on otorhinolaryngeal exam, and 41.4% described improvement in voice quality. After 12 months, these figures were 92.3% and 38.5%, respectively. After a median follow-up of 42 months, 62.5% of patients reported either no cough or mild cough or hoarseness [91].

A more recent prospective concurrent controlled study in patients with LPR symptoms refractory to PPI therapy did not find Nissen fundoplication to be of benefit. One year after surgery, only 10% of patients noted improvement in laryngeal symptoms, while signs of LPR on laryngoscopy improved in 80% of patients [92]. Recent controversy surrounds the role of surgical fundoplication in patients with PPI-refractory symptoms who have abnormal non-acid reflux by impedance monitoring. A retrospective review assessed patients with chronic cough referred for fundoplication after documentation of an association between their symptoms and reflux disease using multichannel intraluminal impedance and pH testing. In all six patients who underwent surgery, fundoplication was found to eliminate chronic cough due to non-acid reflux [93]. In this subgroup of patients, an uncontrolled telephone survey study suggested symptom improvement in most patients with laparoscopic Nissen fundoplication [61]. However, controlled studies are needed before this practice can be advocated, especially since the most recent surgical study suggests that impedance monitoring is not a predictor of LPR symptom response to fundoplication [65]. Based on published data, the role of fundoplication is best delineated in those who have a positive symptom response to PPI therapy and caution should be exercised in referring patients who do not respond to aggressive acid suppression, especially those with extraesophageal complaints.

Summary

Gastroesophageal reflux disease is associated with laryngeal signs and symptoms but the frequency of the association between these two entities is not firmly established. Improvement in the specificity of laryngeal examination would be an important goal in improving the accuracy of diagnosis of gastroesophageal reflux laryngitis. pH or impedance pH studies can serve as diagnostic tools in patients whose symptoms are refractory to an empiric trial of PPIs. If these tests are normal on PPI

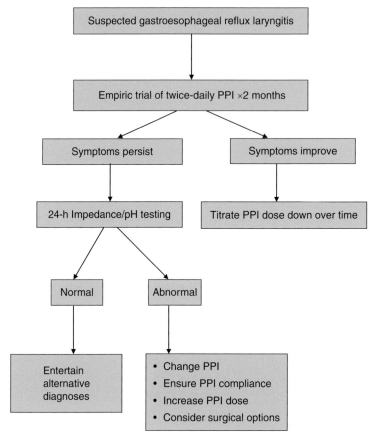

Figure 10.2 Suggested algorithm for evaluation and treatment of suspected laryngopharyngeal reflux. PPI, proton pump inhibitor.

therapy despite persistence of symptoms, other etiologies for abnormal laryngeal signs and symptoms should be investigated [1]. It is prudent to remember that patients with suspected extraesophageal GERD syndromes, including those with LPR, may have GERD as a contributing etiology but rarely as the sole cause of their complaints [18].

Based on our experiences in treating patients with reflux-suspected chronic laryngitis, we suggest a treatment algorithm as illustrated in Figure 10.2. Initial empiric therapy with twice-daily PPI for 2 months is a reasonable starting point for patients with suspected GERD-related laryngitis and no ominous symptoms or signs. If symptoms improve then acid suppression should be tapered to the minimum dose for symptom control. If symptoms persist despite twice-daily PPI therapy, diagnostic testing with pH monitoring "off or on" PPIs or impedance pH monitoring on therapy is recommended. In patients with normal test results, a search for an alternative explanation for symptoms should be pursued. In the infrequent cases of abnormal test results on therapy, clinical judgment should be exercised regarding the role of surgical fundoplication given the lack of controlled studies in this area.

CASE STUDY

A 46-year-old woman presents on a referral from her ENT physician for evaluation and treatment of her throat clearing and chronic cough. She has a history of asthma and postnasal drip from seasonal allergies and has been treated aggressively by her pulmonary and allergy physician for the past 3 years. She had already undergone laryngoscopy by her ENT physician, which showed "laryngeal irritation that suggested GERD." The patient is on once-daily proton pump inhibitor intermittently which has only minimally helped her symptoms. She does have heartburn and occasional regurgitation, especially at night when in the supine position. The patient is inquiring about undergoing fundoplication.

References

1 Vaezi MF, Hicks DM, Abelson TI, Richter JE. Laryngeal signs and symptoms and gastroesophageal reflux disease (GERD): a critical assessment of cause and effect association. Clin Gastroenterol Hepatol 2003;1(5):333–44.

2 Koufman JA Wiener GJ, Wallace CW, *et al.* Reflux laryngitis and its sequelae: the diagnostic role of ambulatory 24-h pH monitoring. J Voice 1988;2:78–9.

3 Gaynor EB. Otolaryngologic manifestations of gastroesophageal reflux. Am J Gastroenterol 1991;86(7):801–8.

4 Graser A. Gastroesophageal reflux and laryngeal symptoms. Aliment Pharmacol Ther 1994;8:265–72.

5 Koufman J, Sataloff RT, Toohill R. Laryngopharyngeal reflux: consensus conference report. J Voice 1996;10(3):215–16.

6 Koufman JA. The otolaryngologic manifestations of gastroesophageal reflux disease (GERD): a clinical investigation of 225 patients using ambulatory 24-hour pH monitoring and an experimental investigation of the role of acid and pepsin in the development of laryngeal injury. Laryngoscope 1991;101(4 Pt 2 Suppl 53):1–78.

7 Richter JE. Typical and atypical presentations of gastroesophageal reflux disease. The role of esophageal testing in diagnosis and management. Gastroenterol Clin North Am 1996;25(1):75–102.

8 Toohill RJ, Kuhn JC. Role of refluxed acid in pathogenesis of laryngeal disorders. Am J Med 1997;103(5A):100S–6S.

9 Ward PH Hanson DG. Reflux as an etiological factor of carcinoma of the laryngopharynx. Laryngoscope 1998;98:1195–9.

10 Freije JE, Beatty TW, Campbell BH, Woodson BT, Schultz CJ, Toohill RJ. Carcinoma of the larynx in patients with gastroesophageal reflux. Am J Otolaryngol 1996;17(6):386–90.

11 Morrison MD. Is chronic gastroesophageal reflux a causative factor in glottic carcinoma? Otolaryngol Head Neck Surg 1988;99(4):370–3.

12 Vaezi MF, Qadeer MA, Lopez R, Colabianchi N. Laryngeal cancer and gastroesophageal reflux disease: a case–control study. Am J Med 2006;119(9):768–76.

13 Qadeer MA, Colabianchi N, Strome M, Vaezi MF. Gastroesophageal reflux and laryngeal cancer: causation or association? A critical review. Am J Otolaryngol 2006;27(2):119–28.

14 Coffin L. The relationship of upper airway passages to diseases of gastrointestinal tract. Ann Otol Rhinol Laryngol 1903;12:521–6.

15 Jackson C MS. Contact ulcer of larynx. Ann Otol Rhinol Laryngol 1928;37:227–30.

16 Cherry J, Margulies SI. Contact ulcer of the larynx. Laryngoscope 1968;78(11):1937–40.

17 Vakil N, van Zanten SV, Kahrilas P, Dent J, Jones R. The Montreal definition and classification of gastroesophageal reflux disease: a global evidence-based consensus. Am J Gastroenterol 2006;101(8):1900–20; quiz 1943.

18 Kahrilas PJ, Shaheen NJ, Vaezi MF. American Gastroenterological Association Institute technical review on the management of gastroesophageal reflux disease. Gastroenterology 2008;135(4):1392–413.

19 Locke GR 3rd, Talley NJ, Fett SL, Zinsmeister AR, Melton LJ 3rd. Prevalence and clinical spectrum of gastroesophageal reflux: a population-based study in Olmsted County, Minnesota. Gastroenterology 1997;112(5):1448–56.

20 El-Serag HB, Sonnenberg A. Comorbid occurrence of laryngeal or pulmonary disease with esophagitis in United States military veterans. Gastroenterology 1997; 113(3):755–60.

21 Sontag SJ, O'Connell S, Khandelwal S, et al. Asthmatics with gastroesophageal reflux: long term results of a randomized trial of medical and surgical antireflux therapies. Am J Gastroenterol 2003;98(5):987–99.

22 Kahrilas PJ, Shaheen NJ, Vaezi MF, et al. American Gastroenterological Association Medical Position Statement on the management of gastroesophageal reflux disease. Gastroenterology 2008;135(4):1383–91.

23 Shaker R, Castell DO, Schoenfeld PS, Spechler SJ. Nighttime heartburn is an underappreciated clinical problem that impacts sleep and daytime function: the results of a Gallup survey conducted on behalf of the American Gastroenterological Association. Am J Gastroenterol 2003;98(7):1487–93.

24 Koufman JA, Aviv JE, Casiano RR, Shaw GY. Laryngopharyngeal reflux: position statement of the committee on speech, voice, and swallowing disorders of the American Academy of Otolaryngology-Head and Neck Surgery. Otolaryngol Head Neck Surg 2002;127(1):32–5.

25 Hanson DG, Jiang JJ. Diagnosis and management of chronic laryngitis associated with reflux. Am J Med 2000;108(Suppl 4a):112S–9S.

26 Loughlin CJ, Koufman JA, Averill DB, et al. Acid-induced laryngospasm in a canine model. Laryngoscope 1996;106(12 Pt 1):1506–9.

27 Adhami T, Goldblum JR, Richter JE, Vaezi MF. The role of gastric and duodenal agents in laryngeal injury: an experimental canine model. Am J Gastroenterol 2004;99(11):2098–106.

28 Vaezi MF. Laryngitis: from the gastroenterologist's point of view. In: Vaezi MF (ed) Extraesophageal reflux. San Diego, CA: Plural Publishing, 2009: pp. 37–47.

29 Sidhu H, Shaker R, Hogan WJ. Gastroesophageal reflux laryngitis. In: Castell DO, Richter JE (eds) The esophagus, 4th edn. Philadelphia: Lippincott, Williams and Wilkins, 2003: pp. 518–29.

30 Hogan WJ, Shaker R. Supraesophageal complications of gastroesophageal reflux. Dis Mon 2000;46(3):193–232.

31 Belafsky PC, Postma GN, Koufman JA. Validity and reliability of the reflux symptom index (RSI). J Voice 2002;16(2):274–7.

32 Park KH, Choi SM, Kwon SU, Yoon SW, Kim SU. Diagnosis of laryngopharyngeal reflux among globus patients. Otolaryngol Head Neck Surg 2006;134(1):81–5.

33 Sataloff RT. *Professional voice: the science and art of clinical care*, 2nd edn. San Diego, CA: Singular Publishing Group, 1997.

34 Ford CN. Evaluation and management of laryngopharyngeal reflux. JAMA 2005; 294(12):1534–40.

35 Weinberger PM, Postma GN. Laryngopharyngeal reflux from the otolaryngologist's perspective. In: Vaezi MF (ed) *Extraesophageal reflux*. San Diego, CA: Plural Publishing, 2009: pp. 49–66.

36 Axford SE, Sharp N, Ross PE, *et al.* Cell biology of laryngeal epithelial defenses in health and disease: preliminary studies. Ann Otol Rhinol Laryngol 2001;110(12): 1099–108.

37 Ahmed TF, Khandwala F, Abelson TI, *et al.* Chronic laryngitis associated with gastro-esophageal reflux: prospective assessment of differences in practice patterns between gastroenterologists and ENT physicians. Am J Gastroenterol 2006;101(3):470–8.

38 Book DT, Rhee JS, Toohill RJ, Smith TL. Perspectives in laryngopharyngeal reflux: an international survey. Laryngoscope 2002;112(8 Pt 1):1399–406.

39 Hicks DM, Ours TM, Abelson TI, Vaezi MF, Richter JE. The prevalence of hypo-pharynx findings associated with gastroesophageal reflux in normal volunteers. J Voice 2002;16(4):564–79.

40 Vaezi MF, Ours TM, Hicks DM, *et al.* Laryngoscopic signs of gastroesophageal reflux disease: science or fiction? Am J Gastroenterol 1999;94:2601.

41 Belafsky PC, Postma GN, Koufman JA. The validity and reliability of the reflux finding score (RFS). Laryngoscope 2001;111(8):1313–17.

42 Mesallam TA, Stemple JC, Sobeih TM, Elluru RG. Reflux symptom index versus reflux finding score. Ann Otol Rhinol Laryngol 2007;116(6):436–40.

43 Milstein CF, Charbel S, Hicks DM, Abelson TI, Richter JE, Vaezi MF. Prevalence of laryngeal irritation signs associated with reflux in asymptomatic volunteers: impact of endoscopic technique (rigid vs. flexible laryngoscope). Laryngoscope 2005; 115(12):2256–61.

44 Park W, Hicks DM, Khandwala F, *et al.* Laryngopharyngeal reflux: prospective cohort study evaluating optimal dose of proton-pump inhibitor therapy and pretherapy predictors of response. Laryngoscope 2005;115(7):1230–8.

45 Merati AL, Lim HJ, Ulualp SO, Toohill RJ. Meta-analysis of upper probe measurements in normal subjects and patients with laryngopharyngeal reflux. Ann Otol Rhinol Laryngol 2005;114(3):177–82.

46 Ahmed T, Vaezi MF. The role of pH monitoring in extraesophageal gastroesophageal reflux disease. Gastrointest Endosc Clin North Am 2005;15(2):319–31.

47 Jacob P, Kahrilas PJ, Herzon G. Proximal esophageal pH-metry in patients with 'reflux laryngitis'. Gastroenterology 1991;100(2):305–10.

48 Oelschlager BK, Eubanks TR, Maronian N, *et al.* Laryngoscopy and pharyngeal pH are complementary in the diagnosis of gastroesophageal-laryngeal reflux. J Gastrointest Surg 2002;6(2):189–94.

49 Hirano I, Richter JE. ACG practice guidelines: esophageal reflux testing. Am J Gastroenterol 2007;102(3):668–85.

50 Wo JM, Jabbar A, Winstead W, Goudy S, Cacchione R, Allen JW. Hypopharyngeal pH monitoring artifact in detection of laryngopharyngeal reflux. Dig Dis Sci 2002;47(11):2579–85.

51 Noordzij JP, Khidr A, Desper E, Meek RB, Reibel JF, Levine PA. Correlation of pH probe-measured laryngopharyngeal reflux with symptoms and signs of reflux laryngitis. Laryngoscope 2002;112(12):2192–5.

52 Ulualp SO, Toohill RJ, Shaker R. Outcomes of acid suppressive therapy in patients with posterior laryngitis. Otolaryngol Head Neck Surg 2001;124(1):16–22.

53 Eubanks TR, Omelanczuk PE, Maronian N, Hillel A, Pope CE 2nd, Pellegrini CA. Pharyngeal pH monitoring in 222 patients with suspected laryngeal reflux. J Gastrointest Surg 2001;5(2):183–90; discussion 190–1.

54 Maldonado A, Diederich L, Castell DO, Gideon RM, Katz PO. Laryngopharyngeal reflux identified using a new catheter design: defining normal values and excluding artifacts. Laryngoscope 2003;113(2):349–55.

55 Shaker R, Bardan E, Gu C, Kern M, Torrico L, Toohill R. Intrapharyngeal distribution of gastric acid refluxate. Laryngoscope 2003;113(7):1182–91.

56 Belafsky PC, Postma GN, Daniel E, Koufman JA. Transnasal esophagoscopy. Otolaryngol Head Neck Surg 2001;125(6):588–9.

57 Vaezi MF, Richter JE, Stasney CR, et al. Treatment of chronic posterior laryngitis with esomeprazole. Laryngoscope 2006;116(2):254–60.

58 Vaezi MF. Reflux-induced laryngitis (laryngopharyngeal reflux). Curr Treat Options Gastroenterol 2006;9(1):69–74.

59 Sifrim D, Blondeau K. Technology insight: the role of impedance testing for esophageal disorders. Nat Clin Pract Gastroenterol Hepatol 2006;3(4):210–19.

60 Mainie I, Tutuian R, Shay S, et al. Acid and non-acid reflux in patients with persistent symptoms despite acid suppressive therapy: a multicentre study using combined ambulatory impedance-pH monitoring. Gut 2006;55(10):1398–402.

61 Mainie I, Tutuian R, Agrawal A, Adams D, Castell DO. Combined multichannel intraluminal impedance-pH monitoring to select patients with persistent gastro-esophageal reflux for laparoscopic Nissen fundoplication. Br J Surg 2006;93(12):1483–7.

62 Shay S, Tutuian R, Sifrim D, et al. Twenty-four hour ambulatory simultaneous impedance and pH monitoring: a multicenter report of normal values from 60 healthy volunteers. Am J Gastroenterol 2004;99(6):1037–43.

63 Vaezi MF, Hicks DM, Ours TM, Richter JE. ENT manifestation of GERD: a large prospective study assessing treatment outcome and predictors of response. Gastroenterology 2001;120:A636.

64 Pritchett JM, Aslam M, Slaughter JC, Ness RM, Garrett CG, Vaezi MF. Efficacy of esophageal impedance/pH monitoring in patients with refractory gastroesophageal reflux disease, on and off therapy. Clin Gastroenterol Hepatol 2009;7(7):743–8.

65 Fletcher KC GM, Slaughter JC, Garrett CG, Vaezi MF. Significance and degree of reflux in patients with primary extraesophageal symptoms. Laryngoscope 2011;121(12):2561–5.

66 Sun G, Muddana S, Slaughter JC, et al. A new pH catheter for laryngopharyngeal reflux: normal values. Laryngoscope 2009;119(8):1639–43.

67 Wiener GJ, Tsukashima R, Kelly C, et al. Oropharyngeal pH monitoring for the detection of liquid and aerosolized supraesophageal gastric reflux. J Voice 2009;23(4):498–504.

68 Reichel O, Keller J, Rasp G, Hagedorn H, Berghaus A. Efficacy of once-daily esomeprazole treatment in patients with laryngopharyngeal reflux evaluated by 24-hour pH monitoring. Otolaryngol Head Neck Surg 2007;136(2):205–10.

69 Field SK, Sutherland LR. Does medical antireflux therapy improve asthma in asthmatics with gastroesophageal reflux? A critical review of the literature. Chest 1998;114(1):275–83.

70 Charbel S, Khandwala F, Vaezi MF. The role of esophageal pH monitoring in symptomatic patients on PPI therapy. Am J Gastroenterol 2005;100(2):283–9.

71 Havas T, Huang S, Levy M, et al. Posterior pharyngolaryngitis: double-blind randomised placebo-controlled trial of proton pump inhibitor therapy. Aust J Otolaryngol 1999;3:243.

72 Wo JM, Koopman J, Harrell SP, Parker K, Winstead W, Lentsch E. Double-blind, placebo-controlled trial with single-dose pantoprazole for laryngopharyngeal reflux. Am J Gastroenterol 2006;101(9):1972–8; quiz 2169.

73 Steward DL, Wilson KM, Kelly DH, et al. Proton pump inhibitor therapy for chronic laryngo-pharyngitis: a randomized placebo-control trial. Otolaryngol Head Neck Surg 2004;131(4):342–50.

74 Qadeer MA, Phillips CO, Lopez AR, et al. Proton pump inhibitor therapy for suspected GERD-related chronic laryngitis: a meta-analysis of randomized controlled trials. Am J Gastroenterol 2006;101(11):2646–54.

75 Reichel O, Dressel H, Wiederanders K, Issing WJ. Double-blind, placebo-controlled trial with esomeprazole for symptoms and signs associated with laryngopharyngeal reflux. Otolaryngol Head Neck Surg 2008;139(3):414–20.

76 El-Serag HB, Lee P, Buchner A, Inadomi JM, Gavin M, McCarthy DM. Lansoprazole treatment of patients with chronic idiopathic laryngitis: a placebo-controlled trial. Am J Gastroenterol 2001;96(4):979–83.

77 Oridate N, Takeda H, Yamamoto J, et al. Helicobacter pylori seropositivity predicts outcomes of acid suppression therapy for laryngopharyngeal reflux symptoms. Laryngoscope 2006;116(4):547–53.

78 Vaezi MF, Hagaman DD, Slaughter JC, et al. Proton pump inhibitor therapy improves symptoms in postnasal drainage. Gastroenterology 2010;139(6):1887–93.

79 Ulualp SO, Toohill RJ. Laryngopharyngeal reflux: state of the art diagnosis and treatment. Otolaryngol Clin North Am 2000;33(4):785–802.

80 Belafsky PC, Postma GN, Koufman JA. Laryngopharyngeal reflux symptoms improve before changes in physical findings. Laryngoscope 2001;111(6):979–81.

81 Bough ID Jr, Sataloff RT, Castell DO, Hills JR, Gideon RM, Spiegel JR. Gastroesophageal reflux laryngitis resistant to omeprazole therapy. J Voice 1995;9(2):205–11.

82 Chiverton SG, Howden CW, Burget DW, Hunt RH. Omeprazole (20 mg) daily given in the morning or evening: a comparison of effects on gastric acidity, and plasma gastrin and omeprazole concentration. Aliment Pharmacol Ther 1992; 6(1):103–11.

83 Kahrilas PJ, Falk GW, Johnson DA, et al. Esomeprazole improves healing and symptom resolution as compared with omeprazole in reflux oesophagitis patients: a randomized controlled trial. The Esomeprazole Study Investigators. Aliment Pharmacol Ther 2000;14(10):1249–58.

84 Shaw GY, Searl JP. Laryngeal manifestations of gastroesophageal reflux before and after treatment with omeprazole. South Med J 1997;90(11):1115–22.

85 Hunter JG, Trus TL, Branum GD, Waring JP, Wood WC. A physiologic approach to laparoscopic fundoplication for gastroesophageal reflux disease. Ann Surg 1996;223(6):673–85; discussion 685–7.

86 Dallemagne B, Weerts JM, Jeahes C, Markiewicz S. Results of laparoscopic Nissen fundoplication. Hepatogastroenterology 1998;45(23):1338–43.

87 Koufman JA, Belafsky PC, Bach KK, Daniel E, Postma GN. Prevalence of esophagitis in patients with pH-documented laryngopharyngeal reflux. Laryngoscope 2002; 112(9):1606–9.

88 Halum SL, Postma GN, Bates DD, Koufman JA. Incongruence between histologic and endoscopic diagnoses of Barrett's esophagus using transnasal esophagoscopy. Laryngoscope 2006;116(2):303–6.

89 Bjornsson E, Abrahamsson H, Simren M, et al. Discontinuation of proton pump inhibitors in patients on long-term therapy: a double-blind, placebo-controlled trial. Aliment Pharmacol Ther 2006;24(6):945–54.

90 Wright RC, Rhodes KP. Improvement of laryngopharyngeal reflux symptoms after laparoscopic Hill repair. Am J Surg 2003;185(5):455–61.

91 Salminen P, Sala E, Koskenvuo J, Karvonen J, Ovaska J. Reflux laryngitis: a feasible indication for laparoscopic antireflux surgery? Surg Laparosc Endosc Percutan Tech 2007;17(2):73–8.

92 Swoger J, Ponsky J, Hicks DM, *et al.* Surgical fundoplication in laryngopharyngeal reflux unresponsive to aggressive acid suppression: a controlled study. Clin Gastroenterol Hepatol 2006;4(4):433–41.

93 Tutuian R, Mainie I, Agrawal A, Adams D, Castell DO. Nonacid reflux in patients with chronic cough on acid-suppressive therapy. Chest 2006;130(2):386–91.

94 Ossakow SJ, Elta G, Colturi T, Bogdasarian R, Nostrant TT. Esophageal reflux and dysmotility as the basis for persistent cervical symptoms. Ann Otol Rhinol Laryngol 1987;96(4):387–92.

95 Wiener GJ, Koufman JA, Wu WC, Cooper JB, Richter JE, Castell DO. Chronic hoarseness secondary to gastroesophageal reflux disease: documentation with 24-h ambulatory pH monitoring. Am J Gastroenterol 1989;84(12):1503–8.

96 Wilson JA, White A, von Haacke NP, *et al.* Gastroesophageal reflux and posterior laryngitis. Ann Otol Rhinol Laryngol 1989;98(6):405–10.

97 Katz PO. Ambulatory esophageal and hypopharyngeal pH monitoring in patients with hoarseness. Am J Gastroenterol 1990;85(1):38–40.

98 Woo P, Noordzij P, Ross JA. Association of esophageal reflux and globus symptom: comparison of laryngoscopy and 24-hour pH manometry. Otolaryngol Head Neck Surg 1996;115(6):502–7.

99 Metz DC, Childs ML, Ruiz C, Weinstein GS. Pilot study of the oral omeprazole test for reflux laryngitis. Otolaryngol Head Neck Surg 1997;116(1):41–6.

100 Vaezi MF, Schroeder PL, Richter JE. Reproducibility of proximal probe pH parameters in 24-hour ambulatory esophageal pH monitoring. Am J Gastroenterol 1997;92(5):825–9.

101 Chen MY, Ott DJ, Casolo BJ, Moghazy KM, Koufman JA. Correlation of laryngeal and pharyngeal carcinomas and 24-hour pH monitoring of the esophagus and pharynx. Otolaryngol Head Neck Surg 1998;119(5):460–2.

102 Ulualp SO, Toohill RJ, Hoffmann R, Shaker R. Pharyngeal pH monitoring in patients with posterior laryngitis. Otolaryngol Head Neck Surg 1999;120(5):672–7.

103 Smit CF, Copper MP, van Leeuwen JA, Schoots IG, Stanojcic LD. Effect of cigarette smoking on gastropharyngeal and gastroesophageal reflux. Ann Otol Rhinol Laryngol 2001;110(2):190–3.

104 Noordzij JP, Khidr A, Evans BA, *et al.* Evaluation of omeprazole in the treatment of reflux laryngitis: a prospective, placebo-controlled, randomized, double-blind study. Laryngoscope 2001;111(12):2147–51.

105 Eherer AJ, Habermann W, Hammer HF, Kiesler K, Friedrich G, Krejs GJ. Effect of pantoprazole on the course of reflux-associated laryngitis: a placebo-controlled double-blind crossover study. Scand J Gastroenterol 2003;38(5):462–7.

CHAPTER 11

Reflux-Related Cough

Etsuro Yazaki, Ryuichi Shimono, and Daniel Sifrim
Wingate Institute for Neurogastroenterology, Barts and the London School of Medicine
and Dentistry, and GI Physiology Unit, Royal London Hospital, London, UK

Key points
- Gastroesophageal reflux disease is now considered to be one of the three most frequent causes of chronic cough along with asthma and upper airways cough syndrome.
- The accurate, objective detection of both gastroesophageal reflux and cough and suitable statistical analysis are required to assess the association between the two phenomena. The development of impedance pH monitoring with simultaneous cough detection allows objective assessment of all types of reflux events and cough and the use of a statistic algorithm to relate both phenomena.
- Careful clinical selection of patients with suspected gastroesophageal reflux disease-related cough is important before starting treatment. These patients might receive either an empirical trial of double-dose proton pump inhibitor or diagnostic reflux-cough monitoring.

Potential pitfalls
- Cough and gastroesophageal reflux disease are very common presentations in a general population, and these two phenomena can co-exist without any causal association.
- The acidity of the refluxate might be unimportant if the esophagobronchial reflex is already sensitized. This would be one of the reasons why acid-suppressing therapy is less effective than anti-reflux surgery.
- Empirical treatment with proton pump inhibitor double dose for at least 3 months is widely used, but it should be noted that this strategy has not been supported by strong scientific evidence.

Introduction

Pathological gastroesophageal reflux (GER) usually results in typical symptoms, i.e. regurgitation and/or heartburn, but can also be associated with extraesophageal symptoms, such as asthma, laryngitis or chronic

---

Practical Manual of Gastroesophageal Reflux Disease, First Edition.
Edited by Marcelo F. Vela, Joel E. Richter and John E. Pandolfino.

cough [1]. According to the Montreal classification, gastroesophageal reflux disease (GERD)-related cough is regarded as one of the established extraesophageal syndromes of GERD [2].

Epidemiology

Gastroesophageal reflux disease is now considered to be one of the three most frequent etiologies of chronic cough together with asthma and upper airways cough syndrome (previously known as postnasal drip syndrome [3–5]. An epidemiological association between GERD and chronic cough has been recognized for many years and a prevalence of "reflux-related cough" has been reported with a wide range from 5% to 41% [6–10]. This large variation in prevalence can be due to differences in patient populations but is mainly due to the methodology used to establish the reflux-cough association, i.e questionnaires, cough during pH-metry, symptom responses to acid reflux therapies. Clinical awareness of GERD-related chronic cough, both from the pneumology and gastroenterology sides, has influenced the prevalence estimation. For example, studies published by Irwin's group have shown that the prevalence of GERD as the cause of chronic cough increased from 10% in 1981 [8], to 21% in 1990 [9] to 36% in 1998 [10].

Pathophysiology

Three main pathophysiological mechanisms have been proposed to explain the relationship between reflux and cough: microaspiration, activation of esophagobronchial vagal reflexes, and reflux-induced airway hypersensitivity.

Microaspiration

Microaspiration can be responsible for chronic cough by stimulating cough receptors directly. Several studies have suggested the possibility of arrival of gastric contents into the proximal airway. Laryngeal acidification has been demonstrated with transcutaneous pH measurements [11] and more recently, a technique developed to study aerosolized acid in the pharynx [12]. Microaspiration of refluxate can be demonstrated by the presence of gastric contents in bronchoalveolar lavage fluid (BALF) and sputum and suggested by their presence in saliva. Detection of lipid-laden macrophages in BALF or sputum has been used as a marker for microaspiration in children. Studies showed that lipid-laden alveolar macrophages were present in 85% of children with chronic respiratory tract disorders and GER

[13,14]. However, recent reports have shown that this method had low specificity and its prevalence in adult patients with chronic unexplained cough was unknown [15,16]. Pepsin and bile acids (BA) are currently assessed in saliva, sputum and BALF in patients with respiratory disorders. While pepsin and BA are clearly increased in patients with cystic fibrosis and lung transplant [17], there is no difference in pepsin concentrations of BALF between chronic cough patients and healthy controls [5]. Recent studies using impedance pH monitoring failed to demonstrate increased numbers of reflux episodes with high proximal extent in patients with chronic cough [18,19]. The current data suggest, therefore, that micro-aspiration is unlikely to be the most important mechanism for cough in these patients.

Esophagobronchial reflex

Esophagus, larynx, and bronchi are all innervated by the vagal nerve. The divergence of vagal afferent neurons in the brainstem may allow vagally mediated reflexes from the distal esophagus by chemical or mechanical stimuli [20]. Ing *et al.* reported that acid perfusion into the distal esophagus of patients with cough and GERD significantly increased cough frequency, when compared with saline infusion [21]. Topical esophageal anesthesia with lidocaine blocked acid-induced cough [21]. In contrast, when the anti-cholinergic agent ipratropium was instilled into the esophagus, there was no effect, whilst inhaled ipratropium inhibited cough, suggesting a vagally mediated esophagobronchial reflex. Such a reflex can be sensitized in patients with GERD and chronic cough [22,23]. These patients have a hypersensitive cough reflex to both capsaicin and citric acid inhalation. Reduced cough threshold due to prolonged acid exposure in the distal esophagus could be an important mechanism for chronic cough [24]. A lowered airway cough threshold becomes stimulus non-specific and any other stimulus, not necessarily reflux, would trigger cough, i.e. cold air, stress, etc. Interestingly, Benini *et al.* demonstrated that treatment with proton pump inhibitors (PPIs) could reverse the bronchial hypersensitivity [22].

Recent studies using multichannel intraluminal impedance pH (MII-pH) and objective cough recordings have shown that both acid and non-acid reflux events can be time associated with cough [18,25]. Furthermore, equal numbers of patients may have a positive reflux-cough association (Symptom Association Probability – SAP) with acid and non-acid reflux events [26]. These findings suggest that the acidity of reflux might be unimportant if the esophagobronchial reflex is already sensitized. Apart from the reflux-cough association, recent studies have shown evidence of cough-reflux sequences [25,26] which might result in a self-perpetuating cycle of reflux-cough-reflux in some patients. For further complexity, Smith *et al.* [26] suggested cough-induced reflux might occur by triggering of transient lower esophageal sphincter relaxation (TLESR). There might be a central sensitization mechanism that cough would induce TLESR.

Taken together, the current information suggests that reflux should not be considered as an independent single cause but rather as a contributing factor to chronic cough [27]. Finally, it should be noted that cough and GERD are very frequent in the general population, and these two phenomena can co-exist without any clinical pathophysiological relationship.

Clinical management

Patients with chronic cough are managed by internists, specialists in respiratory medicine or specialists in ear, nose, and throat (ENT) disorders. More recently, gastroenterologists have been involved to provide or reject evidence for the presence of gastroesophageal reflux that might or might not be related to the patient's cough.

A detailed anamnesis can help to identify increased reflux in patients with cough but up to 75% of patients with GERD-related cough do not have typical reflux symptoms (heartburn or regurgitation) [28]. There are some useful criteria, proposed by Irwin *et al.*, that allow identification of patients with a higher likelihood of having GERD as a cause for cough [4] (Box 11.1). Furthermore, Morice *et al.* recently proposed the Hull Airway Reflux Questionnaire (HARQ), which is self-administered and comprises 14 items with a maximum score of 70 [29]. The questionnaire is responsive to treatment; the minimum clinically significant change was estimated to be 16 points. The authors propose that it can be used as a diagnostic instrument in reflux-related cough [29].

Box 11.1 Criteria allowing identification of patients who are more likely to have GERD as a cause for cough

- Chronic cough (>8 weeks)
- Not on angiotensin-converting enzyme inhibitor
- Not a present smoker or exposed to other environmental irritants
- Chest radiograph is normal (or near normal)
- Symptomatic asthma has been ruled out*
- Upper airway cough syndrome has been ruled out*
- Eosinophilic bronchitis has been ruled out*

* By appropriate tests (e.g. normal sinus computed tomography scan, negative histamine provocation, normal sputum eosinophilia, no improvement on steroids). Modified from Irwin [4].

The clinical questionnaires may help the initial selection of patients. However, to establish an association between reflux and cough is a challenge, and depends upon the accurate detection of both GERD and cough, and also the appropriate statistical analysis used to understand the temporal relationship between these two phenomena. Finally, to establish a causal relationship between reflux and cough in an individual patient, treatment of reflux should improve cough.

Detection of reflux

Detection of reflux is described elsewhere in this book and this chapter briefly summarizes existing technology. Traditionally, acid reflux has been assessed in these patients using single or double pH monitoring [4]. More recently, impedance pH monitoring has been used, because it detects both acid and non-acid refluxes [18,25]. It can also detect presence of gas reflux and assess proximal extent of the refluxate. Since non-acid or weakly acid reflux can be associated with cough, impedance pH measurements might be preferable to pH-metry in patients with suspected GERD-related cough. Furthermore, a special catheter design can be used to detect acid and non-acid laryngopharyngeal reflux [30]. Finally, a pharyngeal pH-metry technique, using a newly designed pH sensor, is proposed to detect aerosolized acid (Restech Dx-pH Measurement System™, Respiratory Technology Corp., San Diego, CA) [12].

Detection of cough

The most widely available method is using a symptom marker on the reflux monitoring data logger, often with a study diary. This is very simple and useful to detect cough events, in particular during the daytime, if the patient's compliance is reasonably good. However, a significant number of cough events could be missed or not recorded, especially in nocturnal periods.

Manometric cough detection can be used during reflux monitoring [18,25,31]. This technique adds a second thin catheter with two pressure sensors positioned in the abdomen and thorax. Coughing provokes a typical pressure pattern. In this way, cough bursts are identified objectively and the presence of reflux before the cough can be recognized in a predetermined preceding time window [18,25]. Figure 11.1 shows an example of bursts of cough preceded by a reflux event using simultaneous monitoring of impedance pH and intraabdominal and thoracic pressure. More recently, microphone-based acoustic cough detection (with automatic cough recognition software) has been used to assess patients with reflux-related cough [26]. This method is very sensitive in detecting single cough events and is able to identify 2–3 times more cough events than the manometric method and 9–12 times more than patients' reported cough [26].

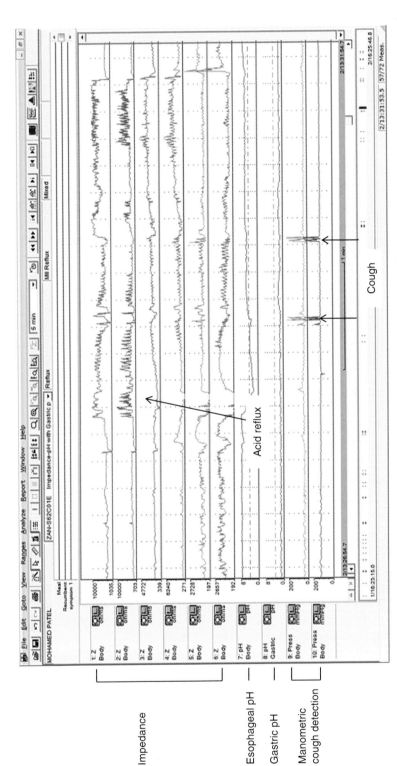

Figure 11.1 Simultaneous monitoring of impedance pH and intraabdominal and thoracic pressure. An acid reflux episode detected by impedance pH monitoring is followed by cough detected by pressure changes.

Finally, using even more advanced technology, Chang *et al.* [32] reported the use of an ambulatory device to measure pH, electromyograph and audio, designed to study reflux-cough in children.

Association between reflux and cough

Several statistical algorithms have been designed in order to analyze the time association between reflux and symptoms [33]. The Symptom Index (SI) has been defined as the percentage of reflux-associated symptom episodes in the total symptoms and is considered positive if >50%. The disadvantage of the SI is that it does not take into account the total number of reflux episodes and symptoms. The Symptom Association Probability (SAP) calculates the statistical relationship between symptoms and reflux episodes using Fischer's exact test, taking into account the number of associated reflux-symptom episodes as well as the total number of reflux and symptom events [34]. The SAP is considered positive when higher than 95% [33]. We and others [26] use a time window of 2 min to assess the association reflux-cough and we identified SAP-positive patients in whom the time association might not occur by chance. It is important to stress, however, that the SI and SAP were designed to study the relationship between reflux and heartburn or chest pain, and not for the reflux-cough association. The optimal time window for GERD-related cough needs further investigation.

Finally, Hersh *et al.* recently reported hierarchical use of parameters from ambulatory pH testing in predicting response to anti-reflux medical therapy in patients with suspected GERD-related cough [35]. The study showed that the highest likelihood of a sustained, durable response (high degree response) to anti-reflux therapy was achieved when acid exposure time, SAP, and SI were all positive.

Treatment

Medical treatment

If increased GER does provoke chronic cough, treatment of GERD should improve cough. Empiric trials with PPI (without investigation of GERD) and lifestyle modifications have been proposed by the American College of Chest Physicians [4] and the British Thoracic Society [36]. This empiric strategy was reported to be effective in a community-based patient population in the US [37]. However, published studies of anti-reflux medical treatments in patients with cough are inconsistent. Kiljander *et al.*, in a prospective, double-blind, placebo-controlled trial, reported significant improvement of cough after 8 weeks of PPI treatment (omeprazole 40 mg o.d.) [38]. Ours *et al.* reported improvement or resolution of cough in 35% of patients with GERD-related cough after 12 weeks of PPI treatment (omeprazole 40 mg b.i.d.) [39]. In contrast, more recent studies have shown no significant improvement of cough after PPI therapy [40,41]. The most recent Cochrane review concluded that: "PPI is not efficacious for cough associated with GORD symptoms in very young children (including infants) and should not be used for cough outcomes. In adults, there is insufficient evidence to conclude definitely that GORD treatment with PPI is universally beneficial for cough associated with GORD. Future paediatric and adult studies should be double-blind, randomized, controlled and parallel design, using treatments for at least 2 months, with validated subjective and objective cough outcomes" [42].

In a subgroup of patients, a possible reason for ineffective PPI therapy could be an association between non-acid reflux and cough. Such association can be assessed using impedance pH monitoring [18,25]. In general, patients presenting with a positive SAP between weakly acidic reflux and cough do not have increased numbers of weakly acidic reflux events, suggesting the possibility of hypersensitivity to such refluxate.

A key mechanism of GER is known to be TLESR. Baclofen is a gamma-aminobutyric acid (GABAB) agonist that reduces the number of reflux episodes by reducing the number of TLESRs. Baclofen was reported to reduce numbers of acid and weakly acidic reflux events and also has an antitussive effect by altering cough reflex [43,44]. However, baclofen is known to have significant side-effects and patient tolerability is relatively low [45]. New GABAB agonists and other medications to reduce TLESRs and reflux with fewer neurological side-effects are currently under development and might be of potential benefit for GERD-related cough.

Prokinetics drugs are frequently used in GERD treatment to accelerate gastric emptying and improve esophageal motility. Their efficacy in GERD-related cough has not been formally tested. Azithromycin (AZI) belongs to the group of macrolide antibiotics, which are known to have prokinetic effects, and often used in lung transplant patients to prevent bronchiolitis obliterans syndrome [46]. In lung transplant patients, standard esophageal pH monitoring revealed an increased acid exposure in 70% [47,48]. Mertens *et al.* studied the effect of AZI on GER in lung transplant patients and found that AZI reduced esophageal acid and volume exposure as well as the number of proximal reflux events [49]. AZI is currently under investigation in patients with reflux-associated cough.

Surgical treatment

Fundoplication is an alternative to medical treatment for GERD. The procedure is known to be highly effective in reducing esophageal acid exposure time and reflux symptoms [50]. Various mechanisms are responsible for a decrease in reflux frequency after fundoplication, i.e. correction of the anatomy with reduction of a hiatus hernia, reduction in number of TLESRs, increased residual pressure during TLESRs, increased basal LES pressure, and possible reduction in volume of refluxate [51,52]. More recently, Broeders *et al.* showed that fundoplication similarly controlled acid and weakly acidic reflux, but gas reflux is reduced to a lesser extent [53].

In patients with clearly demonstrated association between reflux and cough, anti-reflux surgery would be a treatment option. To date, outcomes of uncontrolled studies in surgical treatments are encouraging [54–59]. These studies showed that 56–100% of surgically treated patients with cough had a positive response.

Allen and Anvari [58,59] proposed reported factors predicting good symptom outcome after reflux surgery. The results indicated that a positive Bernstein test, a higher preoperative cough symptom score and a good cough response to PPI therapy were factors predicting good surgical outcome in patients with suspected reflux-induced cough. Mainie showed that a positive SI between non-acid reflux and cough was a good predictor of surgical outcome [54]. Hersh *et al.* [35] showed that 67% of patients who had anti-reflux surgery achieved a long-term high-degree response. Allen and Anvari reported long-term outcomes in 528 surgically treated patients by using a validated cough scale [59]. Over 5-year periods, they found a decrease in the cough response from 83% (6 months post surgery) down to 71% (5 years post surgery).

Although outcomes of uncontrolled surgical studies are encouraging, controlled studies are absolutely necessary to define the real role of anti-reflux surgery in GER-related cough. This is even more important when considering surgery in patients not responding to PPI but with a positive association between non-acid reflux and cough.

Management of patients with suspected gastroesophageal reflux disease-related cough

Management of patients with suspected GERD-related cough is difficult and a real challenge. In our unit we follow the management strategy proposed by Galmiche *et al.* [60] (Figure 11.2). The first step involves careful exclusion of other causes of cough and consideration of clinical criteria that suggest a possible reflux-cough association (see Box 11.1).

There are two possible pathways: empirical trial with PPI and diagnostic investigations, including high-resolution manometry and simultaneous reflux-cough monitoring. We use a pressure-based objective cough-detecting system to assess the temporal reflux-cough association. The SAP plays an important role in our strategy [18,26]. The empirical strategy with PPI

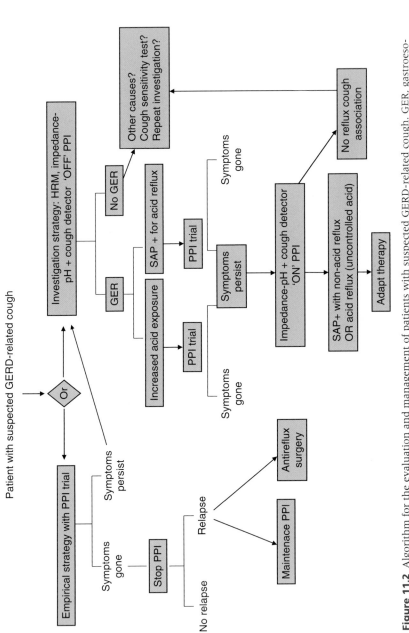

Figure 11.2 Algorithm for the evaluation and management of patients with suspected GERD-related cough. GER, gastroesophageal reflux; GERD: gastroesophageal reflux disease; HRM, high resolution manometry; PPI, proton pump inhibitor; SAP, symptom association probability.

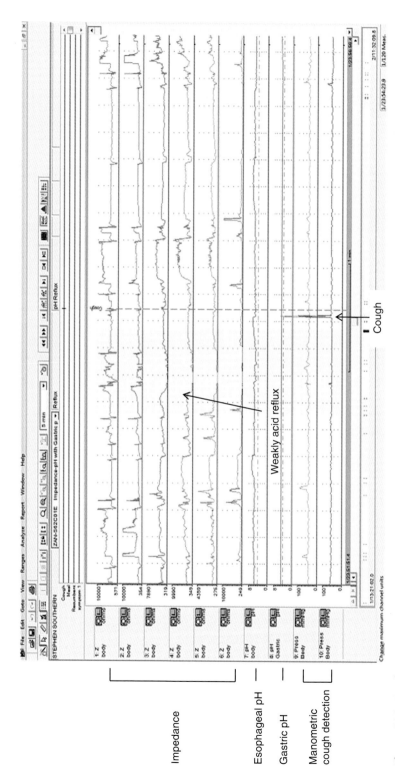

Figure 11.3 Simultaneous monitoring of impedance pH and intra abdominal and thoracic pressure in a patient who is acid suppressed with a proton pump inhibitor (PPI). A weakly acidic reflux episode (reflux detected by impedance, pH remains above 4) detected by impedance pH monitoring is followed by a cough event.

CASE STUDY

A respiratory physician referred a 47-year-old female patient who had been suffering with chronic cough that significantly affected her quality of life. Her cough symptoms were more frequent during the day. She was a non-smoker and investigations excluded asthma and upper airway syndrome. High-resolution manometry showed intermittent hypotensive peristalsis. Simultaneous 24-h impedance pH and cough monitoring "off" PPI showed increased acid exposure (9.2% day, 0.9% night) with positive SAP between cough and acid reflux. The patient had already had an unsuccessful empirical PPI trial but only with single dose. PPI double-dose therapy was initially effective for 3 weeks, but her cough reoccurred and became troublesome. Simultaneous 24-h impedance pH and cough monitoring "on" PPI showed reasonable gastric acid suppression, but positive SAP between cough and weakly acidic reflux (Figure 11.3). The patient was referred to a gastrointestinal surgeon to discuss possible anti-reflux surgery. She decided to have surgery and symptoms improved significantly (6 months post surgery).

---

double dose for at least 3 months is simple and widely used, but it should be noted that this strategy has not been supported by strong scientific evidence. When the empirical trial of PPI is successful, patients should stop taking PPI for further symptom evaluation. If symptoms relapse, maintenance PPI therapy or anti-reflux surgery can be considered but reflux and cough monitoring prior to surgery is strongly recommended.

When the empirical trial of PPI fails, patients should move on to the investigation strategy, including reflux and cough monitoring. We perform high-resolution manometry to assess esophageal motility and prokinetic agents can be added if esophageal hypomotility is associated with liquid retention and proximal retrograde flow (as detected with impedance). Reflux-cough monitoring is performed "off" PPI, with special emphasis given to analyzing the total esophageal acid exposure, a severe supine acid reflux pattern and a temporal relationship between cough and acid reflux episodes at this stage. In patients without evidence of GERD, further investigations to identify underlying problems other than reflux should be performed. Patients with increased esophageal acid exposure and/or positive SAP for acid reflux will receive PPI double dose. If the PPI trial fails to improve cough, a new reflux-cough monitoring is performed "on" PPI. This can identify patients with residual acid reflux (in spite of PPI) or patients with non-acid reflux-related cough.

Summary

Gastroesophageal reflux disease is considered to be one of the three most frequent etiologies of chronic cough along with asthma and upper airways cough syndrome. Different mechanisms can be responsible for GERD-related cough, i.e. microaspiration, esophagobronchial reflex and central sensitization of the cough reflex [26]. The diagnosis and management of reflux-related cough are a difficult challenge. The development of impedance pH monitoring with simultaneous cough detection allows a more objective assessment of all types of reflux events and cough [18,26]. Empirical PPI treatment is widely used. The response rate to PPI treatment appeared to be rather poor. Studies have suggested that acidity of the refluxate is not critical when the esophagobronchial reflex has already been sensitized, which is one of the reasons for failed acid-suppressing treatments. Anti-reflux surgery has been performed successfully on a group of patients with GERD-related cough in uncontrolled trials. However, controlled, prospective studies are necessary to confirm the role of anti-reflux surgery in the management of GERD-related cough.

Management strategies for patients with suspected GERD-related cough include empirical PPI trial and reflux-cough investigation. In our unit, simultaneous monitoring of reflux and cough "off" PPI is performed first. Evidence of GERD and SAP between reflux and cough are important parameters for managing patients further. For patients who do not respond to double-dose PPI trial, simultaneous reflux and cough monitoring is repeated "on" PPI. This identifies patients with a positive SAP between weakly acidic reflux and cough, or patients with PPI resistance.

References

1 Richter JE. Review article: extraoesophageal manifestations of gastro-oesophageal reflux disease. Aliment Pharmacol Ther 2005;22(Suppl 1):70–80.

2 Vakil N, van Zanten SV, Kahrilas P, Dent J, Jones R, Group GC. The Montreal definition and classification of gastroesophageal reflux disease: a global evidence-based consensus. Am J Gastroenterol 2006;101(8):1900–20; quiz 43.

3 Pratter MR. Chronic upper airway cough syndrome secondary to rhinosinus diseases (previously referred to as postnasal drip syndrome): ACCP evidence-based clinical practice guidelines. Chest 2006;129(1 Suppl):63S–71S.

4 Irwin RS. Chronic cough due to gastroesophageal reflux disease: ACCP evidence-based clinical practice guidelines. Chest 2006;129(1 Suppl):80S–94S.

5 Smith J, Woodcock A, Houghton L. New developments in reflux-associated cough. Lung 2010;188(Suppl 1):S81–6.

6 Marchesani F, Cecarini L, Pela R, Sanguinetti CM. Causes of chronic persistent cough in adult patients: the results of a systematic management protocol. Monaldi Arch Chest Dis 1998;53(5):510–14.

7 Palombini BC, Villanova CA, Araújo E, et al. A pathogenic triad in chronic cough: asthma, postnasal drip syndrome, and gastroesophageal reflux disease. Chest 1999;116(2):279–84.

8 Irwin RS, Corrao WM, Pratter MR. Chronic persistent cough in the adult: the spectrum and frequency of causes and successful outcome of specific therapy. Am Rev Respir Dis 1981;123(4 Pt 1):413–17.

9 Irwin RS, Curley FJ, French CL. Chronic cough. The spectrum and frequency of causes, key components of the diagnostic evaluation, and outcome of specific therapy. Am Rev Respir Dis 1990;141(3):640–7.

10 French CL, Irwin RS, Curley FJ, Krikorian CJ. Impact of chronic cough on quality of life. Arch Intern Med 1998;158(15):1657–61.

11 Ledson MJ, Wilson GE, Tran J, Walshaw MJ. Tracheal microaspiration in adult cystic fibrosis. J Roy Soc Med 1998;91(1):10–12.

12 Sun G, Muddana S, Slaughter JC, et al. A new pH catheter for laryngopharyngeal reflux: normal values. Laryngoscope 2009;119(8):1639–43.

13 Ahrens P, Noll C, Kitz R, Willigens P, Zielen S, Hofmann D. Lipid-laden alveolar macrophages (LLAM): a useful marker of silent aspiration in children. Pediatr Pulmonol 1999;28(2):83–8.

14 Parameswaran K, Anvari M, Efthimiadis A, Kamada D, Hargreave FE, Allen CJ. Lipid-laden macrophages in induced sputum are a marker of oropharyngeal reflux and possible gastric aspiration. Eur Respir J 2000;16(6):1119–22.

15 Köksal D, Ozkan B, Simşek C, Köksal AS, Ağaçkýran Y, Saşmaz N. Lipid-laden alveolar macrophage index in sputum is not useful in the differential diagnosis of pulmonary symptoms secondary to gastroesophageal reflux. Arch Med Res 2005;36(5):485–9.

16 Krishnan U, Mitchell JD, Tobias V, Day AS, Bohane TD. Fat laden macrophages in tracheal aspirates as a marker of reflux aspiration: a negative report. J Pediatr Gastroenterol Nutr 2002;35(3):309–13.

17 Blondeau K, Mertens V, Vanaudenaerde BA, et al. Gastro-oesophageal reflux and gastric aspiration in lung transplant patients with or without chronic rejection. Eur Respir J 2008;31(4):707–13.

18 Blondeau K, Dupont LJ, Mertens V, Tack J, Sifrim D. Improved diagnosis of gastro-oesophageal reflux in patients with unexplained chronic cough. Aliment Pharmacol Ther 2007;25(6):723–32.

19 Smith JA, Abdulqawi R, Houghton LA. GERD-related cough: pathophysiology and diagnostic approach. Curr Gastroenterol Rep 2011;13(3):247–56.

20 Irwin RS, Zawacki JK, Curley FJ, French CL, Hoffman PJ. Chronic cough as the sole presenting manifestation of gastroesophageal reflux. Am Rev Respir Dis 1989;140(5):1294–300.

21 Ing AJ, Ngu MC, Breslin AB. Pathogenesis of chronic persistent cough associated with gastroesophageal reflux. Am J Respir Crit Care Med 1994;149(1):160–7.

22 Benini L, Ferrari M, Sembenini C, et al. Cough threshold in reflux oesophagitis: influence of acid and of laryngeal and oesophageal damage. Gut 2000;46(6): 762–7.

23 Javorkova N, Varechova S, Pecova R, et al. Acidification of the oesophagus acutely increases the cough sensitivity in patients with gastro-oesophageal reflux and chronic cough. Neurogastroenterol Motil 2008;20(2):119–24.

24 Benini L, Ferrari M, Talamini G, Vantini I. Reflux associated cough is usually not associated with reflux: role of reduced cough threshold. Gut 2006;55(4):583; author reply 584.

25 Sifrim D, Dupont L, Blondeau K, Zhang X, Tack J, Janssens J. Weakly acidic reflux in patients with chronic unexplained cough during 24 hour pressure, pH, and impedance monitoring. Gut 2005;54(4):449–54.

26 Smith JA, Decalmer S, Kelsall A, et al. Acoustic cough-reflux associations in chronic cough: potential triggers and mechanisms. Gastroenterology 2010;139(3):754–62.

27 Kahrilas PJ. Chronic cough and gastroesophageal reflux disease: new twists to the riddle. Gastroenterology 2010;139(3):716–18.

28 Irwin RS, French CL, Curley FJ, Zawacki JK, Bennett FM. Chronic cough due to gastroesophageal reflux. Clinical, diagnostic, and pathogenetic aspects. Chest 2009;136(5 Suppl):e30.

29 Morice AH, Faruqi S, Wright CE, Thompson R, Bland JM. Cough hypersensitivity syndrome: a distinct clinical entity. Lung 2011;189(1):73–9.

30 Maldonado A, Diederich L, Castell DO, Gideon RM, Katz PO. Laryngopharyngeal reflux identified using a new catheter design: defining normal values and excluding artifacts. Laryngoscope 2003;113(2):349–55.

31 Paterson WG, Murat BW. Combined ambulatory esophageal manometry and dual-probe pH-metry in evaluation of patients with chronic unexplained cough. Dig Dis Sci 1994;39(5):1117–25.

32 Chang AB, Connor FL, Petsky HL, et al. An objective study of acid reflux and cough in children using an ambulatory pHmetry-cough logger. Arch Dis Child 2011; 96(5):468–72.

33 Bredenoord AJ, Weusten BL, Smout AJ. Symptom association analysis in ambulatory gastro-oesophageal reflux monitoring. Gut 2005;54(12):1810–17.

34 Weusten BL, Roelofs JM, Akkermans LM, Van Berge-Henegouwen GP, Smout AJ. The symptom-association probability: an improved method for symptom analysis of 24-hour esophageal pH data. Gastroenterology 1994;107(6):1741–5.

35 Hersh MJ, Sayuk GS, Gyawali CP. Long-term therapeutic outcome of patients undergoing ambulatory pH monitoring for chronic unexplained cough. J Clin Gastroenterol 2010;44(4):254–60.

36 Morice AH, McGarvey L, Pavord I, British Thoracic Society Cough Guideline Group. Recommendations for the management of cough in adults. Thorax 2006;61(Suppl 1):i1–24.

37 Poe RH, Kallay MC. Chronic cough and gastroesophageal reflux disease: experience with specific therapy for diagnosis and treatment. Chest 2003;123(3):679–84.

38 Kiljander TO, Salomaa ER, Hietanen EK, Terho EO. Chronic cough and gastro-oesophageal reflux: a double-blind placebo-controlled study with omeprazole. Eur Respir J 2000;16(4):633–8.

39 Ours TM, Kavuru MS, Schilz RJ, Richter JE. A prospective evaluation of esophageal testing and a double-blind, randomized study of omeprazole in a diagnostic and therapeutic algorithm for chronic cough. Am J Gastroenterol 1999;94(11):3131–8.

40 Poe RH, Harder RV, Israel RH, Kallay MC. Chronic persistent cough. Experience in diagnosis and outcome using an anatomic diagnostic protocol. Chest 1989;95(4):723–8.

41 Shaheen NJ, Crockett SD, Bright SD, et al. Randomised clinical trial: high-dose acid suppression for chronic cough – a double-blind, placebo-controlled study. Aliment Pharmacol Ther 2011;33(2):225–34.

42 Chang AB, Lasserson TJ, Gaffney J, Connor FL, Garske LA. Gastro-oesophageal reflux treatment for prolonged non-specific cough in children and adults. Cochrane Database Syst Rev 2011;1:CD004823.

43 Vela MF, Tutuian R, Katz PO, Castell DO. Baclofen decreases acid and non-acid postprandial gastro-oesophageal reflux measured by combined multichannel intraluminal impedance and pH. Aliment Pharmacol Ther 2003;17(2):243–51.

44 Dicpinigaitis PV, Grimm DR, Lesser M. Baclofen-induced cough suppression in cervical spinal cord injury. Arch Phys Med Rehabil 2000;81(7):921–3.

45 Lehmann A. GABAB receptors as drug targets to treat gastroesophageal reflux disease. Pharmacol Ther 2009;122(3):239–45.

46 Trulock EP, Edwards LB, Taylor DO, et al. Registry of the International Society for Heart and Lung Transplantation: twenty-third official adult lung and heart–lung transplantation report –2006. J Heart Lung Transplant 2006;25(8):880–92.

47 Benden C, Aurora P, Curry J, Whitmore P, Priestley L, Elliott MJ. High prevalence of gastroesophageal reflux in children after lung transplantation. Pediatr Pulmonol 2005;40(1):68–71.

48 D'Ovidio F, Mura M, Ridsdale R, *et al*. The effect of reflux and bile acid aspiration on the lung allograft and its surfactant and innate immunity molecules SP-A and SP-D. Am J Transplant 2006;6(8):1930–8.

49 Mertens V, Blondeau K, Pauwels A, *et al*. Azithromycin reduces gastroesophageal reflux and aspiration in lung transplant recipients. Dig Dis Sci 2009;54(5):972–9.

50 Draaisma WA, Rijnhart-de Jong HG, Broeders IA, Smout AJ, Furnee EJ, Gooszen HG. Five-year subjective and objective results of laparoscopic and conventional Nissen fundoplication: a randomized trial. Ann Surg 2006;244(1):34–41.

51 Lindeboom MA, Ringers J, Straathof JW, van Rijn PJ, Neijenhuis P, Masclee AA. Effect of laparoscopic partial fundoplication on reflux mechanisms. Am J Gastroenterol 2003;98(1):29–34.

52 Bredenoord AJ, Draaisma WA, Weusten BL, Gooszen HG, Smout AJ. Mechanisms of acid, weakly acidic and gas reflux after anti-reflux surgery. Gut 2008;57(2):161–6.

53 Broeders JA, Bredenoord AJ, Hazebroek EJ, Broeders IA, Gooszen HG, Smout AJ. Effects of anti-reflux surgery on weakly acidic reflux and belching. Gut 2011; 60(4):435–41.

54 Mainie I, Tutuian R, Agrawal A, *et al*. Fundoplication eliminates chronic cough due to non-acid reflux identified by impedance pH monitoring. Thorax 2005;60(6):521–3.

55 Mainie I, Tutuian R, Agrawal A, Adams D, Castell DO. Combined multichannel intra-luminal impedance-pH monitoring to select patients with persistent gastro-oesophageal reflux for laparoscopic Nissen fundoplication. Br J Surg 2006; 93(12):1483–7.

56 So JB, Zeitels SM, Rattner DW. Outcomes of atypical symptoms attributed to gastro-esophageal reflux treated by laparoscopic fundoplication. Surgery 1998;124(1): 28–32.

57 Irwin RS, Zawacki JK, Wilson MM, French CT, Callery MP. Chronic cough due to gastroesophageal reflux disease: failure to resolve despite total/near-total elimination of esophageal acid. Chest 2002;121(4):1132–40.

58 Allen CJ, Anvari M. Preoperative symptom evaluation and esophageal acid infusion predict response to laparoscopic Nissen fundoplication in gastroesophageal reflux patients who present with cough. Surg Endosc 2002;16(7):1037–41.

59 Allen CJ, Anvari M. Does laparoscopic fundoplication provide long-term control of gastroesophageal reflux related cough? Surg Endosc 2004;18(4):633–7.

60 Galmiche JP, Zerbib F, Bruley des Varannes S. Review article: respiratory manifestations of gastro-oesophageal reflux disease. Aliment Pharmacol Ther 2008;27(6): 449–64.

CHAPTER 12

Relationship between Gastroesophageal Reflux Disease and Sleep

Tiberiu Hershcovici and Ronnie Fass

Neuroenteric Clinical Research Group, Section of Gastroenterology, Department of Medicine, Southern Arizona VA Health Care System and University of Arizona School of Medicine, Tucson, AZ, USA and Division of Gastroenterology and Hepatology, MetroHealth Medical Center, Case Western Reserve University, Cleveland, OH, USA

Key points

- Approximately half the patients with gastroesophageal reflux disease report heartburn that awakens them from sleep during the night.
- Nighttime reflux has been more commonly associated with gastroesophageal reflux disease complications.
- Gastroesophageal reflux disease and sleep demonstrate a bidirectional relationship.
- Nighttime gastroesophageal reflux occurs primarily after patients' arousal from sleep.
- Sleep deprivation due to gastroesophageal reflux disease is markedly improved after treatment with a proton pump inhibitor.

Potential pitfalls

- Nighttime reflux has not been clearly defined in the literature, and may not necessarily denote reflux during sleep (it may reflect reflux while recumbent but awake).
- It is very unusual for gastroesophageal reflux disease patients to have nighttime reflux alone.
- Gastroesophageal reflux may still be associated with awakening from sleep, even if patients report no gastroesophageal reflux disease-related symptoms.
- Proton pump inhibitor therapy has been shown to improve sleep quality using subjective but not objective tools.

Introduction

Gastroesophageal reflux disease (GERD) is a chronic disorder and the most common disease that affects the esophagus. A population-based study estimated that 20% of the US adult population experience GERD-related

---

Practical Manual of Gastroesophageal Reflux Disease, First Edition.
Edited by Marcelo F. Vela, Joel E. Richter and John E. Pandolfino.
© 2013 John Wiley & Sons, Ltd. Published 2013 by John Wiley & Sons, Ltd.

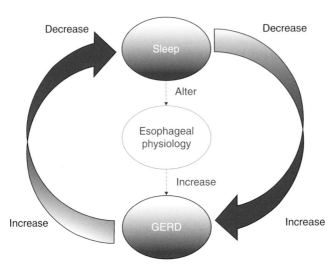

Figure 12.1 The bidirectional relationship between gastroesophageal reflux disease (GERD) and sleep.

symptoms at least once a week [1]. GERD can lead to esophageal mucosal injury in a subset of patients as well as bothersome symptoms, such as heartburn and acid regurgitation, that may affect patients' reported quality of life.

Gastroesophageal reflux (GER) may occur during both daytime and nighttime periods [2]. Studies have demonstrated that up to 79% of GERD patients experience nighttime symptoms. Of all GERD patients, 65% experience both nighttime and daytime symptoms [3–6]. It has been estimated that 13% of GERD patients experience nighttime symptoms only. Of the patients with nocturnal heartburn, 75% reported that the symptoms affected their sleep, and 40% stated that symptoms affected their ability to function the following day.

Recent studies have suggested a bidirectional relationship between GERD and sleep. GERD has been shown to adversely affect sleep by awakening patients from sleep during the night or more commonly by leading to multiple short amnestic arousals, resulting in sleep fragmentation. At the same time, sleep deprivation *per se* can adversely affect GERD by enhancing perception of intraesophageal acid (esophageal hypersensitivity) and potentially by increasing esophageal acid exposure [7]. In fact, there is a potential "vicious cycle" in which GERD leads to poor quality of sleep, which then in turn enhances perception of intraesophageal stimuli that further exacerbates GERD (Figure 12.1) [8].

Nighttime reflux has been demonstrated to be associated with a more aggressive presentation of GERD (erosive esophagitis, complications of GERD, Barrett's esophagus, and adenocarcinoma of the esophagus) [9–15].

In addition, these patients have a higher prevalence of oropharyngeal, laryngeal, and pulmonary manifestations [12, 16]. Poor quality of sleep and a variety of sleep disturbances have been recently added to the growing list of extraesophageal manifestations of GERD [17]. Most importantly, the overall quality of life of patients with nighttime heartburn appears to be significantly worse than the quality of life of patients with daytime heartburn only [5].

Sleep

There is growing evidence that sleep has an important role in maintaining good health. However, at the same time there is evidence that average nightly sleep duration has declined by 2 h in the last century and that many people sleep no more than 5–6 h instead of the needed 7–8 h per night [18]. Approximately 20% of the population regularly experiences fits of irresistible daytime sleepiness, 10–15% have severe or chronic insomnia, and 50–60% of older people report sleep abnormalities.

Sleep deprivation has a profound impact on people's quality of life and has far-reaching implications on subjects' mental and physical health. Sleep deprivation makes people prone to accidents, more irritable, and often listless. It leads to decreased creativity and enthusiasm, memory impairment, and limited comprehension and attention span. In addition, it has been associated with psychiatric disorders, mood impairment, dementia, heart disease, metabolic disorder, and reduced immune function. Recently, studies have shown that sleep deprivation can lead to glucose intolerance, diabetes mellitus, and obesity. Sleep should be considered as one of the pillars of good health, equivalent to diet and exercise.

Polysomnography (PSG) has traditionally been considered the gold standard for objectively assessing sleep. Sleep is scored as non-rapid eye movement (NREM) and rapid eye movement on the basis of the electroencephalogram (EEG) component of PSG. NREM accounts for 75–80% of total sleep time in normal human adults and consists of three stages. Stage N1 involves transition of EEG from alpha-waves (frequently seen in drowsy state or during quiet wakefulness with eyes closed and having a frequency of 8–13 Hz) to theta-waves (frequency 4–7 Hz) along with significant changes in respiration, heart rate, and cerebral blood flow. Stage N2 is a deeper sleep stage characterized by low-amplitude background superimposed with two morphologically distinct waveforms: sleep spindles (11–16 Hz) and K-complexes. Stage N3 or slow-wave sleep is characterized by delta-waves (0.5–2 Hz) and is considered to be the deepest stage of sleep. Beta-waves are seen during awake and alert stages.

Epidemiology

Nighttime heartburn or regurgitation has long been used as a clinical marker for nocturnal reflux. Unfortunately, the literature is devoid of a widely accepted definition for nighttime heartburn. More disconcerting is the fact that almost all studies assessing the prevalence or therapeutic response of patients with nighttime heartburn lacked a clear definition of nocturnal GERD [1,3,19,20]. Farup *et al.* offered the following definition of nighttime GERD: nocturnal awakening by GERD symptoms; nocturnal awakening caused by coughing or choking, regurgitation of fluid or food, and acidic/bitter taste; GERD symptoms while in the supine position; and morning awakening secondary to GERD symptoms [21]. This is an inclusive definition that may include patients who experience GERD-related symptoms in the supine position while still awake. In contrast, Fass *et al.* suggested that nighttime heartburn should be defined as heartburn that awakens patients from sleep during the night [22]. While this is a much more restrictive definition, it underscores the importance of having GERD-related symptoms during sleep physiology.

Overall, the epidemiology of nocturnal gastroesophageal reflux is not well studied. According to a Gallup poll in which 1000 subjects with GERD completed the survey, 75% of the participants reported that GERD symptoms affected their sleep, and 63% believed that heartburn negatively affected their ability to sleep well [19]. Additionally, 42% stated that they were unable to sleep through a full night, 39% had to take naps during the day, and 34% were sleeping in a seated position. Interestingly, 27% reported that their heartburn-induced sleep disturbances kept their spouse from having a good night's sleep. The prevalence of sleep disturbances among respondents increased with increase in frequency of the nighttime heartburn episodes during the week. In a study by Farup *et al.*, 74% of subjects with frequent GERD symptoms reported nocturnal GERD symptoms [21]. In contrast, Locke *et al.* found in a community-based survey that 47% and 34% of GERD sufferers reported nocturnal heartburn and nocturnal acid regurgitation, respectively [1]. However, in the first two studies, only 57% and 54% of the patients, respectively, reported heartburn that awakened them from sleep during the night. Fass *et al.*, in a large prospective, cohort study of subjects evaluated for sleep disturbances, demonstrated that 24.9% reported heartburn during sleep [22]. Recently, it was demonstrated that heartburn that awakens patients from sleep during the night is highly predictive for GERD [23]. This effect was further accentuated in morbidly obese subjects.

In general, sleep disturbances in patients with GERD are poorly recognized and rarely elicited during clinic visits despite the significant impact of these disturbances on patients' quality of life and perception of the severity of their disease. When 759 patients with non-erosive reflux disease (NERD), who were enrolled in the esomeprazole (Nexium) clinical trial program, were assessed by a quality-of-life tool for "sleep disturbances for at least some of the time" (score≤4), 50% reported that symptoms of GERD were responsible for difficulties in getting a good night's sleep [24]. Other indicators of sleep disturbances were "feeling tired/worn out due to lack of sleep" (42%), "failure to wake up feeling fresh/rested" (41%), "having trouble falling asleep" (40%), and "heartburn/acid regurgitation waking the patient and preventing him/her from falling asleep" (35%) [24]. Additionally, nocturnal reflux may present with nighttime cough, wheezing, sore throat, choking, and other symptoms [25]. In one series, it was demonstrated that patients with nighttime heartburn were more likely to report wheezing (odds ratio (OR) 2.5), breathlessness at rest (OR 2.8), and nocturnal breathlessness (OR 2.9). These subjects also had increased peak flow variability compared with subjects without gastroesophageal reflux [26]. Furthermore, insomnia, repeated awakening during the night, snoring, tossing and turning, and even nightmares have all been related to nocturnal GER.

A recent national patient-reported survey quantified the effects of GERD symptoms on sleep difficulties and their effects on outcomes [27]. Of 11,685 survey respondents with GERD, 88.9% experienced nighttime symptoms, 68.3% sleep difficulties, 49.1% difficulty initiating asleep (induction symptoms), and 58.3% difficulty maintaining sleep (maintenance symptoms). Respondents with nighttime GERD symptoms were more likely to experience sleep difficulties (OR 1.53) and difficulties with induction (OR 1.43) and maintenance (OR 1.56) of sleep ($P < 0.001$ for all). Sleep difficulties were associated with a 5.5% increase in overall work impairment, and reductions of 3.1 and 3.6 points in Short Form (SF)-8 physical and mental summary scores, respectively.

Gastroesophageal physiology during sleep

The accentuated noxious effects of nocturnal reflux are driven primarily by decrease in saliva production, swallowing rate, primary and secondary esophageal peristalsis, gastric emptying, and conscious perception of reflux events (Box 12.1) [2]. The normal esophageal defense mechanisms are pivotal for preventing mucosal injury during acid reflux events.

Sleep impairs esophageal acid clearance in both GERD patients and healthy controls [28]. It has been shown that the clearance time is significantly prolonged when sleep was maintained compared with the awakening period. Overall, acid clearance occurs predominantly in association

> **Box 12.1 Physiological changes during sleep that affect gastroesophageal reflux**
>
> • Decreased salivary secretion and flow
> • Decreased swallowing rate
> • Decreased primary esophageal peristalsis
> • Decreased secondary esophageal peristalsis
> • Decreased upper esophageal sphincter pressure
> • Decreased perception of intraesophageal stimuli

with arousals from sleep. Furthermore, esophageal clearance time during sleep remains prolonged regardless of the pH or the volume of the refluxate [29,30]. Sleep, but not body position, is a significant factor for acid migration to the proximal esophagus for even minute volumes of acid reflux and markedly prolongs acid clearance [31].

In the awake state, the contact of esophageal mucosa with acid produces a response characterized by enhanced salivary bicarbonate secretion and flow and increased swallowing frequency. These physiological responses serve to propel the refluxate aborally from the distal esophagus into the stomach as well as neutralizing the pH of the esophageal lumen. However, during sleep, salivary secretion and flow are virtually absent [32] and the swallowing frequency is markedly reduced from 25 per hour during the awake state to approximately five per hour during sleep [33].

Upper esophageal sphincter (UES) pressure progressively declines with deeper stages of sleep, resulting in an increased risk of reflux that can reach the larynx, pharynx, and pulmonary system [34,35]. Transient lower esophageal sphincter (LES) relaxation and gastroesophageal reflux occur primarily during transient arousals from sleep or when the subjects are fully awake [36]. Furthermore, acid reflux events may occur during either prolonged awake periods or brief arousals [37]. Overall, LES basal pressure is not affected during sleep.

Esophageal acid clearance and airway protection are dependent on secondary esophageal peristalsis and the esophago-upper esophageal sphincter contractile reflex (EUCR) [38–40]. The rate of secondary esophageal peristalsis (defined as non-deglutitive esophageal peristalsis initiated by esophageal distension) [41] decreases progressively with deeper sleep stages and is absent during slow-wave sleep [42,43]. EUCR is a reflex contraction of the UES in response to esophageal distension [38]. Bajaj *et al.* evaluated EUCR and secondary esophageal peristalsis elicitation in 13 normal subjects during different sleep stages [44]. EUCR and secondary esophageal peristalsis were elicited by infusion of small volumes of water into the proximal esophagus after sleep confirmation by polysomnography.

It was possible to elicit EUCR and secondary esophageal peristalsis during stage 2 and REM sleep. Their activation occurred before arousal and helped clear the esophagus. However, during slow-wave sleep (stages 3 and 4), EUCR and secondary peristalsis could not be triggered. Instead, the infusion induced arousal and coughing. During these sleep stages, esophageal clearance occurred only during arousals by swallow-induced primary peristalsis.

There is also evidence that gastric emptying is significantly slower for solid food during late evening hours [45]. A decrease in the frequency of gastric slow wave was noted during non-REM sleep, which returned to normal during REM sleep [46]. These sleep changes in gastric emptying may promote nighttime reflux, although their effect was not specifically studied in GERD patients.

Sleep is an altered state of consciousness, resulting in reduced perception of visceral events. Consequently, conscious-dependent defensive behavior against gastroesophageal reflux (antacid consumption, assuming the upright position, initiating a swallow, etc.) is markedly affected during this period [47].

Pathophysiology of nocturnal gastroesophageal reflux disease

Acid reflux episodes are traditionally divided into upright and recumbent reflux. It has been noted that acid reflux during the upright period tends to be more frequent but of shorter duration. In contrast, acid reflux during recumbency is commonly less frequent but of longer duration [48]. Early studies suggested that acid reflux was significantly more frequent during the first half of the recumbent period compared with the second half [49]. However, there was no attempt in these studies to distinguish between the recumbent-awake and the recumbent-asleep periods. Thus, it was unclear if sleep induction or the early sleep period is associated with increase in acid reflux.

In a study by Dickman et al., the authors compared the principal characteristics of acid reflux events during upright, recumbent-awake, and recumbent-asleep periods [50]. Recumbent-awake and recumbent-asleep periods were estimated by using patients as well as their spouses or other family members in documenting the time they went to bed at night, time they fell asleep and time they woke up. The authors demonstrated that the mean percentage of total time pH <4, frequency of acid reflux events, and number of sensed reflux events were similar in the upright and recumbent-awake periods but were significantly higher than those in the recumbent-asleep period. The authors concluded that, due to similar reflux patterns in the upright and recumbent-awake periods, pH data analysis should be divided into awake and asleep periods rather than upright and recumbent periods. The results of this study have been further supported by a recently published study demonstrating that the recumbent period is heterogeneous and clearly divided into recumbent-awake and recumbent-asleep periods [51]. The percent total time pH <4, the mean number of acid reflux events, and the number of symptoms associated with reflux events were significantly greater in the recumbent-awake period compared with the recumbent-asleep period.

The nighttime period is heterogeneous regarding the frequency of reflux events. Dickman *et al.* demonstrated that esophageal acid exposure was the highest during the first 2 h of sleep [52]. This was further accentuated in patients with Barrett's esophagus compared to those with erosive esophagitis or NERD with an abnormal pH test. Patients with Barrett's esophagus had the highest esophageal acid exposure parameters throughout the sleep period. The increase in esophageal acid exposure during the first hours of sleep is likely to be driven, amongst others, by short dinner-to-bed time. It has been shown that dinner-to-bed time less than 3 h significantly increased the risk of subjects experiencing gastroesophageal reflux regardless of their phenotypic presentation of GERD (erosive esophagitis or NERD) [53]. A study by Piesman *et al.* also demonstrated that a meal consumed 2 h before going to bed was significantly more associated with recumbent reflux compared to a meal consumed 6 h prior to bed time [54]. The presence of hiatal hernia, higher Body Mass Index (BMI), and having erosive esophagitis increased the likelihood of developing recumbent reflux. Other factors like alcohol and/or carbonated beverage consumption, and use of benzodiazepines at bed time have all been shown to increase the risk for reported heartburn during sleep time [22,55].

Underlying mechanisms for sleep disturbances

The two pivotal underlying mechanisms for reduced quality of sleep and sleep disturbances in patients with GERD are heartburn that awakens patients from sleep during the night and short, amnestic arousals that lead to sleep deprivation. Whilst nighttime heartburn has been perceived by many investigators as the most important underlying mechanism for sleep disturbances in GERD patients, recent studies have shown that acid reflux events are more commonly encountered and often associated with short, amnestic arousals. These arousals usually last 30 sec and tend to occur during an acid reflux event. Most of the arousals occurred during stage 2 of sleep and rarely during the REM period. When assessing the risks for injury to the esophagus in patients who awake with heartburn versus those with short arousals in response to an acid reflux event, the former

Table 12.1 Different esophageal physiological responses to gastroesophageal reflux during sleep (waking up with heartburn versus short, amnestic arousals).

	Waking up with heartburn	Short, amnestic arousals
Initiating swallows	↑	↓
Saliva production	↑	↓
Primary peristalsis	↑	↓
Gravitation	↑	↓
Esophageal acid contact time	↓	↑
Acute antireflux therapy	↑	↓

Reproduced from Fass R. J Clin Gastroenterol 2007;41 (Suppl 2):S154–S159, with permission from Lippincott Williams & Wilkins.

appears to have an important defensive effect. Patients who awake with heartburn can initiate swallows and thus primary peristalsis, deliver saliva to the distal portion of the esophagus, and consume anti-reflux treatment with an acute ameliorating effect (e.g. antacids, Gaviscon, over-the-counter H2 receptor antagonists). In contrast, patients who respond to gastro-esophageal reflux with only short arousal will be unable to activate these vital esophageal defense mechanisms. leading to prolonged esophageal acid contact time and possibly esophageal mucosal injury (Table 12.1). Surprisingly, there is no difference in relation to the effect on sleep quality between patients with NERD and those with erosive esophagitis [56].

As previously mentioned, the importance of the recumbent position for gastroesophageal reflux was previously suggested. However, none of the aforementioned studies utilized any technique to determine if the reflux occurred primarily during the recumbent-awake or recumbent-asleep periods. Actigraphy is a validated technique that has been shown to be highly comparable to a polysomnographic study in determining sleep duration and awakening in many conditions [57]. The actigraph, a watch-like device worn on the patient's non-dominant wrist, records motion with an accelerometer (Figure 12.2). Subsequently, stored digital information is downloaded and analyzed by proprietary software to yield periods of quiescence that can be inferred as sleep time. Thus, actigraphs can be used to estimate the timing and duration of sleep as well as identifying periods of wakefulness. A novel analysis software (FRIM© analysis) superimposes simultaneously recorded actigraphy raw data over pH-collected data matched by time. For the first time, the new, color-coordinated integrated analysis allows determination of all pH parameters during the awake and asleep periods in addition to the traditional recumbent and upright periods. The integrative analysis can objectively determine recumbent-awake and

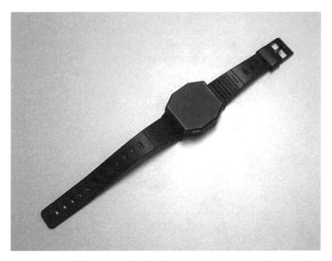

Figure 12.2 The actigraph is a watch-like device that is worn on the non-dominant wrist and records motion with an accelerometer that is stored digitally in the device (Basic Motionlogger, manufactured by Ambulatory Monitoring Inc., Ardsley, NY, USA). Reproduced from Hershcovici *et al.* [58], with permission from Nature Publishing Group.

recumbent-asleep time, frequency and duration of conscious awakenings during sleep, the relationship between conscious awakenings during sleep and reflux events, the relationship between GERD-related symptoms and conscious awakenings, and the presence of patients' recall bias (inaccurate reporting of recumbent and upright information) [58]. Using this analysis software, the principal characteristics of reflux during the recumbent-awake and recumbent-asleep periods were recently reassessed [59–62]. Most acid reflux events observed during the early part of the recumbent period occurred during the recumbent-awake period [62]. There was a significant reduction in the number of acid reflux events during the corresponding recumbent-asleep period. This study suggests that the recumbent-awake period is more commonly associated with increased acid reflux events and symptom reports compared with the recumbent-asleep period, which further supports the need to separate the two periods during esophageal function analysis.

Overall, the recumbent-awake period was noted to be of substantial duration. The mean duration of acid reflux events was similar among the various periods (upright, recumbent-awake, and recumbent-asleep) [59]. However, within the recumbent-asleep period, some of the acid reflux events occurred during conscious awakenings and others during sleep. The mean duration of an acid reflux event that occurred during sleep was significantly longer than the mean duration of an acid reflux event that occurred during a conscious awakening (Figure 12.3). The results of this

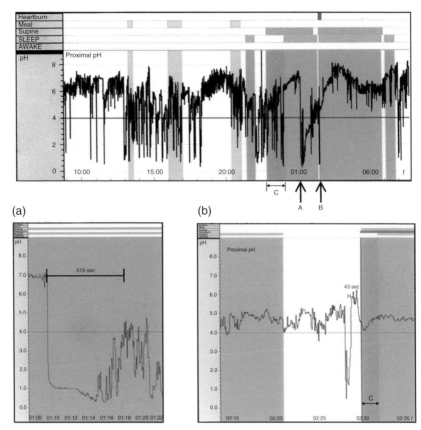

Figure 12.3 Duration of acid reflux events during sleep and during conscious awakenings. In this example, the "A" reflux event during sleep is typically long. However, the "B" reflux event, occurring during conscious awakenings, appears to be of very short duration, comparable to reflux events during the upright (*white background*) or recumbent-awake "C" periods. Reproduced from Poh *et al.* [59] with permission from Elsevier.

study demonstrated that reflux events during the recumbent-asleep period were heterogeneous and that their principal characteristics were dependent upon whether the patient was asleep or consciously awake during the reflux event.

The relationship between acid reflux events and conscious awakenings in GERD patients was further assessed using the integrated actigraphy and pH program [61]. Interestingly, 76% of the patients reported at least one conscious awakening, and 47% of the conscious awakenings were associated with acid reflux events. However, only 18% of the conscious awakenings associated with acid reflux events were also associated with GERD-related symptoms (Figure 12.4). Furthermore, in 83% of the reflux-associated awakenings, the awakening preceded the reflux event. Acid

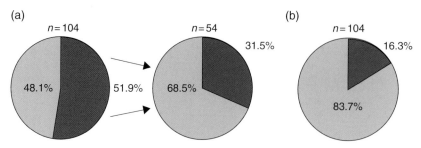

Figure 12.4 The relationship between conscious awakenings and acid reflux events as well as symptoms in the GERD group (*n*=39). (a) The *left pie* demonstrates the percentage of conscious awakenings with (*purple*) and without (*gray*) acid reflux. The *right pie* depicts the percentage of symptomatic (*purple*) and asymptomatic (*gray*) conscious awakenings associated with acid reflux events. (b) The overall percentage of conscious awakenings associated with (*purple*) or without (*gray*) acid reflux events and GERD-related symptoms. Reproduced from Poh *et al.* [61] with permission from Elsevier.

reflux events occurring after awakening were significantly shorter than those that preceded an awakening (occurred during sleep) [63].

The integrated actigraphy and pH testing analysis also allowed the evaluation of acid reflux events that occur during the transition between sleep and awakening [60]. In this study, almost half of the patients experienced an acid reflux event within 20 minutes after waking up in the morning. This is in contrast to only 18% of the patients who experienced a reflux event during the hour of sleep prior to awakening in the morning (Figure 12.5). While changes in body position may potentially explain these reflux events, the actigraphy-based analysis demonstrated that the reflux events were still documented immediately after waking up in the morning by 42% of the patients who remained recumbent after waking up.

Several recent studies were unable to demonstrate differences in sleep architecture (i.e. the patterning of sleep stages and quantification of sleep stages throughout the night), including conventional sleep stage summaries and sleep efficiency (i.e. the percentage of time during the night spent asleep) when comparing the different phenotypes of GERD or when anti-reflux treatment has been instituted [64, 65]. However, it has been demonstrated that spectral analysis of sleep in patients with erosive esophagitis is characterized by a shift in the electroencephalogram (EEG) power spectrum toward higher frequencies compared to patients with functional heartburn (having classic GERD-related symptoms but no reflux events) [65]. The presence of delta activity in the sleep EEG indicates the density of low-frequency slow waves and is considered an established indicator of sleep homeostasis. Consequently, the lower delta-power and higher alpha-power in subjects with erosive esophagitis suggests a specific sleep physiological difference in this group compared with those with functional heartburn.

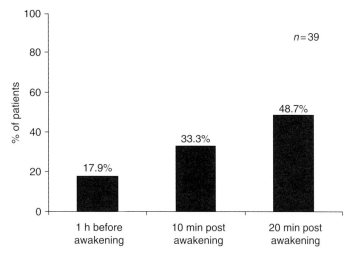

Figure 12.5 Percentage of gastro-oesophageal reflux disease (GERD) patients with acid reflux events in the three evaluative time periods (1 h prior to and 10 min and 20 min after waking up in the morning). Reproduced from Poh *et al.* [60] with permission from Blackwell Publishing.

Sleep deprivation and gastroesophageal reflux disease

In order to explore the mechanism of the association between sleep deprivation and GERD, Schey *et al.* exposed 10 healthy subjects and 10 GERD patients to sleep deprivation (<3 h) and normal sleep (≥7 h) [7]. The authors were able to demonstrate that after sleep deprivation, subjects were significantly more sensitive to esophageal acid perfusion than after a good night's sleep. This study clearly showed that sleep deprivation is likely an important central factor that can exacerbate GERD symptoms by enhancing perception of intraesophageal stimuli.

In another study it was demonstrated that sleep deprivation *per se* can precipitate acid reflux and even result in an abnormal pH test in normal subjects [66]. In this study, a total of 11 normal subjects without evidence of GERD were randomized to either sleep deprivation protocol (4 h of sleep on two consecutive nights) or good sleep protocol (at least 7 h of sleep on two consecutive nights). The mean percentage total time pH <4 was significantly higher after bad sleep compared to good sleep (5.6 versus 2.3, P <0.05). Mean percentage upright and recumbent time pH <4 were also higher after bad sleep compared to good sleep (4.6 versus 1.9 and 5.5 versus 2.6, respectively, P <0.05). Five (45.5%) of the normal subjects developed an abnormal pH test after sleep deprivation (>4.2%). All pH tests after good sleep were within the normal range.

The aforementioned information suggests that sleep deprivation *per se* may adversely affect GERD through two mechanisms. The first is increased esophageal sensitivity and the second is increased esophageal acid exposure. The latter is likely due to increased food consumption observed in sleep-deprived subjects.

Gastroesophageal reflux disease and obstructive sleep apnea

Obstructive sleep apnea (OSA) is a breathing disorder that occurs during sleep in which the patient experiences respiratory pauses lasting at least 10 sec and occurring at least five times per hour of sleep [67]. OSA is characterized by excessive daytime sleepiness, snoring, repeated episodes of upper airway obstruction during sleep, and nocturnal hypoxemia leading to memory problems, irritability, and depression.

The exact association between OSA and GERD remains controversial. Kerr *et al.* have demonstrated that precipitous drops in pH were frequently preceded by arousal (98.4%), movement of the patient (71.9%), and swallowing (80.4%) [68]. In this case, arousal is theorized to be caused by increased ventilatory effort [69]. Arousal and movement may trigger gastroesophageal reflux by causing transient alteration in the pressure gradient across the LES. Additionally, the lowered intrathoracic pressure that accompanies OSA may by itself predispose the patient to gastroesophageal reflux by exacerbating the LES pressure gradient. A recent physiological investigation using concurrent high-resolution manometry, intraluminal impedance + pH sensor, and polysomnography was performed in order to evaluate physiological mechanisms for reflux in patients with OSA [70]. The study demonstrated that despite a decrease in esophageal body pressure during OSA events, compensatory changes in UES and gastroesophageal junction pressure prevented reflux. Specifically, crural diaphragm contractions became increasingly vigorous, augmenting the anti-reflux barrier and preventing reflux during OSA events.

Investigators have suggested that GERD is associated with OSA and that there might be a potential causal link between the two disorders. Continuous positive airway pressure (CPAP) that has been shown to improve breathing mechanics also improved GERD parameters in patients with OSA. In one study, Tawk *et al.* investigated 16 patients with both OSA and GERD [71]. Nasal CPAP treatment (titrated to reduce the Apnea-Hypopnea Index (AHI) to <10/h) was found to normalize the esophageal acid exposure in 81% and reduce the mean percentage esophageal acid exposure time from 12.4% before CPAP to 6.8% on CPAP. In another study, treatment with nasal CPAP showed dramatic reduction in the esophageal acid exposure (the mean percentage time pH <4 dropped significantly from 6.3±2.1 to 0.1±0.1%) by elevating intrathoracic pressure [68]. Thirty-seven of the 52 reflux events which occurred during sleep, either an apnea or a hypopnea, were found prior to the event.

Recent studies have failed to demonstrate a causal relationship between OSA and GERD. In a study of 15 patients with OSA, Penzel *et al.* found that in 37 of 52 reflux events that occurred during sleep, either apnea or hypopnea was documented prior to the reflux event [72]. The sequence in time did not prove a causal relationship between the respiratory and reflux events. In another study, 24-h esophageal pH monitoring was performed in 16 patients with OSA [73]; 80% of the patients had abnormally high esophageal acid exposure time. However, there was no relationship between the number of reflux episodes and the severity of OSA nor a time association between reflux and OSA episodes. Patients subjectively reported that the quality of sleep was affected by the severity of GERD; however, objective correlation between OSA and GERD was lacking. Another study concluded that both conditions are common entities sharing similar risk factors but may not be causally linked [74]. OSA is not influenced by severity of GERD. Additionally, objective measures of disordered sleep had stronger association with age, smoking, and alcohol use than with GERD in men and stronger association with age and BMI than with GERD in women [74]. Similarly, a study by Kim *et al.* could not find a relationship between OSA and GERD symptoms among 123 patients referred to a sleep disorders center [75]. Furthermore, there was no relationship between the severity of OSA and the likelihood of GERD symptoms.

Silent reflux and sleep

It is highly plausible that patients who experience silent reflux might be recognized by the presence of sleep abnormalities, despite lack of reports of typical or atypical manifestations of GERD. Recent studies have shown that even in patients without nighttime heartburn, GER may result in sleep disturbances and reports of reduced quality of sleep [76]. Short, amnestic, reflux-related awakenings are not uncommon in patients with nocturnal GER, resulting in sleep fragmentation and thus poor quality of sleep [77]. In addition, conscious awakenings from sleep during the night associated with acid reflux events are commonly asymptomatic [61]. Hence, sleep abnormalities and reports of poor quality of sleep could potentially be the sole presentation of silent GERD. In a study, 81 subjects with documented sleep abnormalities and without heartburn were evaluated by two simultaneous polysomnographic sleep studies and pH testing, separated by an interval of 10–21 days [78]. They were compared with

39 normal subjects. The mean acid exposure time was significantly higher (3.76 versus 0.56%) among the disturbed-sleep group than the normal sleepers. The disturbed-sleep group required significantly longer time to fall asleep, had less total sleep time, increased wake time after sleep onset, and less deep sleep. There was no significant difference between the study groups with regard to the frequency of arousal responses. The authors speculated that silent reflux may be the cause of sleep disturbances in individuals with unexplained sleep disorders. This study illuminates an area that has been rarely evaluated in the past: sleep disturbances as the sole presentation of GERD. The presence of sleep disturbances and poor quality of sleep could be the necessary clinical clues for diagnosing patients with silent GERD. Further studies are needed to assess the predictive value of sleep abnormalities or poor quality of sleep for silent GERD.

Therapeutic approach

Overall, therapeutic studies using proton pump inhibitors (PPI) have shown good control of nighttime heartburn. The timing of PPI dosing may be important for the control of nighttime GERD-related symptoms. Recently, the effect of different dosing regimens of esomeprazole on daytime and nighttime intragastric pH was evaluated [79]. Esomeprazole 40 mg twice daily (morning and evening) provided the best nighttime intragastric pH control (81.0%) followed by esomeprazole 40 mg prior to dinner (70.6%) (Table 12.2).

A number of studies have examined the effects of anti-reflux therapy on sleep quality as assessed by subjective or objective parameters. In an open label trial, Chand *et al.* treated 18 erosive esophagitis patients with esomeprazole 40 mg once daily for 8 weeks [80]. The authors were only able to document improvement in subjective reports of sleep quality using the Pittsburg Sleep Quality Questionnaire. In a study by Johnson *et al.*, 262 patients with moderate-to-severe nighttime heartburn and GERD-related sleep disturbances received esomeprazole 20 mg or placebo each morning for 4 weeks [81]. Patients receiving esomeprazole achieved significantly greater nighttime heartburn relief than those receiving placebo (34.3% versus 10.4%, $P<0.001$). Sleep quality (assessed by the Pittsburg Sleep Quality Questionnaire), work productivity, and regular daily activities also significantly improved with esomeprazole.

Other studies examined improvement in sleep quality by both objective and subjective parameters. In one study, 42 subjects were randomized to receive either placebo or rabeprazole 20 mg twice daily for 1 week [64]. Subsequently, the patients were crossed over to the other arm. Whilst rabeprazole significantly reduced reflux-related parameters, there was no

Table 12.2 Mean pharmacodynamic findings of different esomeprazole regimens (per-protocol population, $n = 33$).

	24 hour		Daytime		Nighttime	
	Percentage of time with intragastric pH >4	Median pH	Percentage of time with intragastric pH >4	Median pH	Percentage of time with intragastric pH >4	Median pH
20 mg before breakfast	56.5	4.3	68.5	4.6	39.8	3.4
20 mg before dinner	46.3	3.8	46.6	3.7	46.8	3.8
20 mg twice daily	76.5	4.9	86.4	5.0	62.8	4.6
40 mg before breakfast	68.8	4.8	80.9	4.9	51.4	4.3
40 mg before dinner	59.5	4.4	52.3	4.1	70.6	4.8
40 mg at bedtime	55.2	4.2	50.6	3.9	60.5	5.2
40 mg twice daily	87.1	5.2	91.4	5.2	81.0	5.2

Reproduced from Brandt et al. Symptoms, acid exposure and motility in patients with Barrett's esophagus. Can J Surg 2004;47:47–51, with permission from Canadian Medical Association.

difference between the drug and placebo in objective polysomnographic measurements (percentage sleep efficiency, percentage slow-wave sleep, percentage REM sleep, and arousals per hour). However, during rabeprazole treatment patients reported a significantly better quality of sleep and reduced mean number of remembered awakenings. The authors concluded that in GERD patients, anti-reflux treatment improves subjective and not objective sleep parameters. In contrast, Dimarino *et al.* demonstrated that in subjects with documented abnormal pH testing and reports of sleep disorders, standard-dose omeprazole reduced acid reflux-related arousals and awakenings, improved sleep efficiency, increased REM sleep, and increased total sleep time [82]. In a large study that included 635 patients with GERD and reduced quality of sleep, treatment with esomeprazole 40 mg or 20 mg daily markedly improved sleep by reducing (83.2–84.1%) the number of days with GERD-associated sleep disturbances [81]. Additionally, both pantoprazole 40 mg daily and esomeprazole 40 mg daily improved sleep in GERD patients with documented sleep disturbances on the ReQuest™ questionnaire [83].

The efficacy and safety of dexlansoprazole medium release (MR) in controlling daytime and nighttime GERD-related symptoms in patients with NERD were evaluated in a 4-week, double-blind, placebo-controlled trial [27]. A total of 947 NERD patients were randomized to dexlansoprazole MR 30 mg, 60 mg, or placebo once daily. The percentage of nights without heartburn was significantly higher in patients receiving dexlansoprazole MR 60 and 30 mg versus placebo (80.8% and 76.9% versus 51.7%, respectively, $P<0.00001$). A subsequent study specifically evaluated the efficacy of dexlansoprazole MR 30 mg in relieving nocturnal heartburn and GERD-related sleep disturbances [84]. A total of 305 patients with frequent, moderate-to-severe nocturnal heartburn and associated sleep disturbances were randomized in a double-blind fashion to receive dexlansoprazole MR 30 mg or placebo once daily for 4 weeks. Dexlansoprazole MR 30 mg ($n=152$) was superior to placebo ($n=153$) in median percentage of nights without heartburn (73.1 versus 35.7%, respectively, $P<0.001$) and in the percentage of patients with relief of nocturnal heartburn and GERD-related sleep disturbances (47.5 versus 19.6%, 69.7 versus 47.9%, respectively, $P<0.001$) (Figure 12.6). Treatment with dexlansoprazole MR led to significantly greater improvement in sleep quality and work productivity and decreased nocturnal symptom severity.

Several studies specifically evaluated the effect of anti-reflux medical treatment on intragastric pH but without correlation with clinical endpoints, like healing or symptom improvement. Immediate-release (IR) omeprazole, a non-enteric-coated omeprazole mixed with sodium bicarbonate, has been shown in several studies to rapidly control nighttime gastric pH and significantly decrease nocturnal acid breakthrough compared

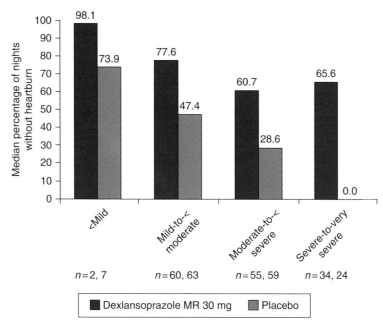

Figure 12.6 Median percentage of nights without heartburn, by baseline nocturnal heartburn severity. $P<0.001$ for overall comparison between treatment groups. Reproduced from Fass *et al.* [84] with permission from Blackwell Publishing.

to esomeprazole, lansoprazole, and pantoprazole [85,86]. A recent study claimed that single-dose rabeprazole increased nighttime intragastric pH significantly higher than single-dose pantoprazole [87]. Again, there was no clinical correlation with these pharmacodynamic findings. Studies evaluating the value of adding a histamine 2 receptor antagonist (H2RA) at bedtime to patients who failed PPI twice daily produced conflicting results [88, 89]. We are still missing a prospective, randomized, placebo-controlled trial that assesses the role of adding H2RA at bedtime in patients who failed PPI twice daily. It is likely that only a subset of these subjects will respond to such a therapeutic strategy. Lastly, patients who require more than one PPI daily to control symptoms demonstrate increase in non-acidic reflux that also occurs during the night [90].

Although generally, PPIs are efficient in the control of nighttime heartburn, there are still patients with predominant nighttime GERD-related symptoms while on twice-daily PPI therapy. It has been hypothesized that nocturnal acid breakthrough (NAB) (defined as the presence of gastric pH <4 for at least 1 h during the night) is the underlying pathophysiological mechanism responsible for refractory nighttime GERD [91]. However, studies have shown that NAB events do not demonstrate a temporal relationship with reflux-related symptoms. Furthermore, 71% of the patients with GERD who did not respond to twice-daily PPI experienced NAB, but only 36% showed a correlation between symptoms and NAB [92]. Furthermore, no relationship between NAB and nocturnal heartburn has ever been established.

The effect of anti-reflux surgery on sleep was evaluated in a small number of GERD patients [93]. The authors primarily demonstrated improvement in subjective reports of quality of sleep but with very little difference in objective sleep parameters between baseline and post fundo-plication. There was a significant increase in the fraction of the night spent in deeper sleep (49.61 versus 58.3%, $P=0.022$).

Another way to treat nighttime heartburn is by addressing sleep. The effect of insomnia treatment on nocturnal GERD was recently examined. Gagliardi *et al.* administered zolpidem 10 mg or placebo to 16 reflux patients and eight control subjects in a cross-over design [94]. Polysomnography combined with esophageal pH testing was performed during each treatment arm to assess nocturnal acid exposure and sleep arousals. Zolpidem was not associated with a significant change in the number of acid reflux events in each group. However, reflux events were associated with arousal or awakening for 40% of the time when zolpidem was administered compared with 89% when subjects received placebo ($P<0.01$). This lack of an arousal response with zolpidem waned after the first 3 h post drug administration. Zolpidem significantly increased the esophageal acid clearance times for individual acid reflux events ($P<0.05$). The results of this study indicate that hypnotic therapy with zolpidem prolongs nocturnal esophageal acid clearance time, probably secondary to the inhibition of the

---

CASE STUDY

A 48-year-old woman, mother of three and busy social worker, is seen by her primary care physician for heartburn that has affected her for the last 4 years. The patient reports almost daily symptoms, primarily after meals and about 3–4 times a week heartburn that awakens her from sleep during the night. Symptoms have worsened in the last 6 months. Besides high blood pressure, which is treated with a calcium channel blocker, the patient's medical history is otherwise unremarkable. The patient's BMI is 30. She is usually very busy during working hours and tends to eat outside her working place. A recent upper endoscopy was unremarkable. The patient is initiated on one PPI per day, taken 30 min before breakfast. Whilst her daytime symptoms completely resolve, breakthrough GERD symptoms during sleep continue to affect her, up to three times a week. A weight loss program is recommended, in addition to other lifestyle modifications. However, the patient is unable to lose weight and continues to report nighttime breakthrough GERD-related symptoms. The patient is instructed to avoid going to bed less than 3 h after the last meal of the day. In addition, she is recommended to eliminate her recumbent-awake period and avoid falling asleep in the right decubitus or supine positions. However, only the introduction of a second PPI 30 min before dinner results in complete resolution of her breakthrough symptoms during sleep.

centrally mediated sleep arousal acid clearance mechanisms. However, the conclusions of this study should be addressed with caution due to the small number of patients evaluated. Moreover, these conclusions may be irrelevant to other classes of hypnotics. Further studies are necessary to evaluate the effect of hypnotic medication on nighttime GERD-related symptoms.

Summary

Nocturnal heartburn is very common, affecting most of the patients with GERD. However, patients may not report nocturnal symptoms, unless specifically asked. In a subset of GERD patients nocturnal symptoms may not be present, but patients may display other manifestations of nocturnal gastroesophageal reflux such as nighttime choking, cough, and wheezing as well as sleep disturbances. The latter may be the sole manifestation of GERD, even in patients who do not report nighttime awakenings due to heartburn.

The recent introduction of the integrated pH testing and actigraphy data analysis program offers better separation of the recumbent-awake and recumbent-asleep periods. Studies using this technique have shown that sleep, and not recumbency, has a greater impact on gastroesophageal reflux during the night. The physiological studies are further supported by clinical trials demonstrating that gastroesophageal reflux characteristics during the recumbent-awake period are similar to those in the upright rather than the recumbent-asleep period. Overall, proton pump inhibitors appear to be an effective therapeutic modality in controlling nocturnal heartburn symptoms and reports of sleep disturbances in most heartburn sufferers.

References

1 Locke G III, Talley NJ, Fett S, Zinsmeister A, Melton L III. Prevalence and clinical spectrum of gastroesophageal reflux: a population-based study in Olmsted County, Minnesota. Gastroenterology 1997;112:1448–56.
2 Orr WC. Review article: sleep-related gastro-oesophageal reflux as a distinct clinical entity. Aliment Pharmacol Ther 2010;31(1):47–56.
3 Gerson LB, Fass R. A systematic review of the definitions, prevalence, and response to treatment of nocturnal gastroesophageal reflux disease. Clin Gastroenterol Hepatol 2009;7(4):372–8; quiz 367.
4 Shaker R, Brunton S, Elfant A, Golopol L, Ruoff G, Stanghellini V. Review article: impact of night-time reflux on lifestyle – unrecognized issues in reflux disease. Aliment Pharmacol Ther 2004;20(Suppl 9):3–13.
5 Farup C, Kleinman L, Sloan S, *et al*. The impact of nocturnal symptoms associated with gastroesophageal reflux disease on health-related quality of life. Arch Intern Med 2001;161(1):45–52.

6 Shaker R, Castell DO, Schoenfeld PS, Spechler SJ. Nighttime heartburn is an under-appreciated clinical problem that impacts sleep and daytime function: the results of a Gallup survey conducted on behalf of the American Gastroenterological Association. Am J Gastroenterol 2003;98(7):1487–93.

7 Schey R, Dickman R, Parthasarathy S, et al. Sleep deprivation is hyperalgesic in patients with gastroesophageal reflux disease. Gastroenterology 2007;133(6): 1787–95.

8 Maneerattanaporn M, Chey WD. Sleep disorders and gastrointestinal symptoms: chicken, egg or vicious cycle? Neurogastroenterol Motil 2009;21(2):97–99.

9 Adachi K, Fujishiro H, Katsube T, et al. Predominant nocturnal acid reflux in patients with Los Angeles grade C and D reflux esophagitis. J Gastroenterol Hepatol 2001;16(11):1191–6.

10 Frazzoni M, de Micheli E, Savarino V. Different patterns of oesophageal acid exposure distinguish complicated reflux disease from either erosive reflux oesophagitis or non-erosive reflux disease. Aliment Pharmacol Ther 2003;18(11–12):1091–8.

11 Lagergren J, Bergstrom R, Lindgren A, Nyren O. Symptomatic gastroesophageal reflux as a risk factor for esophageal adenocarcinoma. N Engl J Med 1999;340(11):825–31.

12 Jacob P, Kahrilas PJ, Herzon G. Proximal esophageal pH-metry in patients with 'reflux laryngitis'. Gastroenterology 1991;100(2):305–10.

13 Pellegrini CA, DeMeester TR, Johnson LF, Skinner DB. Gastroesophageal reflux and pulmonary aspiration: incidence, functional abnormality, and results of surgical therapy. Surgery 1979;86(1):110–19.

14 Harding SM, Guzzo MR, Richter JE. The prevalence of gastroesophageal reflux in asthma patients without reflux symptoms. Am J Respir Crit Care Med 2000; 162(1):34–9.

15 Dean BB, Aguilar D, Johnson LF, et al. Night-time and daytime atypical manifestations of gastro-oesophageal reflux disease: frequency, severity and impact on health-related quality of life. Aliment Pharmacol Ther 2008;27(4):327–37.

16 Cuttitta G, Cibella F, Visconti A, Scichilone N, Bellia V, Bonsignore G. Spontaneous gastroesophageal reflux and airway patency during the night in adult asthmatics. Am J Respir Crit Care Med 2000;161(1):177–81.

17 Fass R. The relationship between gastroesophageal reflux disease and sleep. Curr Gastroenterol Rep 2009;11(3):202–8.

18 Wilson JF. Is sleep the new vital sign? Ann Intern Med 2005;142(10):877–80.

19 Shaker R, Castell DO, Schoenfeld PS, Spechler SJ. Nighttime heartburn is an under-appreciated clinical problem that impacts sleep and daytime function: The results of a Gallup Survey conducted on behalf of the American Gastroenterological Association. Am J Gastroenterol 2003;98(7):1487–93.

20 Castell DO, Richter JE, Robinson M, Sontag SJ, Haber MM. Efficacy and safety of lansoprazole in the treatment of erosive reflux esophagitis. The Lansoprazole Group. Am J Gastroenterol 1996;1996(91):9.

21 Farup C, Kleinman L, Sloan S, et al. The impact of nocturnal symptoms associated with gastroesophageal reflux disease on health-related quality of life. Arch Intern Med 2001;161(1):1448–56.

22 Fass R, Quan SF, O'Connor GT, Ervin A, Iber C. Predictors of heartburn during sleep in a large prospective cohort study. Chest 2005;127(5):1658–66.

23 Fornari F, Madalosso CAS, Callegari-Jacques SM, Gurski RR. Heartburn during sleep: a clinical marker of gastro-oesophageal reflux disease in morbidly obese patients. Neurogastroenterol Motil 2009;21(2):136–42.

24 Fass R. Poorly recognized reflux-induced symptoms. Eur J Gastroenterol Hepatol 2001;13(Suppl 3):S32–S34.

25 Dean BB, Aguilar D, Johnson LF, *et al.* Night-time and daytime atypical manifestations of gastro-oesophageal reflux disease: frequency, severity and impact on health-related quality of life. Aliment Pharmacol Ther 2008;27:327–37.

26 Gislason T, Janson C, Vermeire P, *et al.* Respiratory symptoms and nocturnal gastro-esophageal reflux: a population-based study of young adults in three European countries. Chest 2002;121(1):158–63.

27 Mody R, Bolge SC, Kannan H, Fass R. Effects of gastroesophageal reflux disease on sleep and outcomes. Clin Gastroenterol Hepatol 2009;7(9):953–9.

28 Orr WC, Robinson MG, Johnson LF. Acid clearance during sleep in the pathogenesis of reflux esophagitis. Dig Dis Sci 1981;26(5):423–7.

29 Orr WC, Robinson MG, Johnson LF. The effect of esophageal acid volume on arousals from sleep and acid clearance. Chest 1991;99(2):351–4.

30 Orr WC, Johnson LF. Responses to different levels of esophageal acidification during waking and sleeping. Dig Dis Sci 1998;43(2):241–5.

31 Orr WC, Elsenbruch S, Harnish MJ, Johnson LF. Proximal migration of esophageal acid perfusions during waking and sleep. Am J Gastroenterol 2000;95(1):37–42.

32 Schneyer LH, Pigman W, Hanahan L, Gilmore RW. Rate of flow of human parotid, sublingual, and submaxillary secretions during sleep. J Dent Res 1956;35(1):109–14.

33 Lear CS, Flanagan JB Jr, Moorrees CF. The frequency of deglutition in man. Arch Oral Biol 1965;10:83–100.

34 Eastwood PR, Katagiri S, Shepherd KL, Hillman DR. Modulation of upper and lower esophageal sphincter tone during sleep. Sleep Med 2007;8(2):135–43.

35 Avots-Avotins AE, Ashworth WD, Stafford BD, Moore JG. Day and night esophageal motor function. Am J Gastroenterol 1990;85(6):683–5.

36 Dent J, Dodds WJ, Friedman RH, *et al.* Mechanism of gastroesophageal reflux in recumbent asymptomatic human subjects. J Clin Invest 1980;65(2):256–67.

37 Freidin N, Fisher MJ, Taylor W, *et al.* Sleep and nocturnal acid reflux in normal subjects and patients with reflux oesophagitis. Gut 1991;32(11):1275–9.

38 Shaker R, Hogan WJ. Reflex-mediated enhancement of airway protective mechanisms. Am J Med 2000;108(Suppl 4a):8S–14S.

39 Lang IM, Medda BK, Shaker R. Mechanisms of reflexes induced by esophageal distension. Am J Physiol 2001;281(5):G1246–63.

40 Enzmann DR, Harell GS, Zboralske FF. Upper esophageal responses to intraluminal distention in man. Gastroenterology 1977;72(6):1292–8.

41 Schoeman MN, Holloway RH. Stimulation and characteristics of secondary oesophageal peristalsis in normal subjects. Gut 1994;35(2):152–8.

42 Castiglione F, Emde C, Armstrong D, *et al.* Nocturnal oesophageal motor activity is dependent on sleep stage. Gut 1993;34(12):1653–9.

43 Dent J, Dodds WJ, Friedman RH, *et al.* Mechanism of gastroesophageal reflux in recumbent asymptomatic human subjects. J Clin Invest 1980;65(2):256–67.

44 Bajaj JS, Bajaj S, Dua KS, *et al.* Influence of sleep stages on esophago-upper esophageal sphincter contractile reflex and secondary esophageal peristalsis. Gastroenterology 2006;130(1):17–25.

45 Goo RH, Moore JG, Greenberg E, Alazraki NP. Circadian variation in gastric emptying of meals in humans. Gastroenterology 1987;93(3):515–18.

46 Elsenbruch S, Orr WC, Harnish MJ, Chen JD. Disruption of normal gastric myoelectric functioning by sleep. Sleep 1999;22(4):453–8.

47 Pasricha PJ. Effect of sleep on gastroesophageal physiology and airway protective mechanisms. Am J Med 2003;115(Suppl 3A):114S–118S.

48 Orr WC, Lackey C, Robinson MG, Johnson LF, Welsh JD. Esophageal acid clearance during sleep in patients with Barrett's esophagus. Dig Dis Sci 1988;33(6):654–9.

49 Hila A, Castell DO. Nighttime reflux is primarily an early event. J Clin Gastroenterol 2005;39(7):579–83.

50 Dickman R, Shapiro M, Malagon IB, Powers J, Fass R. Assessment of 24-h oesophageal pH monitoring should be divided to awake and asleep rather than upright and supine time periods. Neurogastroenterol Motil 2007;19(9):709–15.

51 Mizyed I, Allen LM, Navarro-Rodriguez T, et al. Actigraphy is a simple and accurate technique to determine esophageal acid exposure during sleep in patients undergoing pH testing. Gastroenterology 2008;134(4 Suppl 1):T2004, P-284.

52 Dickman R, Parthasarathy S, Malagon IB, et al. Comparisons of the distribution of oesophageal acid exposure throughout the sleep period among the different gastro-oesophageal reflux disease groups. Aliment Pharmacol Ther 2007;26(1):41–8.

53 Fujiwara Y, Machida A, Watanabe Y, et al. Assocation between dinner-to-bed time and gastro-esophageal reflux disease. Am J Gastroenterol 2005;100:2633–6.

54 Piesman M, Hwang I, Maydonovitch C, Wong RKH. Nocturnal reflux episodes following administration of a standardized meal. Does timing matter? Am J Gastroenterol 2007;102:2128–34.

55 Happe MR, Maydonovitch CL, Belle L, Gorske AC, Wong RKH. Not eating close to bedtime – is this good advice? The relationship between dinner and supine reflux. Gastroenterology 2004;126(4 (Suppl 2)):#T1732, A-501.

56 Yi CH, Hu CT, Chen CL. Sleep dysfunction in patients with GERD: erosive versus nonerosive reflux disease. Am J Med Sci 2007;334(3):168–70.

57 Morgenthaler T, Alessi C, Friedman L, et al. Practice parameters for the use of actigraphy in the assessment of sleep and sleep disorders: an update for 2007. Sleep 2007;30(4):519–29.

58 Hershcovici T, Gasiorowska A, Fass R. Advancements in the analysis of esophageal pH monitoring in GERD. Nat Rev Gastroenterol Hepatol 2011;8(2):101–7.

59 Poh CH, Gasiorowska A, Allen L, et al. Reassessment of the principal characteristics of gastroesophageal reflux during the recumbent period using integrated actigraphy-acquired information. Am J Gastroenterol 2010;105(5):1024–31.

60 Poh CH, Allen L, Malagon I, et al. Riser's reflux – an eye-opening experience. Neurogastroenterol Motil 2010;22(4):387–94.

61 Poh CH, Allen L, Gasiorowska A, et al. Conscious awakenings are commonly associated with acid reflux events in patients with gastroesophageal reflux disease. Clin Gastroenterol Hepatol 2010;8(10):851–7.

62 Allen L, Poh CH, Gasiorowska A, et al. Increased oesophageal acid exposure at the beginning of the recumbent period is primarily a recumbent-awake phenomenon. Aliment Pharmacol Ther 2010;32(6):787–94.

63 Poh CH, Allen LM, Gasiorowska A, et al. Acid reflux and arousals: which is the chicken, and which is the egg? Gastroenterology 2009;136(5:Suppl 1):#S1891, A-286.

64 Orr WC, Goodrich S, Robert J. The effect of acid suppression on sleep patterns and sleep-related gastro-oesophageal reflux. Aliment Pharmacol Ther 2005;21(2):103–8.

65 Budhiraja R, Quan SF, Punjabi NM, Drake CL, Dickman R, Fass R. Power spectral analysis of the sleep electroencephalogram in heartburn patients with or without gastroesophageal reflux disease: a feasibility study. J Clin Gastroenterol 2010;44(2):91–6.

66 Hershcovici T, Gasiorowska A, Poh CH, et al. The differential effect of sleep deprivation versus good sleep on esophageal acid exposure in normal subjects. Gastroenterology 2010;138(Suppl 5):S-603.

67 Farmer W, Yaffe J, Santiago T. Managing sleep disorders in military personnel. Federal Pract 2002;19:21–39.

68 Kerr P, Shoenut JP, Millar T, Buckle P, Kryger MH. Nasal CPAP reduces gastroesophageal reflux in obstructive sleep apnea syndrome. Chest 1992;101(6):1539–44.

69 Gleeson K, Zwillch CW, White DP. The influence of increasing ventilatory effort on arousal from sleep. Am Rev Respir Dis 1990;142:295–300.

70 Kuribayashi S, Massey BT, Hafeezullah M, et al. Upper esophageal sphincter and gastroesophageal junction pressure changes act to prevent gastroesophageal and esophagopharyngeal reflux during apneic episodes in patients with obstructive sleep apnea. Chest 2010;137(4):769–76.

71 Tawk M, Goodrich S, Kinasewitz G, Orr W. The effect of 1 week of continuous positive airway pressure treatment in obstructive sleep apnea patients with concomitant gastroesophageal reflux. Chest 2006;130(4):1003–8.

72 Penzel T, Becker HF, Brandenburg U, et al. Arousal in patients with gastro-oesophageal reflux and sleep apnoea. Eur Respir J 1999;14:1266–70.

73 Graf KI, Karaus M, Heinemann S, Korber S, Dorow P, Hampel KE. Gastroesophageal reflux in patients with sleep apnea syndrome. Z Gastroenterol 1995;33(12):689–93.

74 Morse CA, Quan SF, Mays MZ, Green C, Stephen G, Fass R. Is there a relationship between obstructive sleep apnea and gastroesophageal reflux disease? Clin Gastroenterol Hepatol 2004;2(9):761–8.

75 Kim H, Vorona R, Winn M, Doviak M, Johnson D, Ware J. Symptoms of gastro-oesophageal reflux disease and the severity of obstructive sleep apnoea syndrome are not related in sleep disorders center patients. Aliment Pharmacol Ther 2005;21(9):1127–33.

76 Orr WC. Heartburn: another danger in the night? Chest 2005;127(5):1486–8.

77 Dekel R, Green C, Malagon I, et al. Short, spontaneous, anamnestic arousals are the most common sleep abnormality associated with nocturnal esophageal acid exposure. Gastroenterology 2003;124(4 Supplement 1):A-412 (M 2087).

78 Orr WC, Goodrich S, Fernstrom P, Hasselgren G. Occurrence of nighttime gastroesophageal reflux in disturbed and normal sleepers. Clin Gastroenterol Hepatol 2008;6(10):1099–104.

79 Wilder-Smith C, Rohss K, Bokelund Singh S, Sagar M, Nagy P. The effects of dose and timing of esomeprazole administration on 24-h, daytime and night-time acid inhibition in healthy volunteers. Aliment Pharmacol Ther 2010;32(10):1249–56.

80 Chand N, Johnson DA, Tabangin M, Ware JC. Sleep dysfunction in patients with gastro-oesophageal reflux disease: prevalence and response to GERD therapy, a pilot study. Aliment Pharmacol Ther 2004;20(9):969–74.

81 Johnson DA, Orr WC, Crawley JA, et al. Effect of esomeprazole on nighttime heartburn and sleep quality in patients with GERD: a randomized, placebo-controlled trial. Am J Gastroenterol 2005;100(9):1914–22.

82 Dimarino A Jr, Banwait K, Eschinger E, et al. The effect of gastro-oesophageal reflux and omeprazole on key sleep parameters. Aliment Pharmacol Ther 2005;22(4):325–9.

83 DeVault K, Holtmann J, Malagelada J, Schmitt H, Chassany O. Pantoprazole 40 mg (PANTO) is superior to esomeprazole 40 mg (ESO) in resolving sleep disturbances in GERD patients (abstract). Am J Gastroenterol 2006;101(9):S399–S400.

84 Fass R, Johnson DA, Orr WC, et al. The effect of dexlansoprazole MR on nocturnal heartburn and GERD-related sleep disturbances in patients with symptomatic GERD. Am J Gastroenterol 2011;106(3):421–31.

85 Castell D, Bagin R, Goldlust B, Major J, Hepburn B. Comparison of the effects of immediate-release omeprazole powder for oral suspension and pantoprazole delayed-release tablets on nocturnal acid breakthrough in patients with symptomatic gastro-oesophageal reflux disease. Aliment Pharmacol Ther 2005;21(12):1467–74.

86 Katz PO, Koch FK, Ballard ED, *et al.* Comparison of the effects of immediate-release omeprazole oral suspension, delayed-release lansoprazole capsules and delayed-release esomeprazole capsules on nocturnal gastric acidity after bedtime dosing in patients with night-time GERD symptoms. Aliment Pharmacol Ther 2007;25(2): 197–205.

87 Warrington S, Baisley K, Kee D, *et al.* Pharmacodynamic effects of single doses of rabeprazole 20 mg and pantoprazole 40 mg in patients with GERD and nocturnal heartburn. Aliment Pharmacol Ther 2007;25(4):511–17.

88 Rackoff A, Agrawal A, Hila I, Mainie I, Tutuian R, Castell DO. Histamine-2 receptor antagonists at night improve gastroesophageal reflux disease symptoms for patietns on proton pump inhibitor therapy. Dis Esophagus 2005;18:370–3.

89 Janiak P, Thumshirn M, Menne D, *et al.* Clinical trial: the effects of adding ranitidine at night to twice daily omeprazole therapy on nocturnal acid breakthrough and acid reflux in patients with systemic sclerosis – a randomized controlled, cross-over trial. Aliment Pharmacol Ther 2007;26(9):1259–65.

90 Orr WC, Craddock A, Goodrich S. Acidic and non-acidic reflux during sleep under conditions of powerful acid suppression. Chest 2007;131(2):460–5.

91 Peghini PL, Katz PO, Bracy NA, Castell DO. Nocturnal recovery of gastric acid secretion with twice-daily dosing of proton pump inhibitors. Am J Gastroenterol 1998; 93(5):763–7.

92 Nzeako UC, Murray JA. An evaluation of the clinical implications of acid breakthrough in patients on proton pump inhibitor therapy. Aliment Pharmacol Ther 2002;16(7):1309–16.

93 Cohen JA, Harris PA, Byrne DW, Holzman MD, Sharp KW, Richards WO. Surgical trial investigating nocturnal gastroesophageal reflux and sleep (STINGERS). Surg Endosc 2003;17:394–400.

94 Gagliardi GS, Shah AP, Goldstein M, *et al.* Effect of zolpidem on the sleep arousal response to nocturnal esophageal acid exposure. Clin Gastroenterol Hepatol 2009; 7(9):948–52.

CHAPTER 13

Aerophagia and Belching

Albert J. Bredenoord

Department of Gastroenterology, Academic Medical Centre, Amsterdam, The Netherlands

---

Key points

- Two types of belching can be distinguished: gastric and supragastric belching. Both can be detected with impedance monitoring.
- Excessive belching is a behavior disorder in which patients have episodic high-frequency supragastric belching.
- Excessive belching can be treated with speech therapy or behavior therapy.
- Aerophagia is a rare disorder in which too much air is ingested, and the accumulation of air in the stomach and intestines causes abdominal distension and bloating.
- In aerophagia, impedance monitoring shows excessive air swallowing and on a plain abdominal radiograph, distended bowel loops but no air–fluid levels are seen.
- Aerophagia can be treated with lifestyle measures such as avoidance of carbonated drinks and smoking cessation, and with speech therapy.

Potential pitfalls

Excessive belching should be differentiated from other disorders accompanied by belching:

- gastroesophageal reflux disease
- aerophagia
- functional dyspepsia
- irritable bowel syndrome
- acute pancreatitis
- cholecystolithiasis
- peptic ulcer disease.

Aerophagia should be differentiated from other disorders accompanied by gas-related symptoms:

- excessive belching
- functional dyspepsia
- irritable bowel syndrome
- bacterial overgrowth
- paralytic or mechanical ileus
- constipation
- lactose intolerance.

Practical Manual of Gastroesophageal Reflux Disease, First Edition.
Edited by Marcelo F. Vela, Joel E. Richter and John E. Pandolfino.
© 2013 John Wiley & Sons, Ltd. Published 2013 by John Wiley & Sons, Ltd.

Introduction

In normal conditions, a certain volume of air or gas is present in the various compartments of the gastrointestinal tract such as the stomach, intestines and colon, as can be seen in abdominal radiographs. With every swallow, air enters the esophagus and is transported towards the stomach along with the peristaltic wave in the esophagus. Depending on position, gastric and antroduodenal motility and presence of other intragastric factors, this intragastric air is eventually transported towards the small bowel or leaves the stomach through belching. Gas can also be released intragastrically from ingested foods and drinks, such as beverages containing carbon dioxide. In the small intestine and colon, gas is usually the result of bacterial fermentation of luminal contents. Most intragastric gas escapes the gastrointestinal tract proximally in the form of belches and most intestinal and colonic gas leaves the body in the form of flatus.

Although the presence of some gastrointestinal air is thus normal, very large volumes of gastrointestinal gas may lead to symptoms such as bloating and abdominal distension. When this is thought to be related to excessive air swallowing, this disorder is referred to as aerophagia, which in Greek means "air eating." Aerophagia can be accompanied by excessive belching, but excessive belching can also occur as an isolated symptom or in combination with gastroesophageal reflux disease (GERD) and functional dyspepsia.

In this chapter we review the pathophysiology, diagnosis, and treatment of aerophagia and excessive belching and will describe how these syndromes differ from GERD.

Air swallowing and belching

Belching is usually defined as audible escape of air or gas from the esophagus into the throat. Mostly, this air has reached the esophagus from the stomach (gastric belch), but not necessarily so. The air can also come from the throat, reach the esophagus and be expelled from the esophagus in a retrograde direction again. This is referred to as supragastric belching, as the air does not originate from the stomach and does not reach the stomach at all.

Thus, with each swallow, a certain volume of air is ingested [1]. The swallowed air mixed with swallowed saliva and food is pushed towards the stomach by the peristaltic contraction wave and the swallowed mixture moves through the relaxed lower esophageal sphincter (LES) and falls into the stomach [2]. Relaxation of the proximal stomach upon arrival of the bolus ensures accommodation of the swallowed volume without an increase in gastric pressure (receptive relaxation). The ingested air accumulates in the proximal stomach.

When gas or air is swallowed in a soluble state, such as during consumption of carbonated beverages, the gas is released in the stomach and the law of gravity means that it will accumulate in the highest part of the stomach, which is the proximal stomach. This results in dilation of the proximal stomach and subsequent activation of the vagal nerve through stretch receptors in the gastric wall [3–5]. Activation of the dorsal motor nucleus of the vagal nerve activates efferent nerves that follow the vagal and phrenic nerves and result in relaxation of the LES and crural part of the diaphragm [6]. This reflex is called a spontaneous or transient LES relaxation (TLESR) as it is not initiated by a swallow, in contrast to swallow-induced LES relaxations. It is now possible for the intragastric air to escape from the stomach and this air will reach the esophageal body. Rapid dilation of the esophageal body, such as occurs with gaseous reflux, will be followed by relaxation of the upper esophageal sphincter and the intraesophageal content can now escape [7, 8]. It is thought that the velocity and volume of the reflux are important as a slower and larger dilation of the esophageal body, as caused by liquid reflux, will trigger secondary peristalsis, which will push the refluxed material back to the stomach [9].

The escape of air out of the esophagus often causes vibrations of pharyngeal and laryngeal structures and can therefore be audible, but this is not necessarily so. Belching is thus not always audible. In the upright position, the highest point of the stomach is the proximal stomach. However, in the supine position, this is not the case and the majority of stretch receptors in the proximal stomach will not be activated by the swallowed air. Swallowed air will thus not activate the gastric venting reflex and less belching will occur [10]. Swallowed air is more likely to reach the intestines in a recumbent subject.

Belching and reflux

In patients with GERD, belching is a frequent symptom [11]. TLESRs are the underlying mechanism of the majority of both liquid and gas reflux episodes and therefore reflux and belching occur through the same mechanism. When one considers a TLESR mainly as a belch reflex, a consequence would be to consider liquid reflux during TLESRs as an unwanted side-effect of this reflex. Indeed, it has been suggested that liquid reflux is secondary to reflux of gas during a TLESR [12]. From this, it would follow that venting of gastric gas would facilitate acid reflux. With impedance monitoring, transport of gas and liquid in the esophagus can be monitored and with this technique it has been shown that most reflux episodes indeed consist of both a liquid and gaseous component [13].

However, when studying the onset of reflux episodes in patients with GERD, it was observed that liquid followed gas reflux just as frequently as gas followed liquid reflux. This does not support the hypothesis that liquid reflux simply follows gastric venting of air. Furthermore, with impedance monitoring, a accurate estimation can be made of whether a swallow contains a significant volume of air (air swallow) or whether little air is present (Figure 13.1). With this technique, we have studied the relationships between the frequency of air swallowing, the size of the intragastric air bubble, the occurrence of belching, and acid reflux in patients with GERD and healthy volunteers [14,15]. Both the size of the intragastric air bubble and the number of belches were found to be related to the frequency of air swallowing. This implies that more air swallowing leads to more intragastric air and more belching. However, we did not find a relationship between the occurrence of acid reflux and air swallowing, indicating that the intake of air is not related to reflux of acidic liquids. Also, no relationship was found between the occurrence of acid reflux and the size of the intragastric air bubble or the number of belches.

From this it follows that belching and reflux of liquids are not related, at least not directly. A consistent finding, however, is that GERD patients swallow air more often and belch more frequently than asymptomatic controls [14,16,17]. Treatment with a proton pump inhibitor (PPI) reduces the number of swallows in patients with reflux-related symptoms but not in other subjects. Perhaps the unpleasant sensation of heartburn stimulates patients to swallow more and take larger gulps with swallowing [16]. Other explanations for excessive belching in patients with GERD are available. Some patients with GERD report heartburn during reflux episodes of pure gas reflux [18]. It is possible that gastroesophageal reflux of gas causes significant distension of the esophageal body which subsequently can trigger heartburn and chest pain [19,20].

Evaluation and management of belching in gastroesophageal reflux disease patients

There is no guideline or evidence-based approach for the evaluation and management of symptoms of belching in patients with GERD. Ambulatory pH impedance monitoring can confirm the diagnosis of GERD and show increased air swallowing and gaseous reflux. It can also help to distinguish between excessive supragastric belching and regular gastric belching. However, if belching is not excessive and the diagnosis of GERD has been established, no additional testing is required.

Regarding treatment, it seems sensible to advise patients to eat more slowly, reduce the intake of beverages containing carbon dioxide, avoid chewing gum, and stop smoking. Since air swallowing and belching can be secondary to heartburn, a logical first step in medical treatment is to initiate

(a)

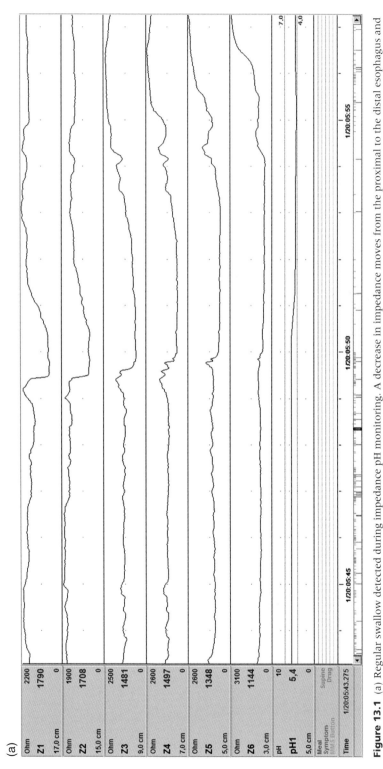

Figure 13.1 (a) Regular swallow detected during impedance pH monitoring. A decrease in impedance moves from the proximal to the distal esophagus and is cleared by the peristaltic wave a few seconds later.

(b)

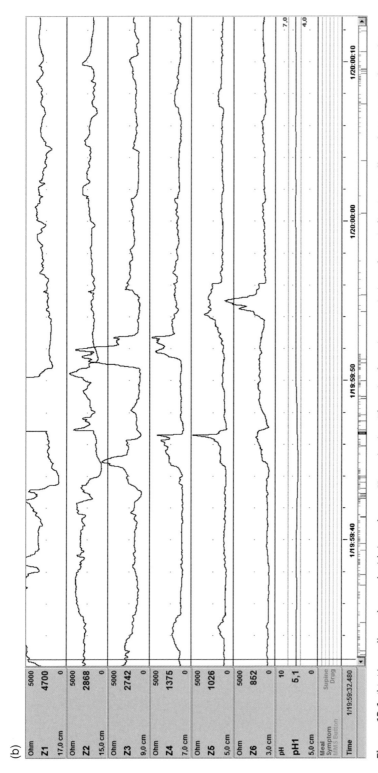

Figure 13.1 (b) Air swallows detected with impedance pH monitoring. There is a large increase in impedance indicating swallowed air, moving from the proximal to the distal esophagus.

test treatment with a PPI. Anti-reflux surgery will reduce the frequency of belching but will induce symptoms of bloating and abdominal distension because of the inability to belch and is therefore relatively contraindicated. A similar effect is likely to result from pharmacological inhibition of TLESRs such as can be induced with the gamma-amino butyric acid (GABA) B receptor agonist baclofen [21].

Belching and functional dyspepsia

Patients with functional dyspepsia often complain of frequent belching. Indeed, these patients swallow air more frequently and have more belches compared to controls, as measured on 24-h impedance monitoring [22–24]. It is suggested that the increased belching frequency is secondary to the observed increase in air swallowing, and in line with GERD, this is a reaction to unpleasant gastrointestinal sensations. Increased belching in organic painful disorders such as acute pancreatitis, peptic ulcer disease, and cholecystolithiasis can also be the result of a reaction to abdominal pain, but this has not been studied so far. In these disorders, one should therefore focus on pain relief and it is likely that the increased prevalence of belching will respond as well.

Isolated excessive belching

Occasionally, patients complain of isolated excessive belching. These patients can belch loudly and repetitively, up to several times a minute, and often demonstrate this in the clinic during consultation. Reflux symptoms and dyspepsia can be present as well but these symptoms are generally not predominant and not spontaneously mentioned by the patient. Isolated excessive belching is accompanied by a pronounced reduction in health-related quality of life, particularly in the domains of social functioning and mental health, which can be explained by the social isolation related to excessive belching. Although it has been suggested that personality and psychiatric disorders are common in these patients, there is little evidence for the presence of depression and anxiety in the majority [25,26].

The belching pattern in patients with isolated excessive belching is distinct from belches in healthy subjects and belches in patients with GERD and other disorders. As mentioned above, normally a belch is the result of the escape of gas from the stomach through the esophagus to the throat, the so-called "gastric belch" (Figure 13.2a). The frequency of these gastric belches is not increased in patients with isolated excessive belching. However, they demonstrate an increase in so-called "supragastric belches" which are belches that result from a rapid inflow of air from the pharynx into the esophagus where it is expelled again in the oral direction within a second [27]. The air thus does not originate from the stomach and does not reach the stomach and therefore these belches are referred to as

(a)

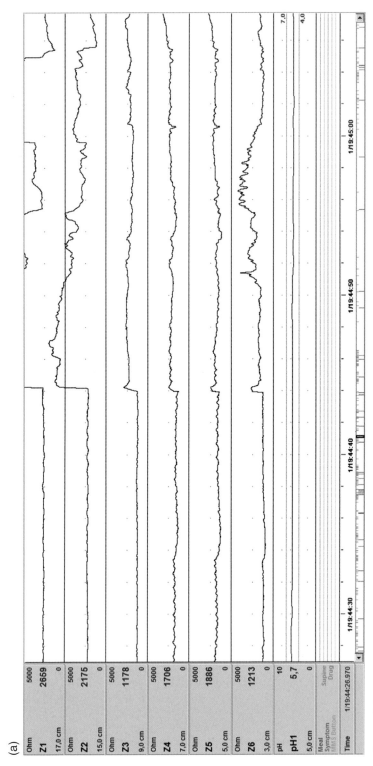

Figure 13.2 (a) Example of a gastric belch. An increase in impedance starts in the distal esophagus (19:44:44) and moves rapidly in a proximal direction, indicating air moving upwards.

(b)

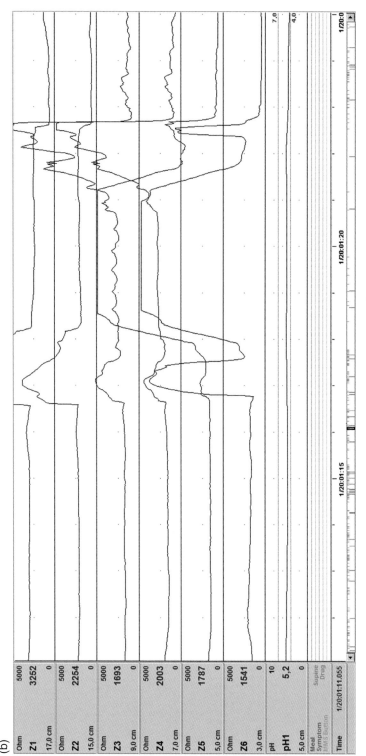

Figure 13.2 (b) Example of a supragastric belch. An increase in impedance can first be seen in the proximal esophagus (20:01:16) and moves rapidly towards the distal esophagus. Less than a second later, the impedance returns to baseline again, starting from the distal esophagus. This indicates air moving rapidly in the esophagus from the pharynx and expelled in an oral direction again.

"supragastric" or "esophageal" belches [28]. These belches are not the result of air swallowing; instead, the mechanism of belching is different and does not initiate the peristaltic contraction that usually follows swallowing. First, air is injected into the esophagus through contraction of pharyngeal muscles or suction into the esophagus through contraction of the diaphragm with opening of the upper esophageal sphincter. After the air has entered the esophageal body, straining is initiated to expel the trapped air in a retrograde direction (Figure 13.2b). While this behavior can be performed intentionally, it is currently believed that patients with isolated excessive belching have somehow lost control of their belching behavior. It thus seems that belching behavior, often initiated purposely to relieve sensations of bloating, becomes involuntary and excessive.

Impedance monitoring can be used to demonstrate supragastric belches and confirm the diagnosis of isolated excessive belching. When this is combined with esophageal manometry, the mechanism of air introduction into the esophagus (injection or suction) can be visualized as well but this is not required to make a diagnosis.

Sometimes this disorder of excessive belching is referred to as aerophagia, which in Greek means "air eating." However, since the air is not "eaten" or swallowed, this is not a correct term for this disorder. In the Rome III criteria, a distinction has been made between excessive belching and true aerophagia, in which air is really swallowed and transported to the stomach and more distally to the intestines [29].

As mentioned above, it is thought that excessive belching is a behavior disorder, and that patients have somehow lost control over an initially voluntary action. One hypothesis is that patients initially used supragastric belching as a futile effort to vent gastric air, for example to relieve symptoms of bloating. The patients who consult for excessive belching have lost control over this behavior. This is supported by a study in which the effect of distraction and stimulation on the frequency of belching was investigated [30]. When the patients were unaware of being monitored, the frequency of belching was significantly lower than during the period after which they were informed of being measured. During distraction, the frequency of belching decreased again. This study thus supports the hypothesis that suction and injection of air into the esophagus during supragastric belching is a behavior disorder.

Evaluation and management of isolated excessive belching.

Excessive belching disorder can be a clinical diagnosis, based on the history and observation of excessive belching in the clinic. In the presence of other symptoms such as dysphagia, gastroscopy can be useful to exclude other diseases. In the case of diagnostic uncertainty, impedance monitoring can be helpful to distinguish between gastric and supragastric belching.

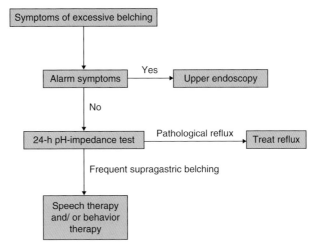

Figure 13.3 Algorithm for excessive belching.

Therapy for excessive (supragastric) belching is difficult and little evidence exists to support the various treatment strategies reported in the literature. We suggest the following approach (Figure 13.3), in which reassurance by explaining the cause of belching is the first step. In addition to this, some physicians demonstrate to patients that they can belch intentionally themselves, in order to show the patients that supragastric belching can be controlled [31]. A second step would be behavior therapy, given that excessive belching is suggested to be a behavior disorder. During behavior therapy, it is explained to patients that excessive belching is a self-induced learned behavior and that it is therefore possible to gain control of this behavior again [32, 33].

Speech therapy may be an alternative to behavior therapy. After a laryngectomy, it becomes impossible to speak as the vocal cords are resected. These patients are taught to speak by means of belching which is called esophageal speech. In order to learn to belch intentionally, speech therapists teach these patients the above described suction and injection methods [34]. As it is possible to use speech therapy to teach laryngectomized patients to perform supragastric belches, it would perhaps also be possible for patients with excessive belching to "unlearn" this behavior. We referred 11 patients to a speech therapist who is familiar with the concept of supragastric belching [35]. A visual analog scale completed before and after 10 sessions of therapy showed that patients significantly benefitted from this therapy. Six patients reported a large decrease in symptoms and four reported a modest decrease.

Prescription of gas-reducing drugs such as simethicone and dimethicone seems not useful for the treatment of excessive belching given that the volume of gastrointestinal gas is not thought to play a role in excessive supragastric belching. Therefore, avoiding beverages containing gas is not very helpful either. Anecdotal reports describe promising results with hypnosis and biofeedback therapy [36,37]. In cases where excessive belching is secondary to a psychiatric disorder, it seems advisable to treat this first [38].

Inability to belch

The importance of the belch reflex is illustrated by the consequences that follow the inability to belch that can occur in certain situations. During anti-reflux surgery such as a Nissen fundoplication, the gastric fundus is wrapped around the distal esophagus. This makes dilation by air of the proximal stomach impossible and results in a very large reduction of the TLESR frequency. Sometimes, belching will become completely impossible [39–41]. This results in the desired reduction of reflux episodes but also in an unwanted total reduction of the capacity of the stomach to vent excessive intragastric air, which results in bloating, abdominal distension and increased flatulence (see Chapter 6).

It has been shown that a self-reported ability to belch does not guarantee that a patient can truly vent gastric air [42]. Often, symptomatic patients develop supragastric belching in a futile effort to evacuate gastric air and to find relief of their symptoms, and gastric belches do not occur. It also happens that patients report that belching has become impossible after surgery but impedance monitoring shows a reduced rate but not total absence of gastric belching. Only the presence or absence of gaseous gastroesophageal reflux found with impedance monitoring is reliable in making a diagnosis here. Treatment of these symptoms is difficult and pneumatic dilation is not effective. In very severe cases dismantling of the fundoplication wrap can be required.

Aerophagia

Aerophagia is the syndrome in which patients swallow air in too frequent and/or in too large quantities, resulting in an excessive volume of gas in the stomach, small bowel, and colon. Extreme aerophagia, even with fatal consequences, has been reported in mentally retarded children but aerophagia also occurs in otherwise healthy adults [43,44]. Usually, symptoms of abdominal distension, bloating, abdominal pain, flatulence, and belching are reported. A high percentage of patients suffer from constipation, although it is unclear how this is related to the aerophagia. On plain abdominal radiographs, a large volume of gas is seen in the gastrointestinal tract in the absence of airfluid levels or other signs of ileus [29] (Figure 13.4).

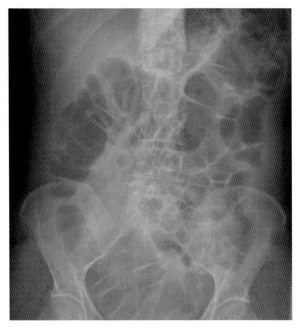

Figure 13.4 Abdominal radiograph of a patient with aerophagia showing a large volume of intestinal air but no air–fluid levels.

Evaluation and management of aerophagia

A diagnosis of aerophagia can be made with esophageal impedance monitoring, in which excessive air swallowing and a high frequency of gastric belching are observed but no supragastric belching [45]. Sometimes, the onset of the air swallowing in aerophagia is acute and transient, for example induced by an emotional event [46]. Not infrequently, patients with such episodes undergo multiple exploratory laparotomies, driven by the suspicion that an ileus or acute abdomen is present.

Similar to excessive belching, an evidence-based treatment approach is lacking. A logical treatment for these patients would be speech therapy, with a different approach compared to the patients with excessive supragastric belching. The aim of therapy for patients with aerophagia would be to reduce the frequency of air swallowing, in contrast to the intended reduction of supragastric belches in patients with excessive belching. Although avoiding gas-containing beverages will not solve the underlying disorder, it may help to reduce the volume of intraintestinal gas and alleviate symptoms. Drugs such as simethicone and dimethicone reduce the surface tension and therefore reduce gas formation in the intestines. These drugs can thus theoretically be helpful in patients with true aerophagia, although this has never been tested in a systematic way. Furthermore, since smoking is suggested to increase air swallowing, it is advisable to stop this habit (Figure 13.5).

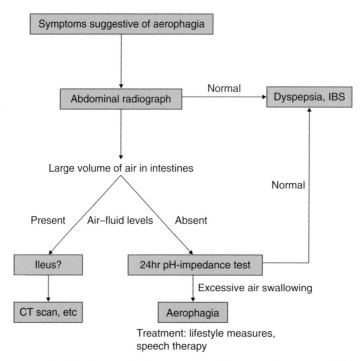

Figure 13.5 Algorithm for aerophagia. CT, computed tomography; IBS, irritable bowel syndrome.

Besides patients with true aerophagia, intestinal gas can cause symptoms of distension and bloating in other subjects. In 90% of patients with irritable bowel syndrome, bloating and abdominal distension are reported. It has been suggested that at least part of this problem is caused by intestinal air [47,48]. An increased volume of air, hypersensitivity to intestinal distension and a different distribution of intestinal air are found. The underlying mechanisms are heterogeneous and differences in intestinal transit, sensitivity, food intolerance, bacterial overgrowth, and sugar malabsorption are suggested to play a role [47,49]. Air swallowing is not suspected to play an important role in irritable bowel syndrome and speech therapy is thus not useful for these patients.

Summary

Belching is a physiological phenomenon and is defined as sometimes audible gastroesophagopharyngeal reflux of gas. Belching is only pathological when it becomes bothersome or excessive. Excessive belching is a common symptom, which is often seen in patients with functional dyspepsia, choledocholithiasis, and GERD. In these disorders, other symptoms are usually predominant. A small group of patients complain of isolated excessive and repetitive belching. These patients suffer from a behavior disorder, as they involuntary apply suction or inject air into the esophagus from the pharynx and expel this air immediately afterwards in a retrograde direction. This behavior is called supragastric belching and can be treated by a well-informed speech pathologist.

Although the presence of intestinal gas plays a role in various disorders, including irritable bowel disorder, the term "aerophagia" should only be used for patients with objectively demonstrable excessive air swallowing and excessive amounts of intestinal gas visualized on a plain abdominal radiograph. The primary symptoms of patients with aerophagia are bloating and abdominal distension, while belching is less predominant. It is important to differentiate aerophagia from a mechanical or paralytic ileus, and avoid unnecessary surgery in these patients. Treatment of aerophagia is with speech therapy and the prognosis is generally good.

CASE STUDY

A 43-year-old office worker presented at our outpatient clinic with symptoms of episodic belching. He mentioned that these belch attacks never occurred during work time but mostly started when he was driving home after work. He admitted that he considered his job very stressful, although he denied a direct relationship between stress and his symptoms. There was some epigastric fullness as well but no heartburn, regurgitation or dysphagia. A few years ago he was diagnosed with fibromyalgia but further history was negative.

The patient's general practitioner prescribed omeprazole 20 mg and domperidone but both were not considered very useful by the patient and he took these medicines only occasionally. A recently performed upper endoscopy was negative and an ultrasound scan of the abdomen revealed no abnormalities.

The patient underwent an ambulatory 24-h impedance pH monitoring test which revealed a physiological esophageal acid exposure time (time pH $<4 = 3.1\%$) and no statistical relationship between his symptoms and acid or weakly acidic reflux. However, manual analysis of the tracings showed several periods with repetitive supragastric belching. In total, more than 100 supragastric belches were detected in a 2-h period.

The patient was diagnosed with excessive supragastric belching and referred to a dedicated speech therapist. Although he gained more control over his belching behavior in the following months, there was no complete resolution of the belching episodes.

References

1 Pouderoux P, Ergun GA, Lin S, Kahrilas PJ. Esophageal bolus transit imaged by ultra-fast computerized tomography. Gastroenterology 1996;110(5):1422–8.

2 Johnson HD, Laws JW. The cardia in swallowing, eructation, and vomiting. Lancet 1966;2(7476):1268–73.

3 Zerbib F, des Varannes SB, Ropert A, Lamouliatte H, Quinton A, Galmiche JP. Proximal gastric tone in gastro-oesophageal reflux disease. Eur J Gastroenterol Hepatol 1999;11(5):511–15.

4 Penagini R, Carmagnola S, Cantu P, Allocca M, Bianchi PA. Mechanoreceptors of the proximal stomach: role in triggering transient lower esophageal sphincter relaxation. Gastroenterology 2004;126(1):49–56.

5 McNally EF, Kelly E, Ingelfinger F. Mechanism of belching: effects of gastric distention with air. Gastroenterology 1964;46:254–9.

6 Mittal RK, Fisher MJ. Electrical and mechanical inhibition of the crural diaphragm during transient relaxation of the lower esophageal sphincter. Gastroenterology 1990;99(5):1265–8.

7 Kahrilas PJ, Dodds WJ, Dent J, Wyman JB, Hogan WJ, Arndorfer RC. Upper esophageal sphincter function during belching. Gastroenterology 1986;91(1):133–40.

8 Enzmann DR, Harell GS, Zboralske FF. Upper esophageal responses to intraluminal distention in man. Gastroenterology 1977;72(6):1292–8.

9 Shaker R, Ren J, Kern M, Dodds WJ, Hogan WJ, Li Q. Mechanisms of airway protection and upper esophageal sphincter opening during belching. Am J Physiol 1992;262(4 Pt 1):G621–G628.

10 Wyman JB, Dent J, Heddle R, Dodds WJ, Toouli J, Downton J. Control of belching by the lower oesophageal sphincter. Gut 1990;31(6):639–46.

11 Klauser AG, Schindlbeck NE, Muller-Lissner SA. Symptoms in gastro-oesophageal reflux disease. Lancet 1990;335(8683):205–8.

12 Straathof JW, Ringers J, Lamers CB, Masclee AA. Provocation of transient lower esophageal sphincter relaxations by gastric distension with air. Am J Gastroenterol 2001;96(8):2317–23.

13 Sifrim D, Silny J, Holloway RH, Janssens JJ. Patterns of gas and liquid reflux during transient lower oesophageal sphincter relaxation: a study using intraluminal electrical impedance. Gut 1999;44(1):47–54.

14 Bredenoord AJ, Weusten BL, Timmer R, Akkermans LM, Smout AJ. Relationships between air swallowing, intragastric air, belching and gastro-oesophageal reflux. Neurogastroenterol Motil 2005;17(3):341–7.

15 Bredenoord AJ, Weusten BL, Timmer R, Smout AJ. Air swallowing, belching, and reflux in patients with gastroesophageal reflux disease. Am J Gastroenterol 2006;101(8):1721–6.

16 Hemmink GJ, Weusten BL, Bredenoord AJ, Timmer R, Smout AJ. Increased swallowing frequency in GORD is likely to be caused by perception of reflux episodes. Neurogastroenterol Motil 2009;21(2):143–8.

17 Kamolz T, Bammer T, Granderath FA, Pointner R. Comorbidity of aerophagia in GERD patients: outcome of laparoscopic antireflux surgery. Scand J Gastroenterol 2002;37(2):138–43.

18 Bredenoord AJ, Weusten BL, Curvers WL, Timmer R, Smout AJ. Determinants of perception of heartburn and regurgitation. Gut 2005;55(3):313–18.

19 Barish CF, Castell DO, Richter JE. Graded esophageal balloon distention. A new provocative test for noncardiac chest pain. Dig Dis Sci 1986;31(12):1292–8.

20 Kahrilas PJ, Dodds WJ, Hogan WJ. Dysfunction of the belch reflex. A cause of incapacitating chest pain. Gastroenterology 1987;93(4):818–22.

21 Zhang Q, Lehmann A, Rigda R, Dent J, Holloway RH. Control of transient lower oesophageal sphincter relaxations and reflux by the GABA(B) agonist baclofen in patients with gastro-oesophageal reflux disease. Gut 2002;50(1):19–24.

22 Lin M, Triadafilopoulos G. Belching: dyspepsia or gastroesophageal reflux disease? Am J Gastroenterol 2003;98(10):2139–45.

23 Camilleri M, Dubois D, Coulie B, *et al.* Prevalence and socioeconomic impact of upper gastrointestinal disorders in the United States: results of the US Upper Gastrointestinal Study. Clin Gastroenterol Hepatol 2005;3(6):543–52.

24 Conchillo JM, Selimah M, Bredenoord AJ, Samsom M, Smout AJ. Air swallowing, belching, acid and non-acid reflux in patients with functional dyspepsia. Aliment Pharmacol Ther 2007;25(8):965–71.

25 Bredenoord AJ, Smout AJ. Impaired health-related quality of life in patients with excessive supragastric belching. Eur J Gastroenterol Hepatol 2010;22(12):1420–3.

26 Chitkara DK, Bredenoord AJ, Tucker MJ, Talley NJ. Aerophagia in adults: a comparison of presenting symptoms with functional dyspepsia. Aliment Pharmacol Ther 2005;22(9):855–8.

27 Bredenoord AJ, Weusten BL, Sifrim D, Timmer R, Smout AJ. Aerophagia, gastric, and supragastric belching: a study using intraluminal electrical impedance monitoring. Gut 2004;53(11):1561–5.

28 [No authors listed] Physiology of belch. Lancet 1991;337(8732):23–4.

29 Tack J, Talley NJ, Camilleri M, *et al.* Functional gastroduodenal disorders. Gastroenterology 2006;130(5):1466–79.

30 Bredenoord AJ, Weusten BL, Timmer R, Smout AJ. Psychological factors affect the frequency of belching in patients with aerophagia. Am J Gastroenterol 2006; 101(12):2777–81.

31 Roth JLA. Aerophagia. In: Linder AE (ed) *Emotional factors in gastrointestinal illness.* Amsterdam: Excerpta Medica, 1973: pp.16–36.

32 Cigrang JA, Hunter CM, Peterson AL. Behavioral treatment of chronic belching due to aerophagia in a normal adult. Behav Modif 2006;30(3):341–51.

33 Chitkara DK, Bredenoord AJ, Talley NJ, Whitehead WE. Aerophagia and rumination: recognition and therapy. Curr Treat Options Gastroenterol 2006;9(4): 305–13.

34 Damste PH. Methods of restoring the voice after laryngectomy. Laryngoscope 1975; 85(4):649–55.

35 Hemmink GJ, Ten Cate L, Bredenoord AJ, Timmer R, Weusten BL, Smout AJ. Speech therapy in patients with excessive supragastric belching – a pilot study. Neurogastroenterol Motil 2010;22(1): 24–8.

36 Spiegel SB. Uses of hypnosis in the treatment of uncontrollable belching: a case report. Am J Clin Hypn 1996;38(4):263–70.

37 Bassotti G, Whitehead WE. Biofeedback as a treatment approach to gastrointestinal tract disorders. Am J Gastroenterol 1994;89(2):158–64.

38 Zella SJ, Geenens DL, Horst JN. Repetitive eructation as a manifestation of obsessive-compulsive disorder. Psychosomatics 1998;39(3):299–301.

39 Smith D, King NA, Waldron B, *et al.* Study of belching ability in antireflux surgery patients and normal volunteers. Br J Surg 1991;78(1):32–5.

40 Scheffer RC, Tatum RP, Shi G, Akkermans LM, Joehl RJ, Kahrilas PJ. Reduced tLESR elicitation in response to gastric distension in fundoplication patients. Am J Physiol Gastrointest Liver Physiol 2003;284(5):G815–G820.

41 Bredenoord AJ, Draaisma WA, Weusten BL, Gooszen HG, Smout AJ. Mechanisms of acid, weakly acidic and gas reflux after anti-reflux surgery. Gut 2008;57(2):161–6.

42 Broeders JA, Bredenoord AJ, Hazebroek EJ, Broeders IA, Gooszen HG, Smout AJ. Effects of antireflux surgery on weakly acidic reflux and belching. Gut 2011:60(4): 435–41.

43 Gauderer MW, Halpin TC Jr, Izant RJ Jr. Pathologic childhood aerophagia: a recognizable clinical entity. J Pediatr Surg 1981;16(3):301–5.

44 Hackl H. Pathologische arophagie als todesursache. Med Klin 1973;68(20):667–9.

45 Hemmink GJ, Weusten BL, Bredenoord AJ, Timmer R, Smout AJ. Aerophagia: excessive air swallowing shown by esophageal impedance monitoring. Clin Gastroenterol Hepatol 2009;7(10):1127–9.

46 Fonagy P, Calloway SP. The effect of emotional arousal on spontaneous swallowing rates. J Psychosom Res 1986;30(2):183–8.

47 Serra J, Salvioli B, Azpiroz F, Malagelada JR. Lipid-induced intestinal gas retention in irritable bowel syndrome. Gastroenterology 2002;123(3):700–6.

48 Caldarella MP, Serra J, Azpiroz F, Malagelada JR. Prokinetic effects in patients with intestinal gas retention. Gastroenterology 2002;122(7):1748–55.

49 Houghton LA, Whorwell PJ. Towards a better understanding of abdominal bloating and distension in functional gastrointestinal disorders. Neurogastroenterol Motil 2005;17(4):500–11.

CHAPTER 14

Dysphagia and Gastroesophageal Reflux Disease

Donald O. Castell[1] and Erick R. Singh[2]

[1] Esophageal Disease Program, Medical University of South Carolina, Charleston, SC, USA
[2] Section of Gastroenterology and Hepatology, Georgia Health Sciences University, Augusta, GA, USA

Key points
- Gastroesophageal reflux disease may induce structural and physiological changes in the esophagus which can cause dysphagia.
- Initial evaluation requires thorough history and physical examination in order to identify the etiology of dysphagia.
- Esophagogastroduodenosopy allows direct visual inspection of the esophageal lumen and mucosa, localization of mechanical obstruction, and therapeutic and diagnostic interventions.
- Barium esophagram and esophageal manometry are often necessary for diagnosis of motility and structural causes of dysphagia not identified by esophagogastroduodenosopy.
- Once the underlying cause of dysphagia has been treated, it is important for the patient to remain on treatment to control reflux and prevent recurrence.

Potential pitfalls
- Failing to distinguish between oropharyngeal and esophageal dysphagia, as gastroesophageal reflux disease is a common cause of the latter but not the former.
- Failing to pursue further testing by esophagram or manometry when esophagogas-troduodenosopy is normal, as endocopy may miss proximal structural or motility causes of dysphagia.
- Assuming that therapeutic failure of any single proton pump inhibitor or H2 blocker medication for treatment of gastroesophageal reflux disease means that other similar drugs will not work. Many patients will respond favorably to other drugs in these medication classes.

Practical Manual of Gastroesophageal Reflux Disease, First Edition.
Edited by Marcelo F. Vela, Joel E. Richter and John E. Pandolfino.
© 2013 John Wiley & Sons, Ltd. Published 2013 by John Wiley & Sons, Ltd.

Introduction

Gastroesophageal reflux disease (GERD) is caused by the retrograde flow of stomach contents into the body of the esophagus caused by chronic hypotension or by transient relaxation or effacement of the lower esophageal sphincter. GERD may cause inflammation of the esophagus leading to the typical symptoms of heartburn and acid regurgitation. Some patients with GERD may also develop difficulty with swallowing. Dysphagia refers to the sensation of difficult passage of organic materialfrom the mouth to the stomach. The word "dysphagia" can be traced from the root origins of the Greek words "*dys*" meaning "difficulty" and "*phagia*" meaning "to eat." The sensations described by patients encompass a wide variety of complaints ranging from inability to transfer material from the mouth into the pharynx or esophagus to feeling that food is "getting stuck" in the esophagus. There is also a wide range of co-existing symptoms which may occur with dysphagia such as immediate regurgitation, pain with swallowing (odynophagia), heartburn, or weight loss.

It is estimated that 5–8% of the general population over the age of 50 years may experience dysphagia but the incidence continues to increase with age, as up to 50–60% of patients in nursing homes and other chronic care facilities report this symptom [1]. Dysphagia should be considered as an alarm symptom warranting immediate evaluation, primarily to exclude a malignant etiology.

Dysphagia can be classified into two main types: oropharyngeal and esophageal. Oropharyngeal dysphagia, also known as "transfer dysphagia," refers to an abnormality in the delivery of oral contents to the proximal esophagus. For adequate bolus transfer from mouth to esophagus, the bolus must pass across a relaxed upper esophageal sphincter via coordinated contractile movements of the pharynx. Symptoms of oropharyngeal dysphagia occur almost immediately after swallowing. Patients may describe sensations due to abnormalities of the oral phase (food spillage, drooling) or the pharyngeal phase which may include failure to protect the airway (choking, coughing, gagging). They are also often able to localize the area of the neck or pharynx as the region of their difficulties. The presence of oropharyngeal dysphagia warrants careful structural and neurological evaluation. Residual neurological deficits following a cerebrovascular accident are often the cause of oropharyngeal dysphagia although cranial nerve palsies, myositis, amyotrophic lateral sclerosis (ALS), Parkinson's disease, and muscular dystrophies also remain in the differential diagnosis. With symptoms of regurgitation of undigested food, halitosis, and aspiration, structural abnormalities such as Zenker's diverticulum must also be considered [2].

Esophageal dysphagia refers to difficulty swallowing that is attributable to dysfunction or obstruction within the body of the esophagus. Mechanical causes or motility abnormalities most often lead to this type of dysphagia. This chapter focuses on evaluation and management of GERD-related causes of esophageal dysphagia.

Evaluation

The first and most important aspect in the evaluation of dysphagia is the patient history. It is imperative to enquire about whether the dysphagia is (a) for liquids, solids or both; (b) intermittent or progressive; (c) oropharyngeal as opposed to esophageal. As previously discussed, oropharyngeal dysphagia is usually described as an immediate difficulty of initiating a swallow localized to the pharyngeal region and characterized by choking, coughing or gagging. On the other hand, esophageal dysphagia is more commonly described as the sensation of the bolus "getting stuck behind the breastbone" (in the esophagus) moments after initiating a swallow.

Once esophageal dysphagia is suspected, the type of food producing symptoms should be ascertained. Dysphagia caused by solids is largely attributable to mechanical obstructions whereas dysphagia to solids and/or liquids is more commonly associated with motility disorders. Next, the temporal relationship or progression of symptoms must be determined. Intermittent dysphagia for solids and liquids may be indicative of a motility disorder such as ineffective esophageal motility (IEM), diffuse esophageal spasm (DES) or nutcracker esophagus. Progressive dysphagia with weight loss, regurgitation, and aspiration is a constellation of symptoms seen with motility disorders such as achalasia, which is not associated with GERD. Determining the location of a mechanical obstruction by the patient's description of symptoms is not very accurate. In general, patient perception of obstruction located down the sternum has good localization with a disorder involving the distal esophagus whereas perceived obstruction at or above the suprasternal notch may represent referred sensation from an obstruction anywhere from the pharynx to the distal esophagus [3].

Esophageal rings and webs produce intermittent dysphagia to solids. Progressive solid food dysphagia is encountered with strictures, esophageal and gastric cardia cancers, and occasionally with esophagitis. Esophageal and gastric cardia cancers may be differentiated from strictures in that the solid food dysphagia which occurs with malignancy is often quite rapid in onset, progressive, and associated with marked weight loss. The presence of heartburn may also be helpful in identifying the etiology of dysphagia. Progressive solid dysphagia in a patient with long history of heartburn may be found with both peptic stricture and erosive esophagitis. Eosinophilic esophagitis may be the cause of dysphagia in a young adult which may also present with an initial symptom of food impaction [4].

After the history and physical examination have identified possible causes of dysphagia, the next diagnostic tool must be selected. Esophagogastroduodenoscopy (EGD) is the initial test of choice for esophageal dysphagia in that it allows thorough inspection of the esophagus and mucosa, localization of possible mechanical obstruction, and diagnostic and therapeutic interventions. If EGD is negative, further evaluation includes barium esophagram to rule out subtle causes of obstruction such as rings or webs which may be missed during endoscopic evaluation, along with esophageal manometry to investigate dysmotility. Barium esophagram may also be the preferred initial test in patients with a clinical presentation suggestive of a proximal esophageal lesion (such as previous laryngeal surgery/cancer, Zenker's diverticulum, radiation therapy) or a complex stricture (radiation exposure or caustic injury), as in these cases EGD may be safer once the expected anatomy is delineated by the esophagram. In addition, esophagram findings consistent with achalasia in a patient with history suggestive of this disorder would also warrant an esophageal manometric evaluation for diagnostic confirmation prior to proceeding to EGD. Computed tomographic (CT) and endoscopic ultrasound (EUS) studies may also be of diagnostic benefit in the evaluation of esophageal and gastric cancers (Figure 14.1).

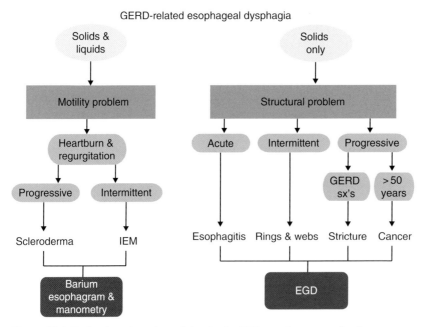

Figure 14.1 Evaluation of esophageal dysphagia. EGD, esophagogastroduodenoscopy; GERD, gastroesophageal reflux disease; IEM, ineffective esophageal motility.

Causes of dysphagia associated with gastroesophageal reflux disease

All GERD-associated causes of dysphagia fall into the category of esophageal dysphagia and the differential diagnosis is as follows.
• Peptic strictures
• Rings and webs
• Esophageal adenocarcinoma
• Esophagitis (erosive and eosinophilic)
• Ineffective esophageal motility (IEM)
• Scleroderma

Peptic stricture

An esophageal peptic stricture is usually a short, focal, and straight narrowing of the esophageal lumen located near the gastroesophageal (GE) junction (Figure 14.2). Although strictures may be produced as a result of many different injuries such as caustic, pill or radiation-induced damage, the vast majority occur as a consequence of long-standing GERD. Approximately 4–20% of patients with GERD undergoing endoscopy are found to have peptic stricture. With the current widespread use of proton pump inhibitors (PPIs), the prevalence of peptic strictures has decreased [5]. The mechanism of stricture formation centers on collagen deposition which occurs during the healing phase of esophageal injury. As acid gastric contents move past the GE junction, they damage the columnar esophageal mucosa, producing an inflammatory state. After this initial injury, collagen is deposited during the healing phase. As healing continues, the esophageal mucosa narrows as the collagen fibers contract to form a peptic stricture. Conditions which may increase the incidence of GERD such as scleroderma, Zollinger–Ellison syndrome, and Heller myotomy in achalasia patients as well as increased age and long duration of GERD symptoms increase the overall incidence of peptic strictures [6].

The most common symptom of peptic stricture is dysphagia. Dysphagia occurs as the esophageal lumen narrows to <13 mm [7]. Patients frequently first experience solid food dysphagia which may progress to liquid dysphagia and possible food impaction if acid control is not obtained. As stricture formation is most commonly associated with long- standing GERD, patients will usually have a history of chronic heartburn, indigestion or acid regurgitation. The initial diagnostic test should be EGD as it enables visual inspection and localization of the injury. This test may also provide the opportunity for treatment through balloon or bougie dilation, which may be repeated if an optimal diameter and symptomatic relief are not achieved after a single dilation. Barium esophagram or

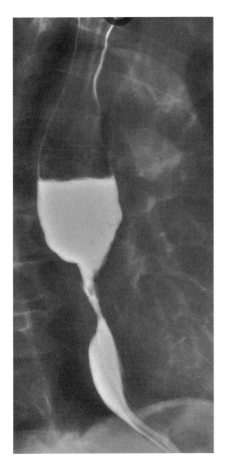

Figure 14.2 Midesophageal peptic stricture.

CT studies may also be of diagnostic utility but they do not provide the benefit of dilation therapy.

Treatment of simple peptic strictures is a two-fold approach which includes endoscopic dilation along with pharmacological acid suppression to maintain healing and prevent recurrence. The pharmacological and surgical treatments for GERD are discussed elsewhere in this book. Dilation may be performed by bougie or balloon-type dilators. Subtypes of mechanical bougie dilators include the Maloney and Savary–Gilliard dilators. The Maloney dilator is tapered and comes in various sizes, and does not require passage over a guidewire. The Savary–Gilliard dilator is the most widely used dilator which is also tapered and available in multiple sizes but does require passage over a guidewire. Both types of mechanical dilators allow for both longitudinal and radial force to be applied to the stricture for stretching [8].

Balloon dilators are passed through the endoscope or over the guidewire but only provide for radial force to be applied to the stricture. The so-called

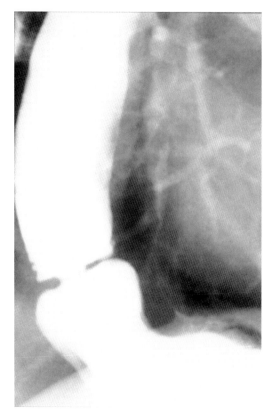

Figure 14.3 Schatzki's ring.

"rule of three" is commonly used in clinical practice as a means of reducing the risk of dilation-related esophageal perforation. Typically, mechanical dilation should be limited to the use of no more than three successively larger dilators, starting with the balloon or bougie size to which resistance is encountered. Dilation sessions may be repeated weekly if the patient remains symptomatic. More complex strictures are often related to conditions such as esophageal tumors, radiation injury, and tracheoesophageal fistula, and may require further intervention such as esophageal stenting, incisional therapy or surgery [9].

Rings and webs

Esophageal rings and webs are thin structures which traverse the esophageal lumen, potentially impeding bolus transit. Rings may be either mucosal or muscular, solitary or multiple. The most common GERD-associated phenomenon of this category is the solitary, mucosal ring first described by Richard Schatzki in the 1950s (Figure 14.3). Schatzki's rings are thin, webbed structures found in the lower esophageal region at the squamocolumnar junction [10]. They are evident in 6–14% of barium esophagrams but may account for >15% of cases of esophageal dysphagia. Rings do not commonly cause dysphagia until the ring diameter constricts to <13 mm. The pathogenesis leading to the formation of these rings is not entirely clear, but GERD may play a role as reduction in esophageal acid exposure in conjunction with dilation procedures has been shown to decrease the risk of recurrence in several studies. Some investigators propose a congenital origin as opposed to that of reactive formation in the setting of chronic GERD. In either case, treatment entails either bougie or balloon dilation along with acid suppressive therapy [11]. Eosinophilic esophagitis may present clinically in a somewhat similar fashion to a Schatzki's ring, but usually multiple rings are present throughout the esophagus [12].

Esophageal webs are web-like structures more commonly found in the proximal esophagus or the hypopharyngeal region. Their origin is less clear than that of esophageal rings. Plummer Vinson syndrome is an entity found in middle-aged women with a triad of symptoms including iron deficiency anemia, glossitis, and dysphagia due to an esophageal web. Possible correlation of esophageal webs with GERD is unclear. Similar to esophageal rings, the mainstay of treatment is esophageal dilation [13].

Esophageal adenocarcinoma

Esophageal and gastric cardia adenocarcinomas are GERD-associated malignancies which cause esophageal dysphagia. Although squamous cell carcinoma is still the most common type of esophageal cancer worldwide, the increasing incidence of adenocarcinoma has led to it becoming the most common esophageal cancer in the Western world. The incidence among white men of 5.69 per 1000,000 person-years in 2000–2004 represents a greater than four-fold increase since the mid-1970s [14].

The pathogenesis of adenocarcinoma involves many steps of transformation which may be attributable to a number of risk factors. These include GERD, obesity, and smoking, as well as race and genetic background as esophageal adenocarcinoma is most common in white males. However, a study of greater than 300 patients with esophageal adenocarcinoma and a similar number of age- and gender-matched controls revealed GERD to be the strongest single risk factor for adenocarcinoma [15]. Although the precise mechanism of carcinogenesis is yet to be fully determined, the initial step involves the metaplastic change known as Barrett's esophagus. This term refers to the transformation of the normal stratified squamous epithelium of the esophagus into intestinal columnar cells. The squamous cells at or near the gastroesophageal junction are damaged by chronic exposure to gastric acid refluxed into the esophagus, and the damaged cells are replaced by aberrantly differentiating squamous cells [16]. Adenocarcinoma manifests once these metaplastic cells neoplastically proliferate after genetic changes are made to their DNA. Such changes are thought to occur due to upregulation and activation of protooncogenes or downregulation of tumor suppressor genes [17].

Unfortunately, many such tumors do not present clinically until they have grown substantially. Rapidly progressive solid dysphagia with accompanying weight loss and tumor-induced cachexia may be an all too common initial presentation. Despite the fact that GERD has been found to be the biggest independent risk factor for the development of esophageal adenocarcinoma, more than 50% of patients diagnosed with this tumor type exhibit no symptoms of GERD [18]. Diagnosis can be suggested with radiographic studies such as barium esophagram or CT imaging, but confirmatory tissue diagnosis is necessary via endoscopy with biopsies. Once tissue diagnosis has been confirmed, staging of the cancer is undertaken with CT imaging and EUS which provide further detail regarding the depth of tumor invasion. EUS may also allow for fine needle aspiration of suspicious-appearing lymph nodes of metastatic potential. Treatment options vary greatly dependent upon the tumor's stage at the time of diagnosis.

Endoscopic therapeutic approaches are reasonable in cases of esophageal cancer which does not reach the submucosa. In such cases, modalities used to treat Barrett's esophagus such as endoscopic mucosal resection (EMR), radiofrequency ablation or cryoablation may be appropriate. Once the depth of the lesion involves the submucosa (T1), esophagectomy is likely necessary although EMR may be used in selected cases. Once tumor depth reaches the muscularis propria (T2) or adventitia (T3), esophagectomy is required [19]. Any patient with T1–T3 tumors being treated with resection should also be considered for chemoradiation therapy with medications most commonly including cisplatin and 5-fluorouracil. The role of curative chemoradiation therapy is controversial and currently reserved for patients thought to be poor surgical candidates due to co-morbidities or inoperable type lesions. Patients with locoregional lymphatic involvement are often treated with neoadjuvant chemoradiation therapy before being restaged and considered for surgery. Chemoradiation and palliation therapy are most common in patients with metastatic disease given their poor overall prognosis, with 5-year survival rate being less than 3% [20].

Esophagitis

Esophagitis refers to the inflammatory changes of the esophageal mucosa in response to a noxious stimulus. In erosive esophagitis, squamous esophageal cells lose their ability to regulate their intracellular pH as they are exposed to acidic gastric secretions. As they acidify, they lose the ability to regulate volume, leading to cellular edema and eventual necrosis [21]. However, GERD-induced esophagitis seems less dependent upon the acidity of the reflux than the persistent exposure of the esophageal mucosa to the acidified medium [22]. Initial symptoms of erosive esophagitis include heartburn, acid regurgitation or bitter taste. Interestingly, the presence of dysphagia is not an accurate clinical predictor of disease severity. However, persistence of dysphagia despite PPI therapy does likely indicate therapeutic failure [23]. The treatment of erosive esophagitis through pharmacological acid suppression is covered elsewhere in this book (see Chapter XX).

Another form of esophagitis linked with dysphagia, especially in the young, is eosinophilic esophagitis. This was first described in the late 1970s with presenting symptoms such as heartburn, regurgitation, and vomiting in children, but more commonly presenting in adults with symptoms of dysphagia and food impaction. Diagnosis requires biopsy evidence of >15 eosinophils per high-power field. Endoscopic findings may include multiple esophageal rings, longitudinal furrows, white spots, and mucosal friability.

Although the exact pathophysiological cause of this disease is unknown, eosinophilic esophagitis is thought to be an antigenic response to food or air-borne allergens [24]. The exclusion of GERD as a cause of esophagitis is a common preliminary stage in the diagnosis of eosinophilic esophagitis. However, many patients are placed on acid-suppressive regimens with high-dose PPI initially in their treatment course. Favorable responses to these trials suggest there may be some relationship between GERD and eosinophilic esophagitis [25]. Eosinophilic esophagitis is discussed elsewhere in this book (see Chapter XX).

Motility disorders

In addition to the structural causes of esophageal dysphagia, several motility disorders related to GERD are also known to contribute to dysphagia (Plate 14.1). Ineffective esophageal motility (IEM) is an entity in which the lower esophageal smooth muscle contracts in a hypotensive manner. More specifically, it is manometrically defined as an esophagus in which 50% or more liquid swallows are found to have amplitude <30 mmHg at positions located 5 or 10 cm above the lower esophageal sphincter (LES) [26].

Many studies have shown an association between GERD and IEM. Ho *et al.* reported the overall prevalence of IEM in a group of 89 GERD patients as 49%, with these patients also exhibiting abnormal esophageal acid exposure compared to GERD patients without motility disorder [27]. The causal relationship as to whether long-standing GERD predisposes the lower esophageal body to continuous injury, prompting the hypotensive contractions found in IEM, or whether the hypotensive contractions of IEM contribute to poor acid clearance and worsened symptoms of GERD is unclear. In either case, patients with IEM often complain of dysphagia, regurgitation, and chronic heartburn.

The mainstays of therapy consist of two options. First, maximal acid suppression is attempted in the hope that the lower esophageal smooth muscle may produce higher amplitude contractions as GERD-induced injury decreases. Second, several drugs have been utilized to preferentially augment the hypotensive contractions. Richter *et al.* first showed that intravenous injection of the short-acting acetylcholinesterase inhibitor edrophonium increased LES resting pressure and distal esophageal amplitudes [28]. Humphries and Castell showed a similar effect in healthy volunteers when given the direct muscarinic agonist bethanechol orally [29]. Given these observations, Blonski *et al.* evaluated the use of oral bethanechol, buspirone, and the longer acting oral acetylcholinesterase inhibitor pyridostigmine amongst 10 healthy volunteers [30]. All three agents had a pro-motility effect, with pyridostigmine seeming to show the most potential to preferentially improve contractility and LES tone. Although further studies regarding the use of the cholinergic agents are necessary, potential therapy with cholinergic agents such as bethanechol and pyridostigmine in IEM patients may be considered [30].

Another motility disorder in which hypotensive or absent contractions of the esophagus may contribute to dysphagia is scleroderma (Plate 14.2). Up to 75% of patients with systemic scleroderma are known to have esophageal dysfunction, and approximately 50% of these patients are symptomatic [31]. Manometric findings commonly found in a scleroderma esophagus include absent or greatly diminished contractile waves in the lower esophageal smooth muscle and decreased tone of the lower esophageal sphincter. The mechanism of dysfunction is likely due to replacement of smooth muscle fibers with collagen and fibrosis, or neuronal abnormalities contributing to an absent smooth muscular contractile and resting tonic response. The diminished resting tone of the LES contributes to the presence of GERD in patients with scleroderma. This hypotensive LES allows acid gastric contents to reflux into the esophageal body, predisposing these patients to esophagitis, stricture formation, ulcers, and possible worsening of already prevalent motility abnormalities [32]. Patients may complain of heartburn, dysphagia, acid regurgitation or respiratory symptoms.

Unlike patients with IEM, scleroderma patients with abnormal peristalsis have been found to have no response to methacholine (a cholinergic agonist) or edrophonium (a cholinesterase inhibitor) which increased contraction amplitudes in scleroderma patients with intact peristalsis [33]. This absence of response strengthens the belief that a dysfunctional neuronal axis may be the basis of dysphagia.

> ## CASE STUDY
>
> A 47-year-old woman with a long-standing history of GERD confirmed by ambulatory reflux monitoring presents with worsening intermittent dysphagia and postprandial regurgitation. She has been treated for GERD characterized by heartburn and acid regurgitation for over 20 years, but symptoms are currently frequent despite acid suppression with a PPI. Her more recent symptoms of dysphagia and postprandial regurgitation have been present for the last 2 years but are now occurring more frequently. She describes dysphagia for solids without oropharyngeal transfer difficulties that was initially intermittent but is now frequent and is often followed by regurgitation. She also reveals occasional difficulty with swallowing liquids, weight loss of 5 pounds over 2 months, and increased time needed to complete meals. Her recent EGD revealed erosive esophagitis (LA Grade A) but was otherwise normal with no signs of obstruction.

The treatment of dysphagia in scleroderma patients may be particularly frustrating due to the lack of therapeutic options. At the current time, treatment consists of maximal pharmacological acid suppression. Fundoplication aimed at augmenting the weakened LES may be counter-productive and generally not recommended, as successful anti-reflux surgery may prevent GERD but may contribute to worsened dysphagia since the hypotensive esophageal smooth muscle may not be able to produce propulsive forces great enough to overcome the resistance produced by fundoplication.

References

1 Lindgren MD, Janzon L. Prevalence of swallowing complaints and clinical findings among 50–70 year old men and women in an urban population. Dysphagia 1991;6:187–92.
2 Katz KO, Anand G. Dysphagia and esophageal obstruction. In: Bope ET, Kellerman R, Rakel RE (eds) *Conn's current therapy*. Philadelphia: Elsevier, 2011: pp.523–6.
3 Wilcox CM, Alexander LN, Clark WS. Localization of an obstructing esophageal lesion. Is the patient accurate? Dig Dis Sci 1995;40:2192–6.
4 Spechler SG. American Gastroenterological Association technical review on treatment of patients with dysphagia caused by benign disorders of the distal esophagus. Gastroenterology 1999;177:233–54.
5 Ruigómez A, García Rodríguez LA, Wallander MA, Johansson S, Eklund S. Esophageal stricture: incidence, treatment patterns, and recurrence rate. Am J Gastroenterol 2006;101:2685–92.
6 Siersema, PD. Strictures, rings, and webs. In: Talley NJ, DeVault KR, Fleischer DE (eds) *Practical gastroenterology and hepatology: esophagus and stomach*. Oxford: Wiley-Blackwell, 2010: pp.276–8.
7 Schatski R. The lower esophageal ring. Long term follow-up of symptomatic and asymptomatic rings. Am J Roentgenol Radium Ther Nucl Med 1963;90:805–10.

8 Piotet E, Escher A, Monnier P. Esophageal and pharyngeal strictures: report of 1,862 endoscopic dilations using the Savary–Gilliard technique. Eur Arch Otorhinolaryngol 2008;265:357–64.

9 Lew RJ, Kochman ML. A review of endoscopic methods of esophageal dilation. J Clin Gastroenterol 2002;35:117–26.

10 Schatzki R, Gary J. Dysphagia due to a diaphragm-like localized narrowing in the lower esophagus ("lower esophageal ring"). Am J Roentgenol 1953;70:911–22.

11 Sgouros SN, Vlachogiannakos J, Karamanolis G, et al. Long-term acid suppressive therapy may prevent the relapse of lower esophageal (Schatzki's) rings: a prospective, randomized, placebo-controlled study. Am J Gastroenterol 2005;100(9):1929–34.

12 Nurko S, Teitelbaum JE, Husain K, et al. Association of Schatzki ring with eosinophilic esophagitis in children. J Pediatr Gastroenterol Nutr 2004;38:436–41.

13 Novacek G. Plummer–Vinson syndrome. Orphanet J Rare Dis 2006;1:36.

14 Thun MJ, Peto R, Lopez AD, et al. Alcohol consumption and mortality among middle-aged and elderly U.S. adults. N Engl J Med 1997;337:1705–14.

15 Zhai R, Chen F, Liu G, et al. Interactions among genetic variants in apoptosis pathway genes, reflux symptoms, body mass index, and smoking indicate two distinct etiologic patterns of esophageal adenocarcinoma. J Clin Oncol 2010;28:2445–51.

16 Morales CP, Souza RF, Spechler SJ. Hallmarks of cancer progression in Barrett's oesophagus. Lancet 2002;360:1587–9.

17 Mendes de Almeida JC, Chaves P, Pereira AD, Altorki NK. Is Barrett's esophagus the precursor of most adenocarcinomas of the esophagus and cardia? A biochemical study. Ann Surg 1997;226:725–33;discussion 733–5.

18 Bytzer P, Christensen PB, Damkier P, Vinding K, Seersholm N. Adenocarcinoma of the esophagus and Barrett's esophagus: a population-based study. Am J Gastroenterol 1999;94:86–91.

19 Smith MS, Lightdale CJ. Esophageal cancer. In: Talley NJ, DeVault KR, Fleischer DE (eds) Practical gastroenterology and hepatology: esophagus and stomach. Oxford: Wiley-Blackwell, 2010: pp.320–3.

20 Cooper JS, Guo MD, Herskovic A, et al. Chemoradiotherapy of locally advanced esophageal cancer: long-term follow-up of a prospective randomized trial (RTOG 85-01). JAMA 1999;281:1623–7.

21 Hirschowitz BI. A critical analysis, with appropriate controls, of gastric acid and pepsin secretion in clinical esophagitis. Gastroenterology 1991;101:1149–58.

22 Little AG, DeMeester TR, Kirchner PT, O'Sullivan GC, Skinner DB. Pathogenesis of esophagitis in patients with gastroesophageal reflux.Surgery 1980;88:101–7.

23 Vakil NB, Traxler B, Levine D. Dysphagia in patients with erosive esophagitis: prevalence, severity, and response to proton pump inhibitor treatment. Clin Gastroenterol Hepatol 2004;2:665–8.

24 Prasad GA, Talley NJ, Romero Y, et al. Prevalence and predictive factors of eosinophilic esophagitis in patients presenting with dysphagia: a prospective study. Am J Gastroenterol 2007 102:2627–32.

25 Spechler SJ, Genta RM, Souza RF. Thoughts on the complex relationship between gastroesophageal reflux disease and eosinophilic esophagitis. Am J Gastroenterol 2007;102:1301–6.

26 Tutuian R, Castell DO. Clarification of the esophageal function defect in patients with manometric ineffective esophageal motility: studies using combined impedance-manometry. Clin Gastroenterol Hepatol 2004;2(3):230–6.

27 Ho SC, Chang CS, Wu CY, Chen GH. Ineffective esophageal motility is a primary motility disorder in gastroesophageal reflux disease. Dig Dis Sci 2002;47:652–6.

28 Richter JE, Hackshaw BT, Wu WC, Castell DO. Edrophonium: a useful provocative test for esophageal chest pain. Ann Intern Med 1985;103:14–21.

29 Humphries TJ, Castell DO. Effect of oral bethanechol on parameters of esophageal peristalsis. Dig Dis Sci 1981;26:129–32.

30 Blonski W, Vela MF, Freeman J, Sharma N, Castell DO. The effect of oral buspirone, pyridostigmine, and bethanechol on esophageal function evaluated with combined multichannel esophageal impedance-manometry in healthy volunteers. J Clin Gastroenterol 2009;43:253–60.

31 Akesson A, Wollheim FA. Organ manifestations in 100 patients with progressive systemic sclerosis: a comparison between the CREST syndrome and diffuse sclero-derma. Br J Rheumatol 1989;28:281–6.

32 D'Angelo WA, Fries JF, Masi AT, Shulman LE. Pathologic observations in systemic sclerosis (scleroderma). A study of fifty-eight autopsy cases and fifty-eight matched controls. Am J Med 1969;46:428–40.

33 Cohen S, Fisher R, Lipshutz W, Turner R, Myers A, Schumacher R. The pathogenesis of esophageal dysfunction in scleroderma and Raynaud's disease. J Clin Invest 1972;51:2663–8.

CHAPTER 15

Eosinophilic Esophagitis: Interactions with Gastroesophageal Reflux Disease

Kumar Krishnan and Ikuo Hirano

Division of Gastroenterology, Feinberg School of Medicine, and Northwestern University, Chicago, IL, USA

Key points

- Suspect eosinophilic esophagitis in younger males with a history of atopy who present with recurrent dysphagia. Heartburn and atypical chest pain are additional symptoms.
- A significant proportion of patients with esophageal eosinophilia may respond symptomatically and histologically to a trial of proton pump inhibitor therapy.
- Given the prevalence of gastroesophageal reflux disease in the general population, invariably a significant proportion of patients with eosinophilic esophagitis will have gastroesophageal reflux disease defined by symptoms or abnormal pH testing.
- Eotaxin-3 expression, eosinophil degranulation proteins and gene expression patterns may be useful biomarkers in the diagnosis of eosinophilic esophagitis.

Potential pitfalls

- Heartburn in the absence of dysphagia is a less common complaint of adult patients with eosinophilic esophagitis.
- In a patient with suspected eosinophilic esophagitis who responds to proton pump inhibitor therapy, it remains to be determined whether the response is indicative of a gastroesophageal reflux disease pathogenesis or proton pump inhibitor-responsive form of eosinophilic esophagitis.
- pH testing cannot reliably distinguish eosinophilic esophagitis from gastroesophageal reflux disease-related esophageal eosinophilia given the complex nature of these two conditions. The predictive value of negative or positive pH testing in eosinophilic esophagitis has not been established.
- Symptoms, reflux testing and even histology can sometimes be misleading in distinguishing eosinophilic esophagitis from gastroesophageal reflux disease as there is no gold standard diagnostic test.

Practical Manual of Gastroesophageal Reflux Disease, First Edition.
Edited by Marcelo F. Vela, Joel E. Richter and John E. Pandolfino.
© 2013 John Wiley & Sons, Ltd. Published 2013 by John Wiley & Sons, Ltd.

Introduction

Eosinophilic esophagitis (EoE) is an increasingly recognized entity amongst both children and adults that is conceptually defined as a chronic, immune/antigen-mediated disease characterized clinically by symptoms related to esophageal dysfunction and histologically by eosinophil-predominant inflammation [1]. The association between gastroesophageal reflux (GERD) and EoE has been the source of growing interest. This interest stems from observations that EoE patients have symptom profiles that can mimic GERD [2–4], eosphageal eosinophilia is seen in both EoE and GERD [5–7], and treatment for GERD may lead to improvement in patients with suspected EoE [8,9]. This chapter will focus on the clinical characteristics of EoE, interactions between GERD and EoE, and evidence for treating GERD in patients with suspected EoE.

Clinical, endoscopic, and manometric manifestations

Clinical presentation

The typical clinical symptoms of EoE in adults are dysphagia and food impaction [10]. It has been reported that 30–50% of food impaction cases in adults are the result of EoE [11]. In larger adult series, 80–90% of EoE patients presented with dysphagia while 20–30% reported heartburn. When present, heartburn is usually not a dominant or frequent primary complaint in EoE. In addition, failure to thrive, abdominal pain, nausea and vomiting are frequently reported in children with EoE, but are uncommon in adults. In pediatrics, a reflux-type phenotype is common, with many children presenting with refractory reflux. This is not the case in adults in whom prospective studies have demonstrated esophageal eosinophilia in only 1–4% of patients with reflux symptoms unresponsive to proton pump inhibition (PPI).

Eosinophilic esophagitis is a disease with a strong male predominance, with most series reporting 75% of afflicted children and adults being male [12]. Between 28% and 86% of adults with EoE also carry a history of allergic disease, including atopic dermatitis, allergic rhinitis, and asthma. Abnormal positive skinprick testing or antigen-specific serum immuno-globulin (Ig)E can be demonstrated in the majority of EoE patients but the clinical significance of such testing in the pathogenesis of EoE remains uncertain [13]. While esophageal eosinophilia is a hallmark of this disease, peripheral eosinophilia is seen in only 10–50% of patients, with a majority of cases revealing only modest increase (<2 times the upper limit of normal) in blood eosinophilia [10]. Interestingly, marked peripheral eosinophilia in patients with EoE has been reported to correlate with disease activity [14,15].

Endoscopic findings

Endoscopically, there are esophageal signs commonly associated with EoE (Plate 15.1) [15]. These include concentric rings, longitudinally oriented, linear furrows, white exudates or plaques, mucosal pallor or edema, and esophageal strictures. While evident in the majority of patients, the endoscopic findings are not specific to EoE [10]. A recent study demonstrated reasonably good interobserver agreement for a classification and grading system for the endoscopically identified, esophageal features of EoE (Table 15.1) [15]. High-frequency, endoscopic ultrasonography in small series revealed expansion of the mucosa and submucosa in patients with EoE, as well as thickening of the muscularis propria [16,17]. Investigations have recently demonstrated significantly diminished esophageal

Table 15.1 Classification and grading system for the endoscopic assessment of esophageal features of eosinophilic esophagitis.

	Gastroesophageal reflux disease	Eosinophilic esophagitis
Dominant symptom	Heartburn	Dysphagia
Food impaction	Uncommon	Common
Gender	M=F	Male predominant (75%)
Atopic history	Normal	70%
Endoscopy	Non-erosive reflux disease Erosive esophagitis Barrett's esophagus	Rings Longitudinal furrows Exudates/plaques
Histology	<7 eos/hpf Basal cell hyperplasia Rete peg elongation Dilated intercellular spaces	≥15 eos/hpf Basal cell hyperplasia Rete peg elongation Dilated intercellular spaces Eosinophilic microabscess Superficial layering of eosinophils Subepithelial fibrosis
Biomarkers	Increased distal esophageal acid exposure ? E-cadherin cleaved products	Eotaxin-3 Eosinophil peroxidase
Primary treatment	Antacids, H2 receptor antagonist, proton pump inhibition	Topical steroids, elimination diet

distensibility in patients with EoE [18]. Reduced distensibility may be an important determinant of impaired bolus transit and dysphagia in EoE.

Manometric findings

There has been considerable investigation into the effect of EoE on esophageal motility. Esophageal dysmotility has been suggested to account for the apparent dissociation between symptoms of dysphagia and the presence of endoscopically evident esophageal strictures. Eosinophil-derived proteins may affect enteric neurons and esophageal smooth muscle function. Investigations using high-resolution manometry with pressure topography demonstrated that the majority of manometric abnormalities identified in EoE are non-specific and overlap significantly with features identified in GERD [18]. Weak and failed peristalsis are frequent findings on high-resolution manometry in both GERD and EoE [19]. Increased esophageal pressurization patterns were identified in 36% of EoE patients and only 12% of GERD patients and may reflect reduced wall compliance. Pediatric investigation using prolonged esophageal manometry also reveals increased frequency of ineffective peristalsis compared to GERD controls [20]. In addition to impaired circular muscle function, as measured by esophageal manometry, Korsapati et al. reported dysfunction in longitudinal muscle function in patients with EoE [21]. Specifically, EoE patients demonstrated decreased amplitude and duration of longitudinal muscle contraction during swallows with dissociation between the timing of circular muscle and longitudinal muscle contractions [21]. Longitudinal muscle dysfunction is a potential mechanism for dysphagia in some patients with EoE. However, it remains unclear as to whether the reduced longitudinal muscle function is the result of a motility defect or increased tissue stiffness related to esophageal mural fibrosis.

Diagnosis of eosinophilic esophagitis

The presence of eosinophils within the esophagus is pathological but not specific for any particular disease state. There are many causes of esophageal eosinophilia, including EoE, GERD, parasitic infection, inflammatory bowel disease, autoimmune disorders, neoplasia, drug hypersensitivity, and caustic injury [22]. Currently, there is no single test for the diagnosis of EoE. Consensus recommendations suggest that EoE is a clinicopathological diagnosis that incorporates symptoms of esophageal dysfunction together with markers of eosinophil-predominant inflammation, with 15 eosinophils per high-power field (hpf) considered the minimum threshold for the diagnosis [1]. Characteristic endoscopic signs raise the suspicion of EoE in the appropriate clinical context, but are not a requirement (see

Table 15.1) [15]. With the exception of GERD, most other secondary causes of esophageal eosinophilia can be excluded through a careful clinical history and endoscopic examination.

Histologically, there are no pathognomonic features of EoE, but several findings have been strongly associated with the diagnosis. The number of eosinophils required to consider the diagnosis has been an area of debate. It is important to note that most studies rely on highest number of eosinophils per hpf, and not average number per hpf [23–25]. There is no study defining the optimal threshold number of eosinophils per hpf for EoE, although the consensus recommendations suggest a minimum threshold of 15/hpf. Higher concentrations of eosinophils may increase the diagnostic specificity for EoE at the expense of sensitivity. Eosinophil microabscesses defined by a cluster of more than four eosinophils, superficial layering of eosinophils, eosinophil degranulation, and subepithelial fibrosis have been suggested to distinguish EoE from GERD in a few small studies [11,26]. Basal zone hyperplasia, rete peg elongation, and dilated intercellular spaces have been associated with EoE, but are also common histological findings in GERD [10,11,24,26].

Distinguishing gastroesophageal reflux disease from eosinophilic esophagitis

Perhaps the most challenging aspect of the diagnosis of EoE is the ability to distinguish it from GERD (Box 15.1). Interestingly, esophageal eosinophilia was characteristically associated with GERD in the 1980s [6,27]. In these early reports, the presence of esophageal eosinophilia correlated with increased esophageal acid exposure and was primarily noted to be in the distal esophagus. In the early 1990s, reports from adult and pediatric centers described a cohort of patients with esophageal eosinophilia in the absence of GERD [24,28,29]. Interestingly, the adult studies revealed a phenotype distinct from that typically seen in GERD. Male predominance and history of atopy were pronounced in comparison to patients with GERD. Symptom presentations were dominated by dysphagia and food impaction, rather than heartburn and regurgitation. Endoscopic findings were not those of erosive esophagitis, and instead revealed concentric rings, exudates, and furrows [15]. In addition, the degree of esophageal eosinophilia was markedly higher compared to that typically associated with GERD. Most importantly, the patients studied had either normal pH testing or had symptoms and histopathology despite acid suppressive therapy.

As clinical recognition and the prevalence of EoE in adults began to increase, further investigation supported the notion that EoE is distinct

---

Box 15.1 Comparison of features of gastroesophageal reflux disease and eosinophilic esophagitis

Major features

Fixed rings (also referred to as concentric rings, corrugated esophagus, corrugated rings, ringed esophagus, trachealization)

Grade 0: None

Grade 1: Mild – subtle circumferential ridges

Grade 2: Moderate – distinct rings that do not impair passage of a standard diagnostic adult endoscope (outer diameter 8–9.5 mm)

Grade 3: Severe – distinct rings that do not permit passage of a diagnostic endoscope

Exudates (also referred to as white spots, plaques)

Grade 0: None

Grade 1: Mild – lesions involving less than 10% of the esophageal surface area

Grade 2: Severe – lesions involving greater than 10% of the esophageal surface area

Furrows (also referred to as vertical lines, longitudinal furrows)

Grade 0: Absent

Grade 1: Present

Edema (also referred to as decreased vascular markings, mucosal pallor)

Grade 0: Absent. Distinct vascularity present

Grade 1: Loss of clarity or absence of vascular markings

Stricture

Grade 0: Absent

Grade 1: Present (include estimate of inner diameter of stricture)

Minor features

Crepe paper esophagus (mucosal fragility or laceration upon passage of diagnostic endoscope but not after esophageal dilation)

Grade 0: Absent

Grade 1: Present

---

from GERD. It was previously thought that eosinophil count alone was sufficient to distinguish EoE from GERD, as early reports revealed that most patients with GERD-related eosinophilia seldom had peak eosinophil counts >10/hpf [26,30]. The utility of the eosinophil count in distinguishing EoE from GERD has recently been challenged. A small case series described three young adults with symptoms and histopathology consistent with EoE but responsive to PPI therapy. Larger, retrospective pediatric and adult studies have confirmed this observation, noting a 28–40% histological response rate after PPI therapy [31–33]. A prospective study by Molina-Infante *et al.* identified 35 adults with esophageal eosinophilia, of whom 75% responded histologically to a 6-week course of PPI therapy [8].

A variety of histological features have been investigated to help distinguish GERD from EoE. Perhaps the most conceptually attractive histological feature distinguishing EoE from GERD is the presence of proximal eosinophilia, the reason being that reflux and reflux-associated injury typically predominantly affect the distal esophagus. Recent investigations have compared the frequency of proximal esophageal eosinophila in patients with EoE compared to those with GERD. In one study, 70% of patients with EoE were noted to have a greater degree of eosinophilia in the proximal esophagus compared to the distal, whereas this was not seen in any patients with GERD. Furthermore, 83% of the EoE patients in this cohort had both proximal and distal eosinophilia compared to 0% in GERD patients [34]. Other histological features that have shown modest utility in favoring a diagnosis of EoE over GERD include superficial localization of eosinophils, eosinophilic microabscesses, and eosinophil degranulation. Unfortunately, none appears to be sensitive or specific enough to aid in diagnosis. The prospective trial by Molina-Infante was unable to demonstrate significant differences in these histological features in distinguishing GERD from EoE as defined by a response to PPI therapy. As a result, the consensus guidelines suggest that the diagnosis of EoE should not be established until acid reflux is excluded with a trial of PPI therapy [1,10].

In addition to its overlap with GERD, EoE can co-exist with conditions that are complications of GERD, specifically Barrett's esophagus (BE). The prevalence of esophageal eosinophilia in patients with BE is not entirely known, but retrospective data from the Mayo Clinic suggest that the prevalence is at least 7%. There was no clear association between dysplastic BE and the presence of esophageal eosinophilia [35]. The relevance of esophageal eosinophilia in patients with BE is not known, but it may be a marker of persistent reflux. There is no evidence to causally link EoE with the development of BE or esophageal cancer. Given the background prevalence of GERD and BE in the general population, BE may be an incidental finding unrelated to EoE.

Complicating our understanding of the interactions between GERD and EoE is the possibility that GERD may predispose to or even cause EoE [36]. This concept emerged not only from the observation that there is considerable overlap between these two conditions, but also from early studies revealing that treatment for acid reflux may improve the clinical and histological manifestations of EoE [9]. From a mechanistic standpoint, it is feasible that acid reflux may predispose to EoE. Though the normal squamous epithelium is rather impermeable to allergenic peptides, erosive or non-erosive acid injury has been shown to cause dilated intercellular spaces. This dilation can allow larger peptides to permeate the esophageal epithelium, thus exposing the stroma and antigen-presenting cells to food-borne allergens [37]. Acid exposure induces release of mast cell mediators and may prolong eosinophil viability. Furthermore, acid exposure to the esophageal epithelium can result in recruitment of eosinophils by increasing expression of vascular cell adhesion molecule (VCAM)-1 on the endothelial surface [36,38].

As a result of the complex relationship between EoE and GERD, and challenges in clinical distinction, there has been increased investigation of identifying molecular and genomic differences. Perhaps the strongest piece of evidence supporting distinct mechanistic pathways in EoE and GERD comes from a genome-wide microarray analysis comparing patients with EoE to those with GERD. This study reveals that the esophageal epithelium in patients with EoE has a unique genomic transcriptional pattern distinct from GERD. This transcriptome pattern is conserved amongst patients despite age and sex. This study revealed that eotaxin-3 was the most highly induced gene compared to controls. Furthermore, a polymorphism at the eotaxin-3 allele indicated disease susceptibility [39]. *Ex vivo* studies comparing esophageal squamous cultures from patients with EoE and those from controls revealed that an acidic environment can augment interleukin (IL)-13-mediated eotaxin-3 expression. Interestingly, there was no difference between EoE patients and controls, suggesting that EoE patients are not more susceptible to acid-related eotaxin-3 expression [40].

Treatment of gastroesophageal reflux disease in eosinophilic esophagitis

Consensus guidelines recommend assessing for GERD with either formal reflux testing or an empiric trial of acid-suppressive medication [1,10]. This recommendation was intended to exclude GERD as a secondary cause of esophageal eosinophilia. Several recent reports, however, have called into question the specificity of the PPI response in distinguishing GERD from EoE.

In a prospective study evaluating the utility of pharmacological acid suppression in patients with EoE, Molina-Infante performed esophageal biopsies in 729 consecutive patients with upper gastrointestinal symptoms referred for endoscopy [8]; 35 patients were found to have eosinophilic esophageal infiltration (>15 eos/hpf). These patients were then given rabeprazole 20mg twice daily for 2 months. Interestingly, 75% achieved clinical and histological remission (defined as <5 eos/hpf) with rabeprazole. Sixty percent of those patients with esophageal eosinophilia also had endoscopic evidence of EoE. Of these patients, 70% achieved clinico-pathological remission with rabeprazole alone. Furthermore, 50% of patients with clinical symptoms and signs consistent with EoE and biopsies with >35 eos/hpf responded to the PPI trial. Importantly, 29 out of the 35 patients with esophageal eosinophilia had evidence of pathological reflux with either formal acid testing or endoscopic findings of reflux esophagitis. Potential mechanisms for reflux-induced esophageal eosinophilia were discussed in the previous section.

It is difficult to discern from this study whether the PPI was treating primary eosinophilic esophagitis or reflux-associated eosinophilia [41]. In pediatric and adult case series, patients with suspected refractory GERD with esophageal eosinophilia underwent fundoplication. Post surgery, these patients had persistent symptoms as well as histological evidence consistent with eosinophilic esophagitis which responded to steroid or dietary therapy [29,42]. This indicates that these patients represent a primary eosinophilic esophagitis that is not reflux mediated. However, acid reflux could theoretically exacerbate or accelerate primary eosinophilic esophagitis via a variety of mechanisms. Alternatively, there may be a pleiotropic effect of proton pump inhibitors on the esophageal epithelium that is independent of acid blockade. *In vitro* data suggest that beyond acid suppression, PPIs may have antiinflammatory properties. Specifically, they have been shown to have antioxidant properties, to inhibit neutrophil degranulation, and decrease epithelial secretion of proinflammatory cytokines and chemotactic factors [43]. Most recently, preliminary data have demonstrated an acid-independent effect of omeprazole on suppression of eotaxin-3 expression from esophageal squamous epithelial cells *in vitro* [44]. Acid-independent, antiinflammatory effects could account for a therapeutic effect of PPIs in primary eosinophilic esophagitis.

In light of this seemingly complex and evolving interplay between acid reflux, PPI therapy and esophageal eosinophilia, a practical approach to patients with suspected eosinophilic esophagitis is suggested [44] (Figure 15.1). When confronted with a patient with symptoms dominated by dysphagia and food impaction, typically male with an atopic history, endoscopic features of rings and furrows and esophageal biopsies demonstrating esophageal eosinophilia, an 8-week therapeutic trial of PPI therapy is recommended. While it is tempting to initiate steroids or dietary elimination at this juncture, the recent reports of high degrees of PPI responsiveness together with the safety profile of PPI therapy argue in favor of empiric PPI therapy. Patients with persistent symptoms and esophageal eosinophilia then meet the consensus recommendation definition of eosinophilic esophagitis. Patients who show symptom and histological response to PPI therapy may have GERD or a PPI-responsive form of eosinophilic esophagitis. Until more specific biomarkers are available to distinguish GERD from EoE, these patients should be designated as having "PPI-responsive esophageal eosinophilia" rather than being given a specific diagnosis. Finally, some patients may demonstrate a partial symptom or histological response to PPI and may benefit from continued PPI therapy together with initiation of topical steroids or anelimination diet.

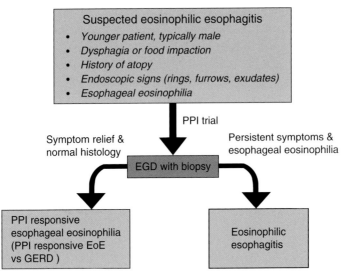

Figure 15.1 Suggested algorithm for evaluation and management of an adult patient with eosinophilic esophagitis (EoE). Eosinophilic esophagitis is suspected based on a clinical profile of symptoms dominated by dysphagia and food impaction in a younger, typically male patient with history of atopy. Features supportive of the diagnosis of EoE include esophageal rings, longitudinal furrows and exudates with histological evidence of esophageal eosinophilia. Following a therapeutic trial of PPI therapy, an EGD differentiates PPI-responsive esophageal eosinophilia from the 2011 consensus recommendation for the diagnosis of primary EoE. It remains controversial whether the PPI-responsive form of esophageal eosinophilia represents GERD or a PPI-responsive subtype of EoE. Patients with persistent symptoms and histopathology of eosinophil-predominant inflammation following PPI therapy meet the current diagnostic criteria for EoE and are offered primary therapy with either elimination diet or topical corticosteroids. Reproduced from Hirano [41] with permission from Elsevier. EGD, esophagogastroduodenoscopy; EoE, eosinophilic esophagitis; GERD, gastroesophageal reflux disease; PPI, proton pump inhibitor.

Summary

Eosinophilic esophagitis is increasingly recognized as a major cause of esophageal dysfunction. The clinical symptoms of EoE in adults include dysphagia and food impaction and less commonly heartburn or chest pain. Endoscopically, the characteristic findings include rings, furrows, exudates, and stricture. Upregulation of eotaxin-3 in response to an environmental trigger is important in the pathogenesis. GERD may predispose to EoE by disrupting the esophageal squamous barrier, resulting in exposure of ingested allergens to antigen-presenting cells. Acid reflux may also increase eosinophil chemotactic factors and eosinophil viability. Consensus recommendations suggest that the diagnosis of EoE should be considered following exclusion of PPI-responsive esophageal eosinophilia. Whether patients with PPI-responsive esophageal eosinophilia have GERD or a PPI-responsive subtype of EoE remains to be determined.

CASE STUDY

A 53-year-old man presents with intermittent dysphagia for 2 years. The patient describes solid food dysphagia occurring on a weekly basis. The dysphagia symptoms are typically relieved by drinking water, but he did have a food impaction that lasted for 36 h. Problem foods include pasta and meat. He has noted heartburn only 1–2 times per month. He denies chest pain, nausea, vomiting, weight loss or blood in stool.

The past medical and surgical history are unremarkable. Family history is negative for allergy or gastrointestinal disease. Social history is significant for social alcohol intake, but is otherwise unremarkable. On physical exam no oral lesions are noted. The neck is supple. The cardiovascular, gastrointestinal, and pulmonary examinations are normal.

Esophagogastroduodenoscopy is performed which reveals concentric rings in the esophagus, linear furrows and white plaques. Distal and proximal esophageal biopsies reveal esophageal eosinophilia (>50 per hpf). The remainder of the upper endoscopy is unremarkable.

The patient is started on omeprazole 40 mg p.o. once daily for 8 weeks. At follow-up, he reports complete relief of his dysphagia. A follow-up EGD reveals rings and furrows, though significantly less pronounced than on the initial endoscopy. Esophageal biopsies do not reveal any pathological change. The patient is maintained on omeprazole 20 mg once daily with no further complaints. On clinic follow-up 6 months later, the patient has no swallowing difficulty, heartburn or food avoidance.

Discussion

This case highlights the difficulty in distinguishing EoE from GERD. As discussed above, there appears to be a complex relationship between acid reflux and EoE. It is unclear whether acid reflux alone or in combination with food allergen can induce the endoscopic and histological changes attributed to eosinophilic esophagitis. The patient described above has intermittent dysphagia for 2 years with minimal reflux symptoms. He does not have the typical atopic history that is common in patients with primary EoE. Futhermore, his endoscopic and histological findings are typical for eosinophilic esophagitis. He has experienced a response to PPI therapy alone, with complete clinical and histological resolution. It is unclear whether he truly has a PPI-responsive form of EoE or an unusual presentation of GERD with secondary esophageal eosinophilia.

References

1 Liacouras CA, Furuta GT, Hirano I, *et al*. Eosinophilic esophagitis: updated consensus recommendations for children and adults. J Allergy Clin Immunol 2011;128(1):3–20.
2 Remedios M, Campbell C, Jones DM, Kerlin P. Eosinophilic esophagitis in adults: clinical, endoscopic, histologic findings, and response to treatment with fluticasone propionate. Gastrointest Endosc 2006;63(1):3–12.

3 Shah A, Kagalwalla AF, Gonsalves N, Melin-Aldana H, Li BU, Hirano I. Histopathologic variability in children with eosinophilic esophagitis. Am J Gastroenterol 2009;104(3):716–21.

4 Teitelbaum JE, Fox VL, Twarog FJ, et al. Eosinophilic esophagitis in children: immunopathological analysis and response to fluticasone propionate. Gastroenterology 2002;122(5):1216–25.

5 Rodrigo S, Abboud G, Oh D, et al. High intraepithelial eosinophil counts in esophageal squamous epithelium are not specific for eosinophilic esophagitis in adults. Am J Gastroenterol 2008;103(2):435–42.

6 Winter HS, Madara JL, Stafford RJ, Grand RJ, Quinlan JE, Goldman H. Intraepithelial eosinophils: a new diagnostic criterion for reflux esophagitis. Gastroenterology 1982;83(4):818–23.

7 Molina-Infante J, Ferrando-Lamana L, Mateos-Rodriguez JM, Perez-Gallardo B, Prieto-Bermejo AB. Overlap of reflux and eosinophilic esophagitis in two patients requiring different therapies: a review of the literature. World J Gastroenterol 7 2008;14(9):1463–6.

8 Molina-Infante J, Ferrando-Lamana L, Ripoll C, et al. Esophageal eosinophilic infiltration responds to proton pump inhibition in most adults. Clin Gastroenterol Hepatol; 9(2):110–17.

9 Ngo P, Furuta GT, Antonioli DA, Fox VL. Eosinophils in the esophagus – peptic or allergic eosinophilic esophagitis? Case series of three patients with esophageal eosinophilia. Am J Gastroenterol 2006;101(7):1666–70.

10 Furuta GT, Liacouras CA, Collins MH, et al. Eosinophilic esophagitis in children and adults: a systematic review and consensus recommendations for diagnosis and treatment. Gastroenterology 2007;133(4):1342–63.

11 Desai TK, Stecevic V, Chang CH, Goldstein NS, Badizadegan K, Furuta GT. Association of eosinophilic inflammation with esophageal food impaction in adults. Gastrointest Endosc 2005;61(7):795–801.

12 Noel RJ, Putnam PE, Rothenberg ME. Eosinophilic esophagitis. N Engl J Med 2004;351(9):940–1.

13 Liacouras CA, Spergel JM, Ruchelli E, et al. Eosinophilic esophagitis: a 10-year experience in 381 children. Clin Gastroenterol Hepatol 2005;3(12):1198–206.

14 Konikoff MR, Blanchard C, Kirby C, et al. Potential of blood eosinophils, eosinophil-derived neurotoxin, and eotaxin-3 as biomarkers of eosinophilic esophagitis. Clin Gastroenterol Hepatol 2006;4(11):1328–36.

15 Hirano I, Moy N, Heckman MG, Thomas CS, Gonsalves N, Achem SR. Endoscopic Assessment of the Esophageal Features of Eosinophilic Esophagitis: Validation of a Novel Classification and Grading System. Gut 2012 In press PMID 22619364.

16 Fox VL, Nurko S, Teitelbaum JE, Badizadegan K, Furuta GT. High-resolution EUS in children with eosinophilic "allergic" esophagitis. Gastrointest Endosc 2003; 57(1):30–6.

17 Stevoff C, Rao S, Parsons W, Kahrilas PJ, Hirano I. EUS and histopathologic correlates in eosinophilic esophagitis. Gastrointest Endosc 2001;54(3):373–7.

18 Kwiatek MA, Hirano I, Kahrilas PJ, Rothe J, Luger D, Pandolfino JE. Mechanical properties of the esophagus in eosinophilic esophagitis. Gastroenterology 2011;140(1):82–90.

19 Roman S, Hirano I, Kwiatek MA, et al. Manometric features of eosinophilic esophagitis in esophageal pressure topography. Neurogastroenterol Motil 2011;23(3):208.

20 Nurko S, Rosen R, Furuta GT. Esophageal dysmotility in children with eosinophilic esophagitis: a study using prolonged esophageal manometry. Am J Gastroenterol 2009;104(12):3050–7.

21 Korsapati H, Babaei A, Bhargava V, Dohil R, Quin A, Mittal RK. Dysfunction of the longitudinal muscles of the oesophagus in eosinophilic oesophagitis. Gut 2009;58(8):1056–62.

22 Rothenberg ME. Biology and treatment of eosinophilic esophagitis. Gastroenterology 2009;137(4):1238–49.

23 Croese J, Fairley SK, Masson JW, et al. Clinical and endoscopic features of eosinophilic esophagitis in adults. Gastrointest Endosc 2003;58(4):516–22.

24 Attwood SE, Smyrk TC, Demeester TR, Jones JB. Esophageal eosinophilia with dysphagia. A distinct clinicopathologic syndrome. Dig Dis Sci 1993;38(1):109–16.

25 Zimmerman SL, Levine MS, Rubesin SE, et al. Idiopathic eosinophilic esophagitis in adults: the ringed esophagus. Radiology 2005;236(1):159–65.

26 Parfitt JR, Gregor JC, Suskin NG, Jawa HA, Driman DK. Eosinophilic esophagitis in adults: distinguishing features from gastroesophageal reflux disease: a study of 41 patients. Mod Pathol 2006;19(1):90–6.

27 Brown LF, Goldman H, Antonioli DA. Intraepithelial eosinophils in endoscopic biopsies of adults with reflux esophagitis. Am J Surg Pathol 1984;8(12):899–905.

28 Straumann A, Spichtin HP, Bernoulli R, Loosli J, Vogtlin J. [Idiopathic eosinophilic esophagitis: a frequently overlooked disease with typical clinical aspects and discrete endoscopic findings]. Schweiz Med Wochenschr 1994;124(33):1419–29.

29 Kelly KJ, Lazenby AJ, Rowe PC, Yardley JH, Perman JA, Sampson HA. Eosinophilic esophagitis attributed to gastroesophageal reflux: improvement with an amino acid-based formula. Gastroenterology 1995;109(5):1503–12.

30 Attwood SE, Fiocca R, Mastracci L, et al. High density eosinophilic infiltration in gastro-esophageal reflux disease is rare and probably not related to primary eosinophilic esophagitis: a cohort study from the Lotus Trial. Paper presented at Digestive Disease Week 2011; Chicago, IL.

31 Dranove JE, Horn DS, Davis MA, Kernek KM, Gupta SK. Predictors of response to proton pump inhibitor therapy among children with significant esophageal eosinophilia. J Pediatr 2009;154(1):96–100.

32 Sayej WN, Patel R, Baker RD, Tron E, Baker SS. Treatment with high-dose proton pump inhibitors helps distinguish eosinophilic esophagitis from noneosinophilic esophagitis. J Pediatr Gastroenterol Nutr 2009;49(4):393–9.

33 Toto E, Garrean C, Hayman A, et al. Differentiation of GERD from EoE (eosinophilic esophagitis): predictive factors and response to PPI trial. Paper presented at Digestive Disease Week 2011; Chicago, IL.

34 Lee S, de Boer WB, Naran A, et al. More than just counting eosinophils: proximal oesophageal involvement and subepithelial sclerosis are major diagnostic criteria for eosinophilic oesophagitis. J Clin Pathol 2010;63(7):644–7.

35 Ravi K, Katzka DA, Smyrk TC, et al. Prevalence of esophageal eosinophils in patients with Barrett's esophagus. Am J Gastroenterol 2011;106(5):851–7.

36 Spechler SJ, Genta RM, Souza RF. Thoughts on the complex relationship between gastroesophageal reflux disease and eosinophilic esophagitis. Am J Gastroenterol 2007;102(6):1301–6.

37 Tobey NA, Hosseini SS, Argote CM, Dobrucali AM, Awayda MS, Orlando RC. Dilated intercellular spaces and shunt permeability in nonerosive acid-damaged esophageal epithelium. Am J Gastroenterol 2004;99(1):13–22.

38 Barthel SR, Annis DS, Mosher DF, Johansson MW. Differential engagement of modules 1 and 4 of vascular cell adhesion molecule-1 (CD106) by integrins alpha4beta1 (CD49d/29) and alphaMbeta2 (CD11b/18) of eosinophils. J Biol Chem 2006;281(43):32175–87.

39 Blanchard C, Wang N, Stringer KF, et al. Eotaxin-3 and a uniquely conserved gene-expression profile in eosinophilic esophagitis. J Clin Invest 2006;116(2):536–47.

40 Blanchard C, Stucke EM, Burwinkel K, *et al.* Coordinate interaction between IL-13 and epithelial differentiation cluster genes in eosinophilic esophagitis. J Immunol 2010;184(7):4033–41.

41 Hirano I. Eosinophilic esophagitis and gastroesophageal reflux disease: there and back again. Clin Gastroenterol Hepatol 2011;9(2):99–101.

42 Dellon ES, Farrell TM, Bozymski EM, Shaheen NJ. Diagnosis of eosinophilic esophagitis after fundoplication for 'refractory reflux': implications for preoperative evaluation. Dis Esophagus 2010;23(3):191–5.

43 Kedika RR, Souza RF, Spechler SJ. Potential anti-inflammatory effects of proton pump inhibitors: a review and discussion of the clinical implications. Dig Dis Sci 2009;54(11):2312–17.

44 Garrean C, Hirano I. Eosinophilic esophagitis: pathophysiology and optimal management. Curr Gastroenterol Rep 2009;11(3):175–81.

CHAPTER 16

Helicobacter pylori and Gastroesophageal Reflux Disease

Maria Pina Dore[1] and David Y. Graham[2]

[1] Instituto di Clinica Medica, University of Sassari, Italy, and Michael E. DeBakey VA Medical Center and Baylor College of Medicine, Houston, TX, USA

[2] Michael E. DeBakey VA Medical Center and Baylor College of Medicine, Houston, TX, USA

Key points

- *Helicobacter pylori* infections and gastroesophageal reflux disease are both common and thus frequently occur together.
- *Helicobacter pylori* does not cause gastroesophageal reflux disease directly or indirectly (i.e. it has no effect on the anti-reflux barrier).
- *Helicobacter pylori* infection does not protect against gastroesophageal reflux disease, Barrett's esophagus or adenocarcinoma of the esophagus.
- Hypochlorhydria or achlorhydria associated with atrophic gastritis prevents symptomatic reflux and gastroesophageal reflux disease sequelae such as erosive esophagitis, Barrett's esophagus, and adenocarcinoma of the esophagus. It is also strongly associated with the risk of gastric cancer.
- Proton pump inhibitor therapy in patients with *Helicobacter pylori* gastritis can result in acceleration of corpus gastritis and thus can theoretically increase the risk of gastric cancer.
- *Helicobacter pylori* eradication does not significantly affect anti-secretory therapy for gastroesophageal reflux disease.
- Patients considered for long-term proton pump inhibitor therapy should be tested for *Helicobacter pylori* and if present, the infection should be eradicated.

Potential pitfalls

- Failure to treat an *Helicobacter pylori* infection because of fear that doing so would increase the patient's risk for gastroesophageal reflux disease and adenocarcinoma of the esophagus.
- Failure to test for *Helicobacter pylori* in a patient in whom long-term proton pump inhibitor therapy is planned.
- Failure to consider transient proton pump inhibitor-induced acid rebound for development of gastroesophageal reflux disease-like symptoms after discontinuing proton pump inhibitors given for a non-gastroesophageal reflux disease indication such as treatment to eradicate *Helicobacter pylori*.

Practical Manual of Gastroesophageal Reflux Disease, First Edition.
Edited by Marcelo F. Vela, Joel E. Richter and John E. Pandolfino.
© 2013 John Wiley & Sons, Ltd. Published 2013 by John Wiley & Sons, Ltd.

Introduction

Prior to the identification of *Helicobacter pylori*, peptic ulcer disease and gastric cancer were both known to be closely associated with the presence of gastritis; the discovery of *H. pylori* provided the link between them. Because *H. pylori* is a bacterial infection, it was thought likely that cure of the infection might result in prevention of gastric cancer and cure of the heretofore incurable peptic ulcer disease.

Helicobacter pylori is now accepted as etiologically related to gastritis and the gastritis-associated diseases: duodenal ulcer, gastric ulcer and gastric cancer, both adenocarcinoma and primary gastric B-cell lymphoma. *H. pylori* infections are typically acquired in childhood with clinical disease occurring typically after a long latent period during which gastric damage occurs silently. The risk of a clinical outcome of the infection is approximately 20% [1]. Different outcomes are associated with different patterns of gastritis: gastric ulcer and gastric cancer with atrophic pangastritis and low acid secretion (hypochlorhydria or achlorhydria), and duodenal ulcer with corpus-sparing gastritis (antral predominant gastritis) and high acid secretion. Because different outcomes are linked to markedly different patterns of gastritis, duodenal ulcer disease and gastric ulcer occur at entirely different ends of the spectrum of gastritis and it can be said that duodenal ulcer "protects" against gastric cancer and vice versa. Protection in this context means "inversely related to" and not any actual involvement (i.e. no one would fear that curing a duodenal ulcer would increase the risk of gastric cancer). This possible misuse of the concept of *H. pylori* infections "protecting" against other diseases will be discussed below.

Within a decade of the culture of *H. pylori*, it was discovered how to reliably eradicate *H. pylori* infections which was also shown to result in the healing of the underlying gastritis. The hypothesis that cure of *H. pylori* infections would also cure peptic ulcer disease was also tested and proven to be correct. However, following *H. pylori* eradication, some patients were reported to have developed gastroesophageal reflux disease (GERD) [2,3]. At the time, the appearance of GERD following the cure of *H. pylori*-related duodenal ulcers was not expected although possibly it should have been. For example, by the mid-20th century it was well known that there was an association between the presence of duodenal ulcer and GERD and this finding was repeatedly confirmed in the West [4–13] and in Japan [14]. During this same time period, it was noted that the incidence of esophageal adenocarcinoma appeared to be increasing. The fact that *H. pylori* caused inflammation, ulcers and cancer in the stomach led to questions about what, if any, was the role of *H. pylori* in GERD and in esophageal adenocarcinoma.

This chapter will discuss whether there is a relationship between *H. pylori* and the frequency and severity of GERD as well as the sequelae of GERD in different populations, attempt to provide an understanding of the pathophysiology involved, and explain the role of *H. pylori*, if any, in "protection" against GERD and its sequelae such as Barrett's esophagus and esophageal adenocarcinoma.

Gastroesophageal reflux disease and *Helicobacter pylori* in the pre-*Helicobacter pylori* era

Interest in GERD became prominent in the late 20th century. However, GERD was not a new problem but rather it became a disease *du jour* [15–17], as dyspepsia had long been recognized as particularly common in America [18] and heartburn, water-brash and pyrosis were all prevalent problems [19]. Antacids were widely and commonly used throughout the 19th and most of the 20th centuries. For example, in the 1970s over-the-counter antacids were used by at least half of US adults, with approximately a quarter of adults taking at least two doses per month and at least 5% of adults using antacids daily [20]. The introduction of H2 receptor antagonists (H2RAs) in the mid-1970s produced the first simple and effective relief of ulcer pain and reliable ulcer healing and it was widely believed that ulcers were finally cured. Clinicians and third-party payers were, however, surprised to find that many patients with duodenal ulcer disease continued to use H2RAs despite healing of their ulcers. Despite the use of fiberoptic endoscopy to identify ulcers and confirm healing, GERD continued to be largely ignored. Evidence that GERD was given short shrift in the major gastroenterology textbooks can be easily found; for example, the major textbooks of gastrointestinal disease in the 1970s in the US did not recognize that GERD was a common manifestation of Zollinger–Ellison syndrome.

The initial focus on GERD and how to study it was in part related to an interest manifested by pharmaceutical companies who saw GERD as a possible way to expand their markets for proton pump inhibitors (PPIs) and to differentiate PPIs from H2RAs which dominated the market at that time. As noted above, over-the-counter antacid use among apparently otherwise healthy individuals was extremely common throughout this period but it was unclear why. In the early 1980s we studied why apparently healthy individuals were frequent users of antacids. We found that the primary reason was GERD [20]. As interest in GERD increased, the gastroenterology community found that the lessons learned in the study of peptic ulcer disease were not directly transferable to GERD. For example, as noted by our forefathers, peptic ulcer was an episodic condition whereas GERD was a chronic disease that required continuous therapy and that therapy was in large part symptomatic and not curative.

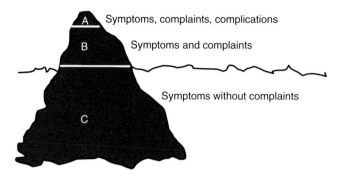

Figure 16.1 The "iceberg" represents the populations of patients with gastroesophageal reflux [22]. The largest group are those with mild disease who self-medicate with over-the-counter drugs and rarely if ever visit doctors because of their symptoms. The smallest group are those who visit gastroenterologists because of severe disease requiring continuous high-dose therapy. A represents those with complications (e.g. symptoms and complications), B those with symptoms who seek medical care (e.g. symptoms and complaints), C those with symptoms who self-medicate and do not seek medical care (e.g. symptoms and no complaints). Adapted from Graham [16] with permission from Blackwell Publishing.

In those days, most patients with GERD did not seek medical attention but rather used over-the counter drugs [20,21]. In contrast, those entering clinical trials were typically from the small subgroup with complicated erosive disease and as such, the results did not necessarily reflect the needs or responses of the average patient [22,23]. We proposed that the population of GERD patients could be visualized as an iceberg or pyramid ranging from those with symptoms who did not seek medical attention (symptoms without complaints), to those with symptoms and complications who tended to get into treatment trials [22] (Figure 16.1). A similar pattern was subsequently noted in Japan [21]. Studies of the relationship between *H. pylori* and GERD led to identification of a fourth group (group D) of asymptomatic reflux which is often the largest group in areas where *H. pylori*-induced atrophic gastritis is common such that, because of low acid secretion, symptoms are infrequent despite a significant reflux [16] (Figure 16.2) (see below).

Helicobacter pylori, gastritis, and acid secretion

Gastric inflammation induced by *H. pylori* can have either positive or negative effects on gastric acid secretory physiology, depending on the pattern of gastritis [16,24,25]. Gastric acid is normally secreted in response to meals and, in the normal and uninfected stomach, the duration of secretion is regulated by a sensitive pH-dependent feedback mechanism (Figure 16.3). Initially, the high pH and proteins in a meal stimulate antral G-cells to secret gastrin which stimulates parietal cells in the gastric corpus to secrete acid.

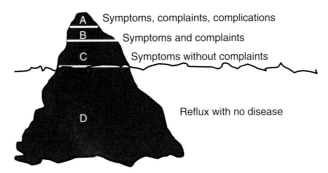

Figure 16.2 This "iceberg" represents the populations of patients with gastroesophageal disease in countries where chronic atrophic gastritis and gastric cancer are common and GERD is rare. A new group (D) is added to depict those with largely non-acid reflux but without symptoms or complaints. In such areas the *H. pylori* gastritis-associated reductions in acid secretion are such that patients have neither symptoms nor endoscopic changes despite the presence of gastroesophageal reflux. Reproduced from Graham [16] with permission from Blackwell Publishing.

When the buffering capacity of the meal is exhausted and the intragastric pH falls below pH 3, antral D-cells secrete somatostatin which downregulates gastrin secretion and turns off the brisk acid secretion. *H. pylori* infection disrupts this regulatory mechanism, resulting in both an exaggerated gastrin response to meals and dysregulation of the normal pH-sensitive downregulatory mechanism. Together, this results in an abnormal prolongation of meal-stimulated acid secretion [26] (see Figure 16.3). Although everyone with an *H. pylori* infection has these abnormalities in the regulation of acid secretion, the end result differs depending on the pattern and severity of gastritis (i.e. antral, corpus or both).

At the beginning of the 20th century, it was recognized that gastric cancer was strongly associated with reduced acid secretion [27]. By 1950, it was recognized that corpus gastritis affected acid secretion and, depending on the degree of destruction of the parietal cell mass, the results could vary from a modest decrease in acid secretion to achlorhydria [27]. Because the degree of reduction in acid secretion was greater than the reduction in parietal cell mass, it was hypothesized that there was an inflammation-related mediator that actually caused the reduction in acid secretion [28]. The discovery of *H. pylori* and studies of acid secretion before and immediately after treatment confirmed that in patients with corpus-sparing gastritis (antral predominant) and duodenal ulcer, *H. pylori* eradication led to a return to the normal mechanisms that controlled acid secretion (elimination of the high prolonged meal-stimulated acid response), but little or no change in maximum secretion (i.e. control of acid secretion was normalized but the parietal cell mass was unchanged).

Gastric inflammation induced by *H. pylori* can have either positive or negative effects on gastric acid secretory physiology, depending on the

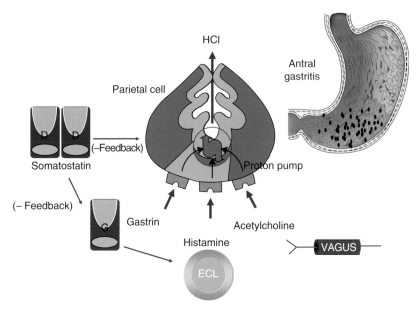

Figure 16.3 Gastric acid secretion is activated throughout the binding of gastrin (secreted by the G-cells), acetylcholine (by vagus), and histamine (by enterochromaffin-like (ECL) cells), and prostaglandins to the specific receptors on the basolateral surface of parietal cells. The ultimate factor in acid secretion is the stimulation of the proton pump (H+, K+−ATPase) to secrete hydrogen ions into the gastric lumen in exchange for potassium ions. After sufficient acid secretion has occurred, a feedback system terminates gastric acid secretion. A decrease of intragastric pH below 3 stimulates somatostatin release from antral D-cells which downregulates gastrin secretion, turning off acid secretion. The presence of an *H. pylori* infection disrupts this mechanism, leading to an exaggerated gastrin response to meals and a delay in the inhibitory effects of somatostatin.

pattern of gastritis [16,24–26] (i.e. the reduction in mucosal acid inhibitory mediators such as interleukin (IL)-1β can result in a marked increase in maximal acid secretion among those with corpus gastritis [20,29,30] whereas in antral-predominant gastritis, the overall effect is a reduction in total acid secretion due to return of the normal acid-related downregulation of acid secretion. Thus, fundamentally, the overall result of *H. pylori* infections correlates with the pattern and severity of gastritis (i.e. antral, corpus or both) [27].

The predominant pattern of *H. pylori* gastritis in any population or patient predicts potential outcomes in terms of *H. pylori* infection (i.e. antral-predominant gastritis leading to duodenal ulcer, and atrophic pangastritis leading to gastric ulcers and/or gastric cancer) [16]. Thus, in countries where gastric cancer is common, the most common pattern of gastritis in adults is pangastritis, and hypochlorhydria and achlorhydria are common. As such, the impaired ability to secrete acid means that irrespective of the status of the individual's gastroesophageal reflux barrier, the average individual will have a low esophageal acid load and erosive reflux will be uncommon [16] (i.e. in countries where atrophic gastritis and gastric cancer are common, such as Japan or Korea, GERD has not been a significant clinical problem) [31]. However, as the pattern of gastritis changes and becomes more like the current pattern in Western countries, the incidence of gastric cancer and gastric ulcer also declines, acid secretion rises and those with abnormal anti-reflux barriers are more likely to experience symptomatic GERD.

Helicobacter pylori infection and its relationship to gastroesophageal reflux

Gastroesophageal reflux refers to the reflux of fluid from the stomach into the esophagus. Occasional reflux is a normal occurrence and is typically asymptomatic and without clinical consequences. Reflux can also cause disease (i.e. symptoms and/or mucosal damage, as in gastroesophageal reflux disease). The lumen of the stomach is separated from that of the esophagus by an anti-reflux barrier that consists of both smooth muscle sphincter (the physiological barrier of the lower esophageal sphincter or LES) and a group of anatomical structures that together constitute a flap valve [32–34]. In addition to the flap valve, the muscular LES normally maintains a pressure gradient between the esophagus and stomach. The three dominant pathophysiological mechanisms causing gastroesophageal junction incompetence are transient lower esophageal sphincter relaxations (TLESRs), a hypotensive LES, and anatomical disruption of the gastroesophageal junction typically associated with the presence of hiatal hernia.

Helicobacter pylori infection *per se* is not thought to have a deleterious effect on the anti-reflux barrier as it has no effect on the LES, the frequency of TLESRs [35–38], esophageal peristaltic function or acid clearance [35,38]. Although *H. pylori* can occasionally be found on the esophageal mucosa, *H. pylori* is only trophic for gastric mucosa and its presence in the esophagus is likely to be transient and related to reflux from the stomach (i.e. an epiphenomenon) [39,40].

As noted above, indigestion and heartburn have been common symptoms throughout the recorded history of mankind. However, the role of the esophagus as a cause of these symptoms was overlooked until recently [15]. While it is commonly believed that there has been a great increase in incidence of GERD in the last 30 years, the data to support this hypothesis are slim at best and we believe that the data better support increased recognition as the most important factor. One only has to think back a few years to the pre-PPI era which was a time when antacid use was extremely common and large numbers of outpatients were being treated for esophageal strictures, which is a "tip of the iceberg" manifestation of GERD [41–43]. As noted above, the textbooks in use before this current "epidemic" of GERD largely ignored GERD despite its high prevalence.

The clinical outcome of an individual with gastroesophageal reflux is determined by the severity and duration of reflux, the causticity of the refluxate, and the ability of the esophageal mucosa to withstand and clear what is refluxed from the stomach. The pH of the refluxate is a major determinant and can vary from alkaline to strongly acidic. Alkaline reflux, especially of intestinal contents, may produce both symptoms and mucosal damage but the majority of patients with GERD have intact stomachs and acid-peptic reflux. Abnormalities of the anti-reflux barrier are, however, only half of the story of GERD as there are important environmental factors as evidenced by the fact that the prevalence of GERD and GERD-related diseases differs geographically and can change rapidly even within a population. Some of these differences may be related to *H. pylori* infections because, although *H. pylori* is not directly involved in alterations of anti-reflux barrier function, it can have a profound effect on acid secretion and thus on esophageal acid load.

One way to conceptualize the risk of a clinical outcome of reflux is in terms of the esophageal acid load [16]. This concept takes into account both the acidity and the duration of reflux (e.g. acidity×duration) (Table 16.1). As shown in Figures 16.4 and 16.5, for a given degree of acidity, the severity of esophageal damage will be a function of the duration of reflux. In contrast, for a given amount and duration of reflux, the degree of damage becomes a function of the acidity and thus, clinically, both are important. Excess acid secretion of any cause is associated with symptomatic reflux (Box 16.1) [16,24,44–50].

Table 16.1 Esophageal acid load before and after cure of *H. pylori* infection.

	H. pylori	Cured
Time pH <4	60 min	60 min
Average pH	3.5	2.2
H+ (mEq/L)	0.55	8.25
Acid load ([H+]×time)	33	495
Load	1	15-fold increase

This shows the effect of cure of an active *H. pylori* infection with corpus gastritis. The slight change in average pH results in no change in the measured time that the esophageal pH is below 4 yet the esophageal acid load has increased 15-fold. Reproduced from Graham [16] with permission from Blackwell Publishing.

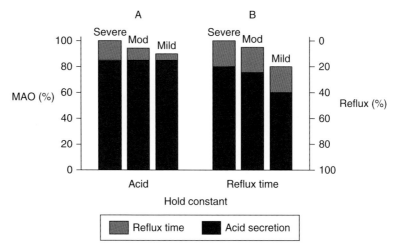

Figure 16.4 The effects of changing acid secretion and percentage reflux time (esophageal acid load) on the severity of gastroesophageal reflux disease. Acid secretion is represented as percentage of pentagastrin-stimulated maximal acid output (MAO) and reflux as the proportion of time that gastric contents reflux into the esophagus. The data are presented as a concept model showing that the severity of gastroesophageal reflux is related to the esophageal acid load and can be dominated by the amount of acid secretion on the amount of reflux time. If the acid secretion is held constant (*left panel*), the esophageal acid load is related directly to the duration of the reflux time. The right panel shows that when the reflux time is held constant and acid secretion is varied, the severity of GERD is then related to the amount of acid secretion. Reproduced from Graham [16] with permission from Blackwell Publishing.

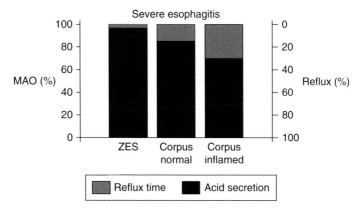

Figure 16.5 This plot illustrates that patients with different acid secretion and reflux times can experience the same outcome (severe esophagus). The key is that esophagitis will occur when the threshold for esophageal acid load is exceeded and this can occur with markedly different patterns of acid secretion which in turn can reflect the patterns of gastritis, especially the severity of corpus gastritis. The threshold for development of GERD likely varies for any particular patients. Reproduced from Graham [16] with permission from Blackwell Publishing. ZES, Zollinger–Ellison syndrome.

> **Box 16.1 Causes of acid hypersecretion often associated with symptomatic GERD**
>
> - Zollinger–Ellison syndrome
> - Antral gastritis *H. pylori* positive
> - Mastocytosis
> - Retained antrum following partial gastrectomy
> - Duodenal ulcer disease
> - Idiopathic gastric acid hypersecretion
> - Rebound hypersecretion related to discontinuation of PPIs

Helicobacter pylori eradication and gastroesophageal reflux disease

As noted above, it has long been recognized that there is a relationship between duodenal ulcer disease and GERD and in retrospect, this was likely responsible for the desire of many patients with duodenal ulcer to continue H2RA therapy even after their ulcer was healed. The fact that some patients complained of GERD after *H. pylori* eradication initially led to confusion about whether *H. pylori* eradication might actually cause GERD [2,3]. The effect of *H. pylori* eradication on GERD can vary from new onset of symptoms, no change in existing symptoms, to amelioration of existing symptoms [16,17,51]. The different outcomes are related to posteradication changes in acid secretion. For example, it is possible for *H. pylori* eradication to make preexisting asymptomatic reflux more acidic and thus turn asymptomatic reflux into clinical GERD or to increase the severity of mild GERD [16]. On the other hand, it could be associated with a reduction in the severity of GERD by reducing the duration of the meal-stimulated acid response.

Most often, eradication has no consistent effect on GERD symptoms or management. The actual outcome depends in part on the patient's ability to secrete acid (e.g. pattern of gastritis) and the status of the anti-reflux barrier mechanism (Figure 16.6) [16]. One also must consider the effects of acid rebound associated with stopping PPI therapy, which is commonly used as a part of the eradication therapy [48,49]. Considering that anti-*H. pylori* therapy is generally of short duration (i.e. 1–2 weeks), rebound is generally self-limited but in other patients who have been on longer term anti-secretory therapy for maintenance of ulcer remission, it may last considerably longer.

A number of double-blind controlled trials have looked into whether *H. pylori* eradication results in new-onset GERD, worsening or improved GERD, as well as whether *H. pylori* eradication makes the management of

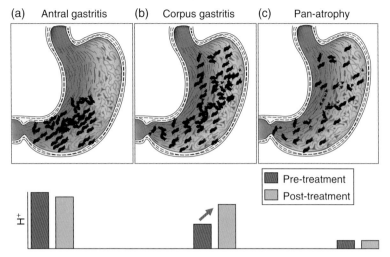

Figure 16.6 The different patterns of gastritis and gastric acid secretion before and following *H. pylori* eradication. Patients with antral-predominant disease (e.g. those with duodenal ulcer) would be expected to have minimal changes in maximum acid secretion although the duration of acid secretion would likely decrease (a). Those with corpus gastritis would be expected to recover acid secretion in proportion to the remaining parietal cells which were released from inhibition (b). This is the group at risk for developing symptomatic reflux as the esophageal acid load of those with asymptomatic reflux would increase. Those with atrophy would have little or no change in acid secretion and the risk of developing posteradication reflux symptoms would be very low (c).

GERD more difficult. Systematic reviews and metaanalyses of these studies have been repeated as new data have become available [52,53]. Overall, these studies have shown that *H. pylori* eradication in those with preexisting GERD is not associated with a change in the frequency of GERD symptoms or endoscopic esophagitis, at least during follow-up for 6 months or 12 months post eradication [52,53]. The data on severity of symptoms and on the effect on pH are as yet insufficient to make a judgment about a consistent effect. For example, one study found that the total time for which the esophageal pH was less than 2 and 3 was increased whereas another did not [54,55]. In reality, our ability to assess change, whether it be in terms of symptoms, endoscopic or acid load, is relatively crude. In addition, few studies have attempted to assess results in terms of a reliable assessment of the pattern of gastritis, changes in acid secretion, and baseline antireflux barrier function [47–49].

Measurement of acid exposure uses the arbitrary pH of 4 as an indicator of acid exposure whereas acid load would require an accurate measurement of pH. The metaanalyses available have primarily related to data from Western countries and showed similar results on GERD symptoms following *H. pylori* eradication in the US and Europe. For example, a *post hoc* analysis of eight double-blind prospective trials of *H. pylori* eradication for duodenal ulcer disease failed to confirm the hypothesis that eradication of *H. pylori* resulted in the development of erosive esophagitis or new symptomatic GERD [56]. Similarly, an analysis of 27 observational studies found no evidence that *H. pylori* eradication in duodenal ulcer disease either provoked reflux esophagitis or worsened heartburn [52]. In contrast, in Japan, on average those with preexisting GERD most typically experienced improvement of GERD symptoms following *H. pylori* eradication [14]. In Japan, when reflux developed post eradication, it was likely to be mild and transient and associated with higher Body Mass Index (BMI) and younger age [57]. One study reported that in duodenal ulcer patients, absence of hiatal hernia and lower BMI were associated with improvement of GERD after *H. pylori* eradication [57].

In areas of Asia (e.g. Japan and Korea) where atrophic gastritis is common and erosive GERD is rare, *H. pylori* eradication in a patient with corpus gastritis may result in an increase in gastric acidity, making those with abnormal anti-reflux barriers and asymptomatic reflux susceptible to development of GERD symptoms [14,16,17,51] (see Figure 16.6). Such a finding would be the result of the increase in esophageal acid load and turning asymptomatic reflux into symptomatic GERD [14,16,17,51].

Clinically, there is no group in which the trade-offs that occur following *H. pylori* eradication do not strongly favor eradication. The management of those with preexisting GERD is typically unchanged. A few with corpus gastritis will develop reflux symptoms but these are generally mild, easily controlled and often transient and the natural progression of their corpus gastritis to more severe atrophic gastritis is halted, thus reducing, if not eliminating, their risk of developing gastric cancer [27,58–60]. Parenthetically, those with atrophic gastritis and low acid secretion are at high risk for gastric cancer with annual risks of more than 500–1000/ 100,000 per year. In countries where atrophic gastritis and gastric cancer are infrequent and duodenal ulcer is common among those with *H. pylori* infection, the overall effect of *H. pylori* eradication would be expected to be little change or a decrease in acid secretion and either no change or a reduction in symptoms (see Figure 16.6). New GERD would not be expected except in those with corpus gastritis [38] or as a consequence of post-PPI acid rebound.

Barrett's esophagus and adenocarcinoma

Although the incidence of adenocarcinoma of the esophagus has increased, it remains a rare problem (i.e. it changed from a very rare to a rare disease) [61].

However, it is important because it is associated with Barrett's esophagus, which is a high-risk, easily recognizable precursor lesion. Barrett's esophagus allows for screening and surveillance programs for detection of early cancer and for cancer prevention programs [62].

Barrett's esophagus is not a new disease; even in 1961, authors were able to bring together series of 200 patients with Barrett's esophagus [63]. It was recognized that:

* Barrett's esophagus and esophageal adenocarcinoma were most common among white men (a group that in the US first experienced a decline in *H. pylori* prevalence) [61]
* Barrett's esophagus was associated with GERD and higher rates of acid secretion [64]
* absence of *H. pylori* infection allowed the stomach to express its full potential for acid secretion (i.e. higher acid loads among those that refluxed) [65].

Together, these data suggested that the rise in Barrett's might be, in part, related to the decline in the prevalence of *H. pylori* infection. This inverse association was, as noted earlier, a form of "protection" but this protection was often construed as not simply an association but rather a risk that might be controlled. This hypothesis resulted in a series of dire consequence hypotheses related to *H. pylori* eradication (discussed in references 66 and 67). The inverse relationship between *H. pylori* and Barrett's esophagus and adenocarcinoma of the esophagus was extended to be most important among those with infecting *H. pylori* that expressed the cytotoxin-associated antigen CagA, a putative virulence factor of *H. pylori* associated with more severe inflammation, ulcer disease, and gastric cancer [65]. Authors describing the importance of CagA in protection have ignored the fact that CagA-positive *H. pylori* infections are strongly associated with duodenal ulcer which, as noted above, is strongly associated with an increased risk of GERD. The low frequency of CagA-positive *H. pylori* among patients with Barrett's esophagus is relative, and not absolute, and as previously discussed, the "protective" feature is the presence of atrophic gastritis. This low prevalence of CagA positivity is also present in individuals from countries in which Barrett's is rare, most patients have CagA-positive infections, and atrophic gastritis and gastric cancer are common [68].

Overall, these data are consistent with the hypothesis that the inverse relationship (inappropriately called protection) is related to the fact that *H. pylori*-induced corpus gastritis can act as a biological anti-secretory agent and reduce or prevent GERD and it sequelae [69]. CagA-containing *H. pylori* does not protect against anything; rather, it is atrophic gastritis that "protects" against GERD and Barrett's esophagus [67,70]. Unfortunately, atrophic gastritis is recognized as the precursor lesion for gastric cancer, the fourth most common cancer worldwide. As noted previously, adenocarcinoma of the esophagus remains a rare disease with a prevalence similar to that of small bowel cancer. Any "protection" against Barrett's esophagus afforded by atrophic gastritis comes with a many hundred-fold increase in risk for gastric cancer and is thus a rather poor trade-off.

The change in the pattern of gastritis in the 20th century (i.e. a fall in the prevalence of atrophic gastritis) in the US resulted in a marked decline in the incidence of gastric cancer and a concomitant increase in the incidence of duodenal ulcer, each of which "protects" against the other. The programs to eradicate H. pylori are based on the fact that H. pylori is an important human pathogen responsible for much morbidity and mortality. Among chronic infectious diseases, H. pylori infection has a higher risk of a serious clinical outcome than either latent syphilis or tuberculosis which, if one looked closely, would both probably "protect" against some other diseases [71]. As noted previously, at least 20% of those with an H. pylori infection will experience a symptomatic clinical illness (e.g. typically peptic ulcer or gastric cancer) and 25% of those with peptic ulcers will experience a life-threatening complication such as a major gastrointestinal bleed, perforation or obstruction [1]. Unfortunately, the dire consequences that have been described in relation to H. pylori eradication have led some to forego H. pylori eradication and to suffer even more the dire consequences of that decision.

In epidemiology, when one variable is associated with a reduction of another (e.g. a disease), it is said to be "protective". For example, populations with limited sanitation, high rates of malnutrition, and early mortality have a low incidence of age-related diseases such as diabetes, stroke, and cancer. One could conclude that from an epidemiological standpoint, poor sanitation "protects" against those diseases. H. pylori can no more be credited with a clinically important protection against esophageal cancer than poor sanitation can be credited with protecting against diseases associated with aging. H. pylori is a proven cause of gastric cancer; one does not keep a King cobra in one's house to protect against mice.

Helicobacter pylori, proton pump inhibitors and atrophic gastritis

Many, if not most, patients with symptomatic GERD who visit physicians will receive anti-secretory drug therapy, typically a PPI. Anti-secretory drug therapy changes the intragastric milieu and, as a consequence, H. pylori, which is normally restricted to the surface of the gastric corpus of a highly acidic stomach, can infect deeper within the mucosa [72,73]. This change in localization is associated with an increase in the severity and depth of corpus gastritis which includes the proliferative zone [72]. In clinical trials it was noticed that PPI use could result in the aggravation of *H. pylori*-induced corpus gastritis [72,74,75]. The natural history of *H. pylori* gastritis is for the inflamed area to advance from the antrum into the corpus, resulting in a reduction in acid secretion and eventually loss of parietal cells and development of atrophy [76] and, as noted above, atrophic pangastritis is the precursor lesion for development of gastric cancer. The fact that PPI therapy was associated with the acceleration of corpus gastritis development led to the suggestion that it may also increase the risk of gastric cancer. Follow-up data of up to 10 years subsequently showed that the annual incidence of gastric corpus mucosal atrophy was higher in *H. pylori*-positive patients receiving PPI therapy than those not receiving it (4.7% versus 0.7%) [75]. Recent long-term follow-up studies from Europe also showed that the annual incidence of gastric corpus mucosal atrophy among *H. pylori*-infected PPI users increased compared with *H. pylori*-uninfected patients [77].

Yang *et al.* studied an Asian population in which atrophic gastritis and gastric cancer were both increased compared with European populations [78]. They compared cohorts with typical reflux symptoms after *H. pylori* eradication therapy ($n = 105$) to *H. pylori*-positive patients without eradication ($n = 105$) and *H. pylori*-negative GERD controls ($n = 115$). Participants were randomized to receive esomeprazole 40 mg daily until sustained symptomatic response and were then switched to on-demand therapy. Endoscopy with antral and corpus biopsies was done initially and at the end of the first and second years. Important changes in gastric inflammation features among the study groups were observed in the first year of follow-up with a persistently high score in the *H. pylori*-positive non-eradicated group compared to the *H. pylori*-positive eradicated group ($P < 0.001$). Extension of atrophy upward to the corpus was only seen in the two *H. pylori*-positive groups and more importantly in the second year of follow-up, the prevalence rates of atrophy and intestinal metaplasia were lower in the *H. pylori*-positive eradicated group than in the non-eradicated controls (i.e. atrophy 72.3% versus 56.6% and intestinal metaplasia 36.1% versus 21.7 %; $P < 0.05$ for both).

Controlled trials have demonstrated that *H. pylori* eradication in patients with reflux esophagitis decreases inflammation and reverses corpus gastritis despite long-term PPI therapy [79]. As noted above, it has clearly been shown that *H. pylori* eradication does not make GERD therapy more complicated or difficult, leading European consensus guidelines to recommend an *H. pylori* test and treat strategy for patients requiring long-term acid suppression therapy [80]. We agree that a test and treat strategy should be employed for all patients for whom long-term anti-secretory, especially PPI, therapy is indicated.

CASE STUDY

Gastric biopsy from a 57-year-old man with erosive GERD was reported to show acute
and chronic inflammation of the antral mucosa and Giemsa stain showed organisms
consistent with *H. pylori*. The primary care physician asks whether the *H. pylori*
infection should be treated, and expresses concern that eradication may result in
worsening of GERD symptoms or an increase in the risk of esophageal adenocarcinoma.

References

1 Axon A, Forman D. *Helicobacter* gastroduodenitis: a serious infectious disease. BMJ 1997;314:1430–1.
2 Schutze K, Hentschel E, Dragosics B, Hirschl AM. *Helicobacter pylori* reinfection with identical organisms: transmission by the patients' spouses. Gut 1995;36:831–3.
3 Labenz J, Blum AL, Bayerdorffer E, Meining A, Stolte M, Borsch G. Curing *Helicobacter pylori* infection in patients with duodenal ulcer may provoke reflux esophagitis. Gastroenterology 1997;112:1442–7.
4 Winkelstein A, Wolf BS, Som ML, Marshak RH. Peptic esophagitis with duodenal or gastric ulcer. JAMA 1954;154:885–9.
5 Winkelstein A. Peptic esophagitis with duodenal ulcer. Am J Surg 1957;93:234–7.
6 Cruze K, Byron FX, Hill JT. The association of peptic ulcers and asymptomatic hiatal hernia. Surgery 1959;46:664–8.
7 Moraes-Filho JP, Zaterka S, Pinotti HW, Bettarello A. Esophagitis and duodenal ulcer. Digestion 1974;11:338–46.
8 Moraes-Filho JP. Lack of specificity of the acid perfusion test in duodenal ulcer patients. Am J Dig Dis 1974;19:785–90.
9 Flook D, Stoddard CJ. Gastro-oesophageal reflux and oesophagitis before and after vagotomy for duodenal ulcer. Br J Surg 1985;72:804–7.
10 Behar J, Biancani P, Sheahan DG. Evaluation of esophageal tests in the diagnosis of reflux esophagitis. Gastroenterology 1976;71:9–15.
11 Goldman MS Jr, Rasch JR, Wiltsie DS, Finkel M. The incidence of esophagitis in peptic ulcer disease. Am J Dig Dis 1967;12:994–9.
12 Earlam RJ, Amerigo J, Kakavoulis T, Pollock DJ. Histological appearances of oesophagus, antrum and duodenum and their correlation with symptoms in patients with a duodenal ulcer. Gut 1985;26:95–100.
13 Boyd EJ. The prevalence of esophagitis in patients with duodenal ulcer or ulcer-like dyspepsia. Am J Gastroenterol 1996;91:1539–43.
14 Fujiwara Y, Arakawa T. Epidemiology and clinical characteristics of GERD in the Japanese population. J Gastroenterol 2009;44:518–34.
15 Dent J. Review article: from 1906 to 2006 – a century of major evolution of understanding of gastro-oesophageal reflux disease. Aliment Pharmacol Ther 2006;24:1269–81.
16 Graham DY. The changing epidemiology of GERD: geography and *Helicobacter pylori*. Am J Gastroenterol 2003;98:1462–70.
17 Liu Y, Akiyama J, Graham DY. Current understandings of *Helicobacter pylori*, peptic ulcer and gastroesophageal reflux disease. Minerva Gastroenterol Dietol 2006;52:235–48.
18 Latrobe CJ. *Travels in North America. The American Quarterly Review*. Philadelphia: Lydia R. Bailey, 1835: pp.390–422.

19 West T. *treatise on pyrosis idiopathica or water-brash as contrasted with certain forms of indigestion and of organic lesions of the abdominal organs, together with the remedies dietetic and medicinal.* London: Longman, Orme, Brown, Green and Longmans, 1841.

20 Graham DY, Smith JL, Patterson DJ. Why do apparently healthy people use antacid tablets? Am J Gastroenterol 1983;78:257–60.

21 Watanabe T, Urita Y, Sugimoto M, Miki K. Gastroesophageal reflux disease symptoms are more common in general practice in Japan. World J Gastroenterol 2007;13:4219–23.

22 Graham DY. Categories of patients with gastroesophageal reflux. Arch Intern Med 1991;151:2476.

23 Graham DY, Patterson DJ. Double-blind comparison of liquid antacid and placebo in the treatment of symptomatic reflux esophagitis. Dig Dis Sci 1983;28:559–63.

24 Graham DY. *Helicobacter pylori* and perturbations in acid secretion: the end of the beginning. Gastroenterology 1996;110:1647–50.

25 Graham DY, Dixon MF. Acid secretion, *Helicobacter pylori*, and peptic ulcer disease. In: Graham DY, Genta RM, Dixon MF (eds) *Gastritis*. Philadelphia: Lippincott Williams and Wilkins, 1999: pp.177–88.

26 Liu Y, Vosmaer GD, Tytgat GN, Xiao SD, ten Kate FJ. Gastrin G. cells and somatostatin D. cells in patients with dyspeptic symptoms: *Helicobacter pylori* associated and non-associated gastritis. J Clin Pathol 2005;58:927–31.

27 Graham DY, Asaka M. Eradication of gastric cancer and more efficient gastric cancer surveillance in Japan: two peas in a pod. J Gastroenterol 2010;45:1–8.

28 Comfort MW. Gastric acidity before and after development of gastric cancer: its etiologic, diagnostic and prognostic significance. Ann Intern Med 1951;36:1331–48.

29 Gutierrez O, Melo M, Segura AM, Angel A, Genta RM, Graham DY. Cure of *Helicobacter pylori* infection improves gastric acid secretion in patients with corpus gastritis. Scand J Gastroenterol 1997;32:664–8.

30 Graham DY, Shiotani A, El-Zimaity HM. Chromoendoscopy points the way to understanding recovery of gastric function after *Helicobacter pylori* eradication. Gastrointest Endosc 2006;64:686–90.

31 Malaty HM, Kim JG, El-Zimaity HM, Graham DY. High prevalence of duodenal ulcer and gastric cancer in dyspeptic patients in Korea. Scand J Gastroenterol 1997;32:751–4.

32 Ellis FH Jr, Lyons WS, Olsen AM. The gastroesophageal sphincter mechanism: a review. Mayo Clin Proc 1956;31:605–14.

33 Hill LD, Kozarek RA. The gastroesophageal flap valve. J Clin Gastroenterol 1999;28:194–7.

34 Hill LD, Kozarek RA, Kraemer SJ, *et al*. The gastroesophageal flap valve: in vitro and in vivo observations. Gastrointest Endosc 1996;44:541–7.

35 Shirota T, Kusano M, Kawamura O, Horikoshi T, Mori M, Sekiguchi T. *Helicobacter pylori* infection correlates with severity of reflux esophagitis: with manometry findings. J Gastroenterol 1999;34:553–9.

36 Wong WM, Lai KC, Hui WM, *et al*. Pathophysiology of gastroesophageal reflux diseases in Chinese – role of transient lower esophageal sphincter relaxation and esophageal motor dysfunction. Am J Gastroenterol 2004;99:2088–93.

37 Zerbib F, Bicheler V, Leray V, *et al*. *H. pylori* and transient lower esophageal sphincter relaxations induced by gastric distension in healthy humans. Am J Physiol Gastrointest Liver Physiol 2001;281:G350–G356.

38 Tanaka I, Tatsumi Y, Kodama T, *et al*. Effect of *Helicobacter pylori* eradication on gastroesophageal function. J Gastroenterol Hepatol 2004;19:251–7.

39 Graham DY. *Campylobacter pylori* and Barrett's esophagus. Mayo Clin Proc 1988;63:1258–60.

40 Rugge M, Russo V, Busatto G, *et al*. The phenotype of gastric mucosa coexisting with Barrett's oesophagus. J Clin Pathol 2001;54:456–60.

41 Lanza FL, Graham DY. Bougienage is effective therapy for most benign esophageal strictures. JAMA 1978;240:844–7.

42 Patterson DJ, Graham DY, Smith JL, *et al*. Natural history of benign esophageal stricture treated by dilatation. Gastroenterology 1983;85:346–50.

43 Benedict EB, Sweet RH. Benign stricture of the esophagus. Gastroenterology 1948;11:618–28.

44 Collen MJ, Lewis JH, Benjamin SB. Gastric acid hypersecretion in refractory gastro-esophageal reflux disease. Gastroenterology 1990;98:654–61.

45 Collen MJ, Johnson DA, Sheridan MJ. Basal acid output and gastric acid hypersecretion in gastroesophageal reflux disease. Correlation with ranitidine therapy. Dig Dis Sci 1994;39:410–17.

46 Collen MJ, Jensen RT. Idiopathic gastric acid hypersecretion. Comparison with Zollinger–Ellison syndrome. Dig Dis Sci 1994;39:1434–40.

47 Gillen D, Wirz AA, Ardill JE, McColl KE. Rebound hypersecretion after omeprazole and its relation to on-treatment acid suppression and *Helicobacter pylori* status. Gastroenterology 1999;116:239–47.

48 Reimer C, Sondergaard B, Hilsted L, Bytzer P. Proton-pump inhibitor therapy induces acid-related symptoms in healthy volunteers after withdrawal of therapy. Gastroenterology 2009;137:80–7.

49 McColl KE, Gillen D. Evidence that proton-pump inhibitor therapy induces the symptoms it is used to treat. Gastroenterology 2009;137:20–2.

50 Graham DY, Dore MP. Perturbations in gastric physiology in *Helicobacter pylori* duodenal ulcer: are they all epiphenomena? Helicobacter 1997;2(Suppl 1):S44–9.

51 Nakajima S, Hattori T. Active and inactive gastroesophageal reflux diseases related to *Helicobacter pylori* therapy. Helicobacter 2003;8:279–93.

52 Raghunath A, Hungin AP, Wooff D, Childs S. Prevalence of *Helicobacter pylori* in patients with gastro-oesophageal reflux disease: systematic review. BMJ 2003;326:737–9.

53 Qia B, Ma S. Effects of *Helicobacter pylori* eradication on gastroesophageal reflux disease: evidence from eleven studies. Helicobacter 2011;16(4):255–65.

54 Moayyedi P, Bardhan C, Young L, Dixon MF, Brown L, Axon AT. *Helicobacter pylori* eradication does not exacerbate reflux symptoms in gastroesophageal reflux disease. Gastroenterology 2001;121:1120–6.

55 Schwizer W, Thumshirn M, Dent J, *et al*. *Helicobacter pylori* and symptomatic relapse of gastro-oesophageal reflux disease: a randomised controlled trial. Lancet 2001;357:1738–42.

56 Laine L, Sugg J. Effect of Helicobacter pylori eradication on development of erosive esophagitis and gastroesophageal reflux disease symptoms: a post hoc analysis of eight double blind prospective studies. Am J Gastroenterol 2002;97:2992–7.

57 Ishiki K, Mizuno M, Take S, *et al*. *Helicobacter pylori* eradication improves pre-existing reflux esophagitis in patients with duodenal ulcer disease. Clin Gastroenterol Hepatol 2004;2:474–9.

58 Asaka M, Kato M, Graham DY. Strategy for eliminating gastric cancer in Japan. Helicobacter 2010;15:486–90.

59 Asaka M, Kato M, Graham DY. Prevention of gastric cancer by *Helicobacter pylori* eradication. Intern Med 2010;49:633–6.

60 Graham DY. Gastric cancer surveillance or prevention plus targeted surveillance. Jap J Helicobacter Res 2009;10:9–14.

61 El-Serag HB. The epidemic of esophageal adenocarcinoma. Gastroenterol Clin North Am 2002;31:421–40.

62 El-Serag HB, Graham DY. Routine polypectomy for colorectal polyps and ablation for Barrett's esophagus are intellectually the same. Gastroenterology 2011;140:386–8.

63 Hayward J. The lower end of the oesophagus. Thorax 1961;16:36–41.

64 Lagergren J, Bergstrom R, Nyren O. Association between body mass and adenocarcinoma of the esophagus and gastric cardia. Ann Intern Med 1999;130:883–90.

65 Rokkas T, Pistiolas D, Sechopoulos P, Robotis I, Margantinis G. Relationship between *Helicobacter pylori* infection and esophageal neoplasia: a meta-analysis. Clin Gastroenterol Hepatol 2007;5:1413–17.

66 Graham DY. *Helicobacter pylori* is not and never was "protective" against anything, including GERD. Dig Dis Sci 2003;48:629–30.

67 Kudo M, Gutierrez O, El-Zimaity HM, *et al*. CagA in Barrett's oesophagus in Colombia, a country with a high prevalence of gastric cancer. J Clin Pathol 2005;58:259–62.

68 Graham DY, Yamaoka Y. *H. pylori* and cagA: relationships with gastric cancer, duodenal ulcer, and reflux esophagitis and its complications. Helicobacter 1998; 3:145–51.

69 Graham DY. The only good *Helicobacter pylori* is a dead *Helicobacter pylori*. Lancet 1997;350:70–1.

70 Graham DY. Can therapy ever be denied for *Helicobacter pylori* infection? Gastroenterology 1997;113 6(Suppl):S113–17.

71 Graham DY, Opekun AR, Yamaoka Y, Osato MS, El-Zimaity HM. Early events in proton pump inhibitor-associated exacerbation of corpus gastritis. Aliment Pharmacol Ther 2003;17:193–200.

72 Graham DY, Genta RM. Long-term proton pump inhibitor use and gastrointestinal cancer. Curr Gastroenterol Rep 2008;10:543–7.

73 Kuipers EJ, Lundell L, Klinkenberg-Knol EC, *et al*. Atrophic gastritis and *Helicobacter pylori* infection in patients with reflux esophagitis treated with omeprazole or fundoplication. N Engl J Med 1996;334:1018–22.

74 Kuipers EJ, Klinkenberg-Knol EC, Vandenbroucke-Grauls CM, Appelmelk BJ, Schenk BE, Meuwissen SG. Role of *Helicobacter pylori* in the pathogenesis of atrophic gastritis. Scand J Gastroenterol 1997;223(Suppl):28–34.

75 Graham DY. *Campylobacter pylori* and peptic ulcer disease. Gastroenterology 1989;96:615–25.

76 Lundell L, Havu N, Miettinen P, *et al*. Changes of gastric mucosal architecture during long-term omeprazole therapy: results of a randomized clinical trial. Aliment Pharmacol Ther 2006;23:639–47.

77 Lundell L, Havu N, Miettinen P, Myrvold HE, Wallin L, Julkunen R, *et al*. Changes of gastric mucosal architecture during long-term omeprazole therapy: results of a randomized clinical trial. Aliment Pharmacol Ther 2006;23:639–47.

78 Yang HB, Sheu BS, Wang ST, Cheng HC, Chang WL, Chen WY. H. *pylori* eradication prevents the progression of gastric intestinal metaplasia in reflux esophagitis patients using long-term esomeprazole. Am J Gastroenterol 2009;104:1642–9.

79 Kuipers EJ, Nelis GF, Klinkenberg-Knol EC, *et al*. Cure of *Helicobacter pylori* infection in patients with reflux oesophagitis treated with long term omeprazole reverses gastritis without exacerbation of reflux disease: results of a randomised controlled trial. Gut 2004;53:12–20.

80 Malfertheiner P, Megraud F, O'Morain C, *et al*. Current concepts in the management of *Helicobacter pylori* infection: the Maastricht III Consensus Report. Gut 2007;56: 772–81.

PART 3
Barrett's Esophagus

CHAPTER 17

Barrett's Esophagus: Diagnosis and Surveillance

Gary W. Falk

Division of Gastroenterology, Perelman School of Medicine at the University of Pennsylvania, Philadelphia, PA, USA

Key points

- Barrett's esophagus is defined as a metaplastic change in the lining of the esophagus accompanied by intestinal metaplasia on biopsy.
- The risk for progression to cancer in patients without dysplasia is low and may in fact be lower than previously estimated.
- Most patients with Barrett's esophagus succumb to a disease other than adenocarcinoma.
- Optimal endoscopic surveillance involves careful inspection of the columnar-lined esophagus with high-quality white light endoscopy accompanied by a systematic four-quadrant biopsy protocol.
- Surveillance intervals in the absence of dysplasia are lengthening.

Potential pitfalls

- A normal-appearing gastroesophageal junction should not be biopsied.
- Screening for Barrett's esophagus remains controversial and repeated screening in the absence of erosive esophagitis should be avoided.
- A diagnosis of dysplasia warrants confirmation by an expert gastrointestinal pathologist.

Introduction

Barrett's esophagus is an acquired condition resulting from severe esophageal mucosal injury. It remains unclear why some patients with gastroesophageal reflux disease (GERD) develop Barrett's esophagus whereas others do not. The diagnosis of Barrett's esophagus is established if the squamocolumnar junction is displaced proximal to the gastroesophageal

---

Practical Manual of Gastroesophageal Reflux Disease, First Edition.
Edited by Marcelo F. Vela, Joel E. Richter and John E. Pandolfino.

junction and intestinal metaplasia is detected by biopsy, although controversy now exists regarding the need for intestinal metaplasia for the diagnosis. Diagnostic inconsistencies remain a problem in Barrett's esophagus, especially in differentiating short segment Barrett's esophagus from intestinal metaplasia of the gastric cardia. Barrett's esophagus would be of little importance if not for its well-recognized association with adenocarcinoma of the esophagus. Fortunately, the overall disease burden of esophageal cancer remains low and cancer risk for a given patient with Barrett's esophagus may now be lower than previously estimated [1,2]. The diagnosis of Barrett's esophagus affects a patient's quality of life and as such, it is essential to be certain that the diagnosis is made by currently acceptable criteria.

Definition

Barrett's esophagus is defined as a metaplastic change in the lining of the distal tubular esophagus that replaces the normal squamous epithelium. Endoscopically, this is characterized by displacement of the squamocolumnar junction proximal to the gastroesophageal junction defined by the proximal margin of gastric folds. If the squamocolumnar junction is above the level of the esophagogastric junction, biopsies should be obtained for confirmation of columnar metaplasia. There is an ongoing debate regarding the requirement that intestinal metaplasia is present in the metaplastic lining of the esophagus in order to diagnose an individual with Barrett's esophagus [3]. Consensus professional society guidelines from North America require intestinal metaplasia for the diagnosis of Barrett's esophagus whereas the British Society of Gastroenterology and a global consensus group require only columnar metaplasia with or without intestinal metaplasia for the diagnosis [4–8].

Diagnosis

Clinical presentation

Patients with Barrett's esophagus are difficult to distinguish clinically from patients with GERD uncomplicated by a columnar-lined esophagus. Observational studies suggest that features such as the development of reflux symptoms at an earlier age, increased duration of reflux symptoms, increased severity of nocturnal reflux symptoms, and increased complications of GERD such as esophagitis, ulceration, stricture, and bleeding may distinguish Barrett's esophagus patients from GERD patients without Barrett's esophagus [9]. Identification of Barrett's esophagus patients may be hampered by the paradox that despite Barrett's esophagus being the most severe complication of GERD, these patients have an impaired sensitivity to esophageal acid perfusion compared to patients with uncomplicated GERD, which may be related to the fact that many Barrett's esophagus patients are elderly, and there may be an age-related decrease in acid sensitivity [10,11]. A subset of Barrett's esophagus patients may have an inherited predisposition, as studies have reported on families with multiple affected relatives over successive generations and recent work has found several germline mutations associated with Barrett's esophagus and esophageal adenocarcinoma [12,13]. These reports suggest an autosomal dominant pattern of inheritance in selected individuals with Barrett's esophagus.

Endoscopy

Endoscopically, Barrett's esophagus is characterized by displacement of the squamocolumnar junction proximal to the gastroesophageal junction defined by the proximal margin of gastric folds. At the time of endoscopy, landmarks should be carefully identified, including the diaphragmatic pinch, the gastroesophageal junction as best defined by the proximal margin of the gastric folds seen on partial insufflation of the esophagus and level of the squamocolumnar junction. The proximal margin of the gastric folds remains the most useful landmark for defining the junction of the stomach and the esophagus [14]. However, the precise junction of the stomach and the esophagus may be challenging to determine endoscopically due to the presence of a hiatal hernia, inflammation, and the dynamic nature of the gastroesophageal junction, all of which may make targeting of biopsies problematic. Unfortunately, endoscopists identify landmarks necessary for the diagnosis of the columnar lined esophagus inconsistently [15]. The new Prague classification scheme provides the most reliable way to describe a Barrett's segment greater than 1 cm in length and guidelines now encourage the use of this system [6,16]. The Prague classification describes the circumferential extent (C value) and maximum extent (M value) of columnar mucosa above the proximal margin of the gastric folds (Figure 17.1). However, even the Prague classification is suboptimal for reliably recognizing segments of columnar metaplasia less than 1 cm in length and it does not account for columnar islands.

If the squamocolumnar junction is above the level of the esophagogastric junction, biopsies should be obtained for confirmation of columnar metaplasia. Biopsies of the squamocolumnar junction should not be routinely obtained in clinical practice if it is at the level of the gastroesophageal junction. There is ongoing debate regarding the requirement of intestinal metaplasia for the diagnosis of Barrett's esophagus. Recent evidence suggests that the non-goblet columnar metaplasia demonstrates DNA content abnormalities indicative of neoplastic risk similar to those

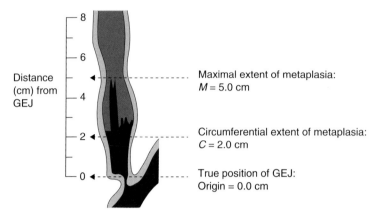

Figure 17.1 Schematic representation of the Prague classification for Barrett's esophagus classified as a C2M5. Note that C is the circumferential extent of metaplasia which extends up 2 cm whereas M is the maximal extent of metaplasia which extends up 5 cm from the gastroesophageal junction (GEJ). Reproduced from Sharma *et al.* [16] with permission from Elsevier.

encountered in intestinal metaplasia [17]. Furthermore, the risk of developing esophageal adenocarcinoma has been described as similar among patients with and without intestinal metaplasia and more than 70% of early adenocarcinomas detected by endoscopic mucosal resection have cardia and fundic-type mucosa adjacent to the cancer instead of intestinal metaplasia [18,19]. Currently, the issue of intestinal metaplasia versus columnar metaplasia as a diagnostic criterion remains unsettled. However, the magnitude of cancer risk associated with non-goblet columnar metaplasia remains unclear and the 2011 American Gastro-enterological Association (AGA) Medical Position Statement notes that there are currently insufficient data to make meaningful recommenda-tions regarding non-goblet columnar metaplasia [6].

The ability to detect intestinal metaplasia in the columnar-lined esoph-agus is related to a number of factors, including location of biopsies, length of columnar-lined segment, number of biopsies obtained, male gender and increasing age [20]. Intestinal metaplasia is more commonly found in biopsies obtained in the proximal portion of the columnar-lined esophagus where goblet cell density is also greater [21]. The optimal yield for intestinal metaplasia comes with taking eight biopsies, whereas taking more than eight biopsies does not seem to enhance the yield of intestinal metaplasia further [22].

Pathology

The columnar-lined esophagus is characterized by a mosaic of three differ-ent types of columnar epithelium above the gastroesophageal junction: fundic-type epithelium characterized by parietal and chief cells similar to that found in the gastric fundus, cardiac-type mucosa characterized by mucous glands and no parietal cells, and specialized columnar epithelium characterized by a villiform surface and intestinal-type goblet cells [23]. In most cases, goblet cells are easily identified on routine hematoxylin and eosin preparations, and special stains such as Alcian blue/periodic acid-Schiff (PAS) are not necessary. Alcian blue/PAS stain can help avoid overinterpretation of pseudogoblet cells characterized by distended surface foveolar-type cells that stain for PAS but do not contain Alcian blue-positive acid mucins [24].

Pathological interpretation of Barrett's esophagus specimens is problematic in the community as well as in academic centers. In a community study, intestinal metaplasia without dysplasia was recognized correctly by only 35% and gastric metaplasia without intestinal metaplasia was identified as Barrett's esophagus in 38% of the cases [25]. For expert gastrointestinal (GI) pathologists, interobserver reproducibility is substantial at the ends of the spectrum of Barrett's esophagus (negative for dysplasia and high-grade dysplasia/carcinoma) but it is not especially good for low-grade dysplasia or indefinite for dysplasia [26]. Factors that contribute to some of the problems in pathological interpretation include experience of the pathologist, quality of the slides, and size of the specimens [27]. Pathological interpretation of dysplasia is clearly improved by the use of endoscopic mucosal resection specimens [26].

Barrett's esophagus and esophageal adenocarcinoma

Barrett's esophagus is a clearly recognized risk factor for the development of esophageal adenocarcinoma. The incidence of this cancer increased from 3.6 per million in 1973 to 25.6 per million in 2006 [28]. Despite these alarming numbers, the overall burden of esophageal adenocarcinoma remains relatively low. It is estimated that there were 16,980 new cases of esophageal cancer (not all of which were adenocarcinoma) in the United States in 2011 [29]. Based on currently available data, the annual incidence of esophageal adenocarcinoma in Barrett's esophagus patients is estimated to range from approximately 0.1% to 0.5% [1,2,6]. Fortunately, adenocarcinoma is an uncommon cause of death in Barrett's esophagus patients, where most patients die of other causes, the most common being cardiovascular disease (Figure 17.2) [30]. Furthermore, the survival of patients with Barrett's esophagus is similar to that of the general population [31].

Esophageal adenocarcinoma is a lethal disease and survival is stage dependent. Early spread prior to the onset of symptoms is an unfortunate

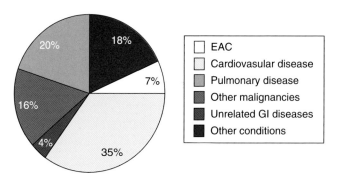

Figure 17.2 Causes of death in patients with Barrett's esophagus. Reproduced from Sikkema *et al.* [30] with permission from Elsevier. EAC, esophageal adenocarcinoma; GI, gastrointestinal.

characteristic of this tumor. Lymph node metastases are a clear prognostic factor for decreased survival and increase with depth of tumor involvement [32]. Thus, the best hope for improved survival of patients with esophageal adenocarcinoma is detection of cancer at an early and potentially curable stage. Two potential strategies to accomplish this are screening and surveillance of Barrett's esophagus patients.

Screening

One potential strategy to decrease the mortality rate of esophageal adenocarcinoma is to identify more patients at risk, namely those with Barrett's esophagus. Population-based studies suggest that in patients with newly diagnosed esophageal adenocarcinoma, a prior endoscopy and diagnosis of Barrett's esophagus is associated with both early-stage cancer and improved survival [33]. Unfortunately, only the minority of patients with esophageal adenocarcinoma have undergone prior endoscopy or have a prior diagnosis of Barrett's esophagus [34].

Current professional society practice guidelines equivocate on screening patients with chronic GERD symptoms for Barrett's esophagus and the 2009 American Cancer Society cancer screening guideline does not include any recommendation for screening of either esophageal cancer or Barrett's esophagus [4–7,35]. The 2011 AGA guidelines provide the most recent clinical recommendations. Screening is recommended as a reasonable approach for individuals with multiple risk factors for esophageal adenocarcinoma, including age greater than or equal to 50 years, male gender, Caucasian race, chronic GERD symptoms, elevated body mass index (BMI) and male-pattern abdominal obesity [6] (Figure 17.3). On the other hand, the current AGA guidelines recommend against screening of the general population of GERD patients without risk factors.

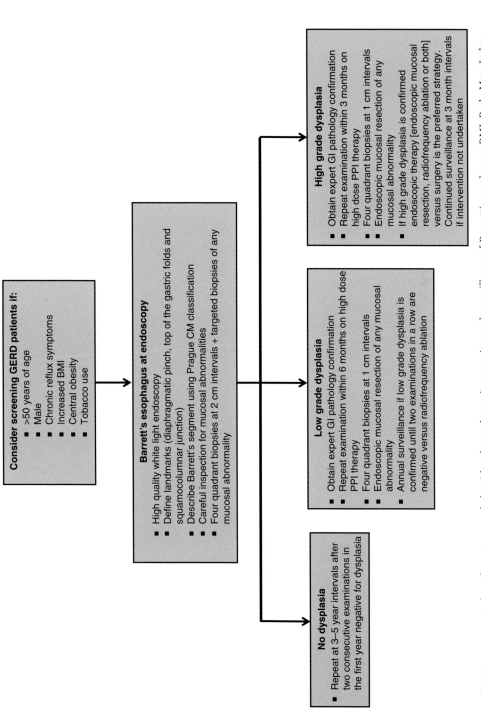

Consider screening GERD patients if:
- >50 years of age
- Male
- Chronic reflux symptoms
- Increased BMI
- Central obesity
- Tobacco use

Barrett's esophagus at endoscopy
- High quality white light endoscopy
- Define landmarks (diaphragmatic pinch, top of the gastric folds and squamocolumnar junction)
- Describe Barrett's segment using Prague CM classification
- Careful inspection for mucosal abnormalities
- Four quadrant biopsies at 2 cm intervals + targeted biopsies of any mucosal abnormality

No dysplasia
- Repeat at 3–5 year intervals after two consecutive examinations in the first year negative for dysplasia

Low grade dysplasia
- Obtain expert GI pathology confirmation
- Repeat examination within 6 months on high dose PPI therapy
- Four quadrant biopsies at 1 cm intervals
- Endoscopic mucosal resection of any mucosal abnormality
- Annual surveillance if low grade dysplasia is confirmed until two examinations in a row are negative versus radiofrequency ablation

High grade dysplasia
- Obtain expert GI pathology confirmation
- Repeat examination within 3 months on high dose PPI therapy
- Four quadrant biopsies at 1 cm intervals
- Endoscopic mucosal resection of any mucosal abnormality
- If high grade dysplasia is confirmed endoscopic therapy [endoscopic mucosal resection, radiofrequency ablation or both] versus surgery is the preferred strategy. Continued surveillance at 3 month intervals if intervention not undertaken

Figure 17.3 Management algorithm. Suggested algorithm for endoscopic screening and surveillance of Barrett's esophagus. BMI, Body Mass Index: GERD, gastroesophageal reflux disease; GI, gastrointestinal; PPI, proton pump inhibitor.

Endoscopy with biopsy remains the only widely available clinical technique to diagnose Barrett's esophagus. However, it has clear limitations as a screening tool, including cost, risk, and complexity. If applied to the estimated 20% of the population with regular GERD symptoms, the cost implications would be staggering [36]. A recent study examined the yield of endoscopy in both symptomatic and asymptomatic individuals utilizing the Clinical Outcomes Research Initative (CORI) database. Among white men with GERD symptoms, the yield of Barrett's esophagus increased from 3.3% in the fourth decade of life to 9.3% in the sixth decade prior to reaching a plateau [37]. Interestingly, the yield in symptomatic middle-aged women was comparable to that in asymptomatic males. These findings suggest that screening should not be considered prior to age 50.

Several alternatives to standard upper endoscopy have been explored for screening. Unsedated upper endoscopy using small-caliber instruments still has the potential to change the economics of endoscopic screening, as this technique may decrease sedation-related complications and costs. Unsedated small-caliber endoscopy detects Barrett's esophagus and dysplasia with a sensitivity comparable to conventional endoscopy [38]. While both procedures are well tolerated by patients, a major hurdle for unsedated endoscopy is patient resistance to undergoing a test without sedation. Esophageal capsule endoscopy will likely not become a screening alternative to conventional upper endoscopy due to suboptimal cost and performance characteristics [39,40]. The most recent alternative to endoscopic screening is a non-endoscopic Cytosponge [41]. This technique involves swallowing a gelatin capsule containing a compressed mesh device attached to a string. After the gelatin dissolves, the mesh is withdrawn and retrieved for immunostaining with trefoil factor 3, which is a diagnostic marker for Barrett's esophagus. The sensitivity of this technique in a primary care GERD population is 73% with a specificity of 94%. Given the minimal cost involved, this is an attractive alternative to conventional endoscopic screening.

While endoscopic screening remains a somewhat controversial issue, there is little controversy on the role of repeating endoscopy to assess for the new development of Barrett's esophagus. Studies show consistent results in patients who have already had a normal initial upper endoscopy. In patients with non-erosive reflux disease at the index endoscopy, Barrett's esophagus is rarely found if the repeat endoscopy is performed within 5 years [42,43]. On the other hand, if erosive esophagitis is found at the time of index endoscopy, Barrett's esophagus may be present in 9–12% of these patients on repeat endoscopy, with higher grades of esophagitis associated with a higher case finding rate of Barrett's esophagus [44,45]. As such, screening for Barrett's esophagus in GERD patients should only take place after initial proton pump inhibitor (PPI) therapy. A negative endoscopy at baseline makes it highly unlikely that Barrett's esophagus will be found if endoscopy is repeated.

There are still no data from randomized controlled trials or observational studies to evaluate the strategy of screening. A decision analysis model examined screening of 50-year-old white men with chronic GERD symptoms for Barrett's esophagus, and found that one-time screening is probably cost-effective if subsequent surveillance is limited to patients with dysplasia on initial examination [46]. Thus there is clearly a need to develop either a better profile of patients at high risk for Barrett's esophagus or a far less expensive tool to provide mass population screening. Problems inherent in demonstrating the utility of a screening program such as healthy volunteer bias, lead time bias, and length time bias will all need to be addressed as well.

Surveillance

Candidates for surveillance

Current practice guidelines recommend endoscopic surveillance of patients with a diagnosis of Barrett's esophagus [4–7]. Prior to entering into a surveillance program, patients should be advised about risks and benefits, including the limitations of surveillance endoscopy as well as the importance of adhering to appropriate surveillance intervals. Other considerations include age, co-morbid conditions, likelihood of survival over the next 5 years and ability to tolerate either endoscopic or surgical interventions for early esophageal adenocarcinoma. Patients in poor overall health are not likely to benefit from endoscopic surveillance or tolerate interventions for dysplasia or adenocarcinoma.

Technique

The aim of surveillance is the detection of dysplasia or early carcinoma. Active inflammation makes it more difficult to distinguish dysplasia from reparative changes. As such, surveillance endoscopy should only be performed after any active inflammation related to GERD is controlled with anti-secretory therapy. The presence of ongoing erosive esophagitis is a contraindication to performing surveillance biopsies.

At the time of endoscopy, the esophagus should be carefully examined with high-resolution white light endoscopy, in particular looking for any mucosal abnormality [47]. Current guidelines do not recommend the routine use of advanced imaging techniques as adjuncts to high-quality white light endoscopy, although many show promise for future application. After careful visual inspection, systematic surveillance biopsies should be obtained in four quadrants at 2 cm intervals along the entire length of the Barrett's segment in the absence of known dysplasia and at 1 cm intervals in the presence of known dysplasia [6]. The rationale for this rigorous approach comes from studies that demonstrate that a systematic biopsy protocol detects more dysplasia and early cancer compared to *ad hoc* random biopsies [48,49]. The safety of systematic endoscopic biopsy protocols has been demonstrated as well [50]. Subtle mucosal abnormalities, no matter how trivial, such as ulceration, erosion, plaque, nodule, stricture or other luminal irregularity in the Barrett's segment, should also be extensively biopsied, as there is an association of such lesions with underlying cancer [51]. Mucosal abnormalities, especially in the setting of known high-grade dysplasia, should undergo endoscopic mucosal resection [4]. Endoscopic mucosal resection will change the diagnosis in approximately 50% of patients when compared to endoscopic biopsies, given the larger tissue sample available for review by the pathologist [52]. Interobserver agreement among pathologists is improved as well [52].

There has been considerable debate over the years regarding the need for large particle forceps to obtain biopsies, but current evidence does not support the routine use of the jumbo biopsy forceps [6]. A new large-capacity forceps that can be passed through standard-diameter endoscopes provides larger samples than standard large-capacity forceps and may increase the yield of dysplasia [53].

Intervals

Surveillance intervals, determined by the presence and grade of dysplasia, are based on our limited understanding of the biology of esophageal adenocarcinoma. The most recent recommendations from the AGA are every 3–5 years in patients without dysplasia, every 6–12 months for low-grade dysplasia and every 3 months for high-grade dysplasia if intervention is not performed [6] (see Figure 17.3). Unfortunately, guidelines from the various professional societies are not in agreement on surveillance intervals, leading to considerable confusion in this area.

If low-grade dysplasia is found, the diagnosis should first be confirmed by an expert gastrointestinal pathologist due to the marked interobserver variability in interpretation of these biopsies. These patients should receive aggressive anti-secretory therapy for reflux disease with a PPI to decrease the changes of regeneration that make pathological interpretation of this category so difficult. A repeat endoscopy should then be performed within 6–12 months of the initial diagnosis. Endoscopic mucosal resection should be performed if any mucosal abnormality is present in these patients. The American College of Gastroenterology recommends annual surveillance when low-grade dysplasia is present until two examinations in a row are negative [4]. At that point, surveillance can be lengthened again to every 3–5 years. The AGA recommends surveillance every 6–12 months and makes no recommendation regarding when to subsequently lengthen biopsy intervals [6].

It is important to remember that the natural history of low-grade dysplasia is poorly understood. This may be due in part to the high degree of interobserver variability in establishing this diagnosis and the variable biopsy protocols by which these patients are followed, resulting in issues related to tissue sampling. While the majority of patients with low-grade dysplasia do not progress to adenocarcinoma or high-grade dysplasia, a subset of these patients do progress to a higher grade lesion. A recent Dutch study found that 85% of patients diagnosed with low-grade dysplasia in the community were downgraded to no dysplasia after review by two expert GI pathologists [54]. However, the risk of progression to high-grade dysplasia or adenocarcinoma was 13.4% per year in individuals in whom the diagnosis was confirmed by the expert pathologists. The recent Danish population-based cohort study also suggests an increased risk for individuals with low-grade dysplasia diagnosed at index endoscopy which is five-fold greater than for those with no dysplasia [1]. Other studies suggest that this lesion has a risk of progression that is no greater than that of non-dysplastic Barrett's esophagus [55].

If high-grade dysplasia is found, the diagnosis should first be confirmed by an experienced GI pathologist as well. Both extent of high-grade dysplasia and mucosal abnormalities may be risk factors for adenocarcinoma [56,57]. The presence of any mucosal abnormality warrants endoscopic mucosal resection in an effort to maximize staging accuracy as described above. If high-grade dysplasia is confirmed by repeat endoscopy within 2–3 months, intervention is warranted either endoscopically or surgically. Observational studies suggest that survival and cancer-free survival are comparable in patients treated either surgically or endoscopically for high-grade dysplasia [58]. Continued surveillance should only be reserved for high-risk patients with multiple co-morbidities who are not good candidates for endoscopic or surgical intervention.

Rationale

While no clinical trials have examined the effectiveness of the strategy of endoscopic surveillance, observational studies show that patients with Barrett's esophagus in whom adenocarcinoma was detected in a surveillance program have their cancers detected at an earlier stage, with improved 5-year survival compared to similar patients not undergoing routine endoscopic surveillance (Figure 17.4) [59,60]. Furthermore, lymph node involvement is less likely in surveyed patients compared to

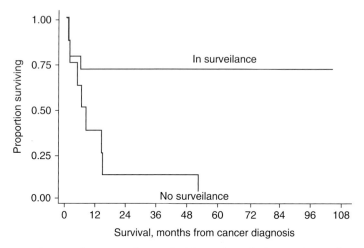

Figure 17.4 Improved postoperative survival in esophageal adenocarcinoma for patients diagnosed during endoscopic surveillance compared to patients diagnosed without prior surveillance. Reproduced from Corley *et al.* [59] with permission from Elsevier.

non-surveyed patients [59]. Since esophageal cancer survival is stage dependent, these studies suggest that survival may be enhanced by endoscopic surveillance. However, since most patients with Barrett's esophagus die of causes other than esophageal adenocarcinoma, endoscopic surveillance remains of uncertain benefit. There are a number of flaws inherent in observational studies that support the concept of surveillance, including selection bias, healthy volunteer bias, lead time bias, and length time bias.

Limitations

Endoscopic surveillance of Barrett's esophagus, as currently practiced, has numerous shortcomings. Dysplasia and early adenocarcinoma are endoscopically indistinguishable from intestinal metaplasia without dysplasia in the absence of mucosal abnormalities. The distribution of dysplasia and cancer is highly variable, and even the most thorough biopsy surveillance program has the potential for sampling error. There are considerable inter-observer variability and quality control problems in the interpretation of dysplasia in both the community and academic settings. Current surveillance programs are expensive and time consuming. A number of studies indicate that while surveillance is widely practiced, there is non-adherence to surveillance guidelines with respect to both the technique of four-quadrant biopsies and interval of surveillance [61,62]. Furthermore, the longer the segment length, the worse the adherence to practice guidelines (Figure 17.5) [61].

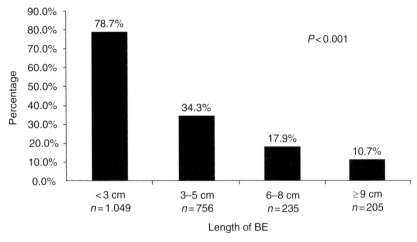

Figure 17.5 Adherence to the Seattle biopsy protocol in the community setting by length of Barrett's esophagus. Reproduced from Abrams *et al.* [62] with permission from Elsevier. BE, Barrett's esophagus.

Potential strategies to enhance surveillance

Most Barrett's esophagus patients do not have dysplasia and will never develop cancer. Thus, it would be highly desirable to make surveillance techniques more effective and efficient by sampling larger areas of Barrett's mucosa, targeting biopsies to areas with a higher probability of having dysplasia or developing risk stratification tools to allow us to concentrate our efforts on individuals at greatest risk while decreasing the frequency and intensity of surveillance in individuals at lower risk. Unfortunately, none of these conceptual paradigms has come to fruition to date despite the obvious intuitive appeal of these approaches.

Advanced imaging technology

A wide variety of endoscopic enhancements to surveillance has been described (Box 17.1), but unfortunately none has really changed clinical practice. Traditional chromoendoscopy with methylene blue is no better than random biopsies for the detection of intestinal metaplasia, high-grade dysplasia or early cancer [63]. Similarly, acetic acid does not appear to increase the detection rate of dysplasia or adenocarcinoma despite initial enthusiasm [64]. Optical contrast endoscopy allows for detailed imaging of the mucosal and vascular surface patterns in Barrett's esophagus without the need for chromoendoscopy. This may be accomplished by either the placement of optical filters that narrow the bandwidth of white light to blue light (narrow band imaging) or by postprocessing software-driven systems to accomplish similar visualization [65]. A recent systematic review found that narrow band imaging

---

Box 17.1 Potential enhancements to white light endoscopic imaging

- Chromoendoscopy
- Magnification endoscopy
- Narrow band imaging
- Photodynamic diagnosis
- Spectroscopy
- Partial wave spectroscopy
- Polarized scanning spectroscopy
- Optical coherence tomography
- Low coherence interferometry
- Autofluorescence endoscopy
- Confocal endomicroscopy
- Molecular imaging

Source: Falk GW. Probe-based confocal endomicroscopy in Barrett's esophagus: the real deal or another tease? Gastrointest Endosc 2011;74:473–6.

---

has a sensitivity of 77–100% and a specificity of 58–100% for the detection of high-grade dysplasia or cancer [66].

Confocal laser endomicroscopy is a targeted imaging technique that allows for subsurface imaging and *in vivo* histological assessment of the mucosal layer during white-light endoscopy [67]. The goal of endomicroscopy is to distinguish neoplastic from non-neoplastic tissue in "real time" by performing virtual "optical biopsies." Optical biopsies could accomplish two important goals: decrease the number of conventional biopsies and allow immediate treatment decisions at the time of endoscopy, thereby decreasing the costs and increasing the efficiency of patient care. Two different endomicroscopy platforms are available: an endoscope-based device that is integrated into the distal tip of the endoscope and a probe-based device that can be inserted through a standard endoscope. Both devices require administration of an intravenous fluorescence agent, fluorescein. Studies suggest that confocal endomicroscopy has the potential to improve the diagnostic yield of endoscopically inapparent neoplasia compared with standard white light endoscopy and surveillance biopsies, while also decreasing the number of biopsies [68,69]. A number of other new techniques to target biopsies, including molecular imaging, angle-resolved low-coherence interferometry, circumferential optical coherence tomography, and nanotechnology, are all under active development, each with enormous promise.

Perhaps the single greatest advance for the detection of dysplasia and early cancer has been the advent of high-definition/high-resolution white light endoscopy. Studies have consistently shown that this technique is as good as or better than more sophisticated methods such as narrow band imaging, chromoendoscopy, autofluorescence endoscopy, and multimodal imaging [64]. The recent AGA position statement does not recommend using advanced imaging techniques for surveillance at this time [6].

Risk stratification

A number of clinical and biological markers may define patients at increased risk for the development of adenocarcinoma. Clinical risk factors for the development of high-grade dysplasia or adenocarcinoma include gender, ethnicity, age, dysplasia, hiatal hernia size, length of the Barrett's segment, BMI, and smoking [70].

Dysplasia is still the best available marker of cancer risk in clinical practice. Dysplasia is recognized adjacent to and distant from Barrett's esophagus-associated adenocarcinoma in resection specimens from patients with Barrett's esophagus. Barrett's esophagus patients progress through a phenotypic sequence of no dysplasia, low-grade dysplasia, high-grade dysplasia and then on to adenocarcinoma, although the time course is highly variable and this step-wise sequence is not preordained [59,71]. Furthermore, some patients may progress directly to cancer without prior detection of dysplasia of any grade [72]. Unfortunately, dysplasia is an imperfect marker of increased cancer risk. It is typically not distinguishable endoscopically and often focal in nature, thereby making targeting of biopsies problematic. Furthermore, there is considerable inter-observer variability in the grading of dysplasia. Therefore, a less subjective marker for cancer risk that could supplement or replace the current dysplasia grading system is still needed.

Biomarkers of increased risk

A number of molecular markers may define patients at increased risk for the development of esophageal adenocarcinoma. Among the most frequently described molecular changes that precede the development of adenocarcinoma in Barrett's esophagus are alterations in p53 (mutation, deletion or loss of heterozygosity (LOH)) p16 (mutation, deletion, promoter hypermethylation, or LOH) and aneuploidy by flow cytometry [73–78]. Neoplastic progression in Barrett's esophagus is accompanied by flow cytometric abnormalities such as aneuploidy or increased G2/tetraploid DNA contents, and these abnormalities may precede the development of high-grade dysplasia or adenocarcinoma. An alternative method for the detection of DNA ploidy abnormalities is image cytometry, which can analyze formalin-fixed tissue with automated analysis algorithms. Image cytometry may be comparable to flow cytometry for the detection of ploidy [79]. Another technique with potential clinical applicability for the detection of abnormal DNA content is fluorescent *in situ* hybridization (FISH) which may also be simpler to apply in clinical practice [80].

Mutations of p53 and 17p LOH have been reported in up to 92% and 100%, respectively, of esophageal adencocarcinomas [73]. Furthermore, both abnormalities have been detected in Barrett's epithelium prior to the development of carcinoma [81]. However, techniques to detect p53 mutations and 17p LOH are also labor intensive and have not achieved widespread acceptance in clinical practice to date. Similarly, p16 LOH and inactivation of the p16 gene by promoter region hypermethylation have been reported frequently in esophageal adenocarcinoma [82]. Furthermore, 9p LOH is commonly encountered in premalignant Barrett's epithelium and can be detected over large regions of the Barrett's mucosa [80]. It is hypothesized that clonal expansion occurs in conjunction with p16 abnormalities, creating a field in which other genetic lesions leading to esophageal adenocarcinoma can arise.

Epigenetic changes, in the form of hypo- and hypermethylation and alteration to histone complexes, have also been implicated in the progression of Barrett's esophagus to adenocarcinoma. Hypermethylation of p16, APC, RUNX3 and HPP1 are all independently associated with an increased risk of progression of Barrett's esophagus to high-grade dysplasia or esophageal adenocarcinoma [83,84].

Given the complexity and diversity of alterations observed to date in the metaplasia, dysplasia, carcinoma sequence, it appears that a panel of biomarkers may be required for risk stratification. The combination of 17p LOH, 9p LOH and DNA content abnormality has been shown to predict the 10-year adenocarcinoma risk better than any single biomarker alone [85]. Patients with a combination of these abnormalities had a markedly increased risk of developing cancer compared to those with no baseline abnormalities (relative risk 38.7, 95% confidence interval (CI) 10.8–138.5). In those with no abnormalities of any of these biomarkers at baseline, 12% developed adenocarcinoma at 10 years. In contrast, those with the combination of 17p LOH, 9p LOH and DNA content abnormality had a cumulative incidence of adenocarcinoma of 79% over the same time period. A risk stratification model utilizing a methylation index constructed from the methylation values for p16, HPP1, and RUNX3 also showed potential for prediction of progression to high-grade dysplasia or adenocarcinoma [86].

Thus, while all of these studies demonstrate the potential for biomarkers to predict risk of esophageal adenocarcinoma, none of these biomarkers has been validated in large-scale clinical trials to date and as such they are not yet useful for clinical decision making. It is likely that in the future, the best predictor for the development of high-grade dysplasia or adenocarcinoma will be a combination of clinical, demographic, histological, genetic, and epigenetic data.

CASE STUDY

A 56-year-old white man with no prior history of dysplasia underwent surveillance endoscopy for known Barrett's esophagus. LA Grade B esophagitis was noted in conjunction with a 5 cm segment of columnar-lined esophagus. No biopsies were performed because of ongoing inflammation and the endoscopy was repeated 8 weeks after commencing twice-daily PPI therapy. At that time endoscopy revealed a 3 cm hiatal hernia and a C3M5 segment of Barrett's esophagus with no mucosal abnormalities seen with high-definition white light endoscopy. Four quadrant biopsies were done every 2 cm commencing at the GE junction and proceeding up to the squamocolumnar junction. All biopsies were read as no dysplasia. The patient was counseled that recent data suggest a very low risk of esophageal adenocarcinoma of the order of 0.1–0.5% per year and to return for his next surveillance examination in 3–5 years.

References

1 Hvid-Jensen F, Pedersen L, Drewes AM, *et al*. Incidence of adenocarcinoma among patients with Barrett's esophagus. N Engl J Med 2011;365:1375–83.

2 Wani S, Falk G, Hall M, *et al*. Patients with nondysplastic Barrett's esophagus have low risks for developing dysplasia or esophageal adenocarcinoma. Clin Gastroenterol Hepatol 2011;9:220–7.

3 Riddell RH, Odze RD. Definition of Barrett's esophagus: time for a rethink – is intestinal metaplasia dead? Am J Gastroenterol 2009;104:2588–94.

4 Wang KK, Sampliner RE, Practice Parameters Committee of the American College of Gastroenterology. Updated guidelines 2008 for the diagnosis, surveillance and therapy of Barrett's esophagus. Am J Gastroenterol 2008;103:788–97.

5 Hirota WK, Zuckerman MJ, Adler DG, *et al*. ASGE guideline: the role of endoscopy in the surveillance of premalignant conditions of the upper GI tract. Gastrointest Endosc 2006;63:570–80.

6 Spechler SJ, Sharma P, Souza RF, *et al*. American Gastroenterological Association medical position statement on the management of Barrett's esophagus. Gastroenterology 2011;140:1084–91.

7 British Society of Gastroenterology. Guidelines for the diagnosis and management of Barrett's columnar – lined oesophagus. Available at: www.BSG.org.uk.

8 Vakil N, van Zanten SV, Kahrilas P, *et al*. Global Consensus Group. The Montreal definition and classification of gastroesophageal reflux disease: a global evidence-based consensus. Am J Gastroenterol 2006;101:1900–20.

9 Eisen GM, Sandler RS, Murray S, *et al*. The relationship between gastroesophageal reflux disease and its complications with Barrett's esophagus. Am J Gastroenterol 1997;92:27–31.

10 Johnson DA, Winters C, Spurling TJ, *et al*. Esophageal acid sensitivity in Barrett's esophagus. J Clin Gastroenterol 1987;9:23–7.

11 Grade A, Pulliam G, Johnson C, *et al*. Reduced chemoreceptor sensitivity in patients with Barrett's esophagus may be related to age and not to the presence of Barrett's epithelium. Am J Gastroenterol 1997;92:2040–3.

12 Chak A, Ochs-Balcom H, Falk G, *et al*. Familiality in Barrett's esophagus, adenocarcinoma of the esophagus, and adenocarcinoma of the gastroesophageal junction. Cancer Epidemiol Biomarkers Prev 2006;15:1668–73.

13 Orloff M, Peterson C, He X, *et al.* Germline mutations in MSR1, ASCC1, and CTHRC1 in patients with Barrett esophagus and esophageal adenocarcinoma. JAMA 2011; 306:410–19.

14 McClave SA, Boyce HW, Gottfried MR. Early diagnosis of the columnar-lined esophagus: a new endoscopic criterion. Gastrointest Endosc 1987;33:413–16.

15 Ofman JJ, Shaheen NJ, Desai AA, *et al.* The quality of care in Barrett's esophagus: endoscopist and pathologist practices. Am J Gastroenterol 2001;96: 876–81.

16 Sharma P, Dent J, Armstrong D, *et al.* The development and validation of an endoscopic grading system for Barrett's esophagus: the Prague C & M criteria. Gastroenterology 2006;131:1392–9.

17 Liu W, Hahn H, Odze RD, *et al.* Metaplastic esophageal columnar epithelium without goblet cells shows DNA content abnormalities similar to goblet cell-containing epithelium. Am J Gastroenterol 2009;104:816–24.

18 Kelty CJ, Gough MD, van Wyk Q, *et al.* Barrett's oesophagus: intestinal metaplasia is not essential for cancer risk. Scand J Gastroenterol 2007;42:1271–4.

19 Takubo K, Aida J, Naomoto Y, *et al.* Cardiac rather than intestinal-type background in endoscopic resection specimens of minute Barrett adenocarcinoma. Hum Pathol 2009;4:65–74.

20 Wang A, Mattek NC, Corless CL, *et al.* The value of traditional upper endoscopy as a diagnostic test for Barrett's esophagus. Gastrointest Endosc 2008;68:859–6.

21 Chandrasoma PT, Der R, Dalton P, *et al.* Distribution and significance of epithelial types in columnar-lined esophagus. Am J Surg Pathol 2001;25:1188–93.

22 Harrison R, Perry I, Haddadin W, *et al.* Detection of intestinal metaplasia in Barrett's esophagus: an observational comparator study suggests the need for a minimum of eight biopsies. Am J Gastroenterol 2007;102:1154–61.

23 Paull A, Trier JS, Dalton MD, *et al.* The histologic spectrum of Barrett's esophagus. N Engl J Med 1976;295:476–80.

24 Weinstein WM, Ippoliti AF. The diagnosis of Barrett's esophagus: goblets, goblets, goblets. Gastrointest Endosc 1996;44:91–4.

25 Alikhan M, Rex D, Khan A, *et al.* Variable pathologic interpretation of columnar lined esophagus by general pathologists in community practice. Gastrointest Endosc 1999;50:23–6.

26 Montgomery E, Bronner MP, Goldblum JR, *et al.* Reproducibility of the diagnosis of dysplasia Barrett esophagus: a reaffirmation. Hum Pathol 2001;32:368–78.

27 Mino-Kenudson M, Hull MJ, Brown I, *et al.* EMR for Barrett's esophagus-related superficial neoplasms offers better diagnostic reproducibility than mucosal biopsy. Gastrointest Endosc 2007;66:660–6.

28 Pohl H, Sirovich B, Welch HG. Esophageal adenocarcinoma incidence: are we reaching the peak? Cancer Epidemiol Biomarkers Prev 2010;19:1468–70.

29 Siegel R, Ward E, Brawley O, *et al.* Cancer statistics, 2011: the impact of eliminating socioeconomic and racial disparities on premature cancer deaths. CA Cancer J Clin 2011;61:212–36.

30 Sikkema M, de Jonge PJ, Steyerberg EW, *et al.* Risk of esophageal adenocarcinoma and mortality in patients with Barrett's esophagus: a systematic review and meta-analysis. Clin Gastroenterol Hepatol 2010;8:235–44.

31 Anderson LA, Murray LJ, Murphy SJ, *et al.* Mortality in Barrett's oesophagus: results from a population based study. Gut 2003;52:1081–4.

32 Rice TW, Blackstone EH, Goldblum JR, *et al.* Superficial adenocarcinoma of the esophagus. J Thorac Cardiovasc Surg 2001;122:1077–90.

33 Cooper GS, Kou TD, Chak A. Receipt of previous diagnoses and endoscopy and outcome from esophageal adenocarcinoma: a population-based study with temporal trends. Am J Gastroenterol 2009;104:1356–62.

34 Dulai GS, Guha S, Kahn KL, *et al.* Preoperative prevalence of Barrett's esophagus in esophageal adenocarcinoma: a systematic review. Gastroenterology 2002;122: 26–33.

35 Smith RA, Cokkinides V, Brawley OW. Cancer screening in the United States, 2009: a review of current American Cancer Society guidelines and issues in cancer screening. CA Cancer J Clin 2009;59:27–41.

36 Shaheen NJ, Provenzale D, Sandler RS. Upper endoscopy as a screening and surveillance tool in esophageal adenocarcinoma: a review of the evidence. Am J Gastroenterol 2002;97:1319–27.

37 Rubenstein JH, Mattek N, Eisen G. Age- and sex-specific yield of Barrett's esophagus by endoscopy indication. Gastrointest Endosc 2010;71:21–7.

38 Jobe BA, Hunter JG, Chang EY, *et al.* Office-based unsedated small-caliber endoscopy is equivalent to conventional sedated endoscopy in screening and surveillance for Barrett's esophagus: a randomized and blinded comparison. Am J Gastroenterol 2006;101:2693–703.

39 Gerson L, Lin OS. Cost–benefit analysis of capsule endoscopy compared with standard upper endoscopy for the detection of Barrett's esophagus. Clin Gastroenterol Hepatol 2007;5:319–25.

40 Sharma P, Wani S, Rastogi A, *et al.* The diagnostic accuracy of esophageal capsule endoscopy in patients with gastroesophageal reflux disease and Barrett's esophagus: a blinded, prospective study. Am J Gastroenterol 2008;3:525–32.

41 Kadri SR, Lao-Sirieix P, O'Donovan M, *et al.* Acceptability and accuracy of a non-endoscopic screening test for Barrett's oesophagus in primary care: cohort study. BMJ 2010;341:c4372.

42 Stoltey J, Reeba H, Ullah N, *et al.* Does Barrett's oesophagus develop over time in patients with chronic gastro-oesophageal reflux disease? Aliment Pharmacol Ther 2007;25:83–91.

43 Rodriguez S, Mattek N, Lieberman D, *et al.* Barrett's esophagus on repeat endoscopy: should we look more than once? Am J Gastroenterol 2008;103:1892–7.

44 Hanna S, Rastogi A, Weston AP, *et al.* Detection of Barrett's esophagus after endoscopic healing of erosive esophagitis. Am J Gastroenterol 2006;101:1416–20.

45 Modiano N, Gerson LB. Risk factors for the detection of Barrett's esophagus in patients with erosive esophagitis. Gastrointest Endosc 2009;69:1014–20.

46 Inadomi JM, Sampliner R, Lagergren J, *et al.* Screening and surveillance for Barrett esophagus in high risk groups: a cost–utility analysis. Ann Intern Med 2003;138: 176–86.

47 Spechler SJ, Sharma P, Souza RF, *et al.* American Gastroenterological Association technical review on the management of Barrett's esophagus. Gastroenterology 2011;140:e18–52.

48 Fitzgerald RC, Saeed I, Khoo D, *et al.* Rigorous surveillance protocol increases detection of curable cancers associated with Barrett's esophagus. Dig Dis Sci 2001;46:1892–8.

49 Abela JE, Going JJ, Mackenzie JF, *et al.* Systematic four-quadrant biopsy detects Barrett's dysplasia in more patients than nonsystematic biopsy. Am J Gastroenterol 2008;103:850–5.

50 Levine DS, Blount PL, Rudolph RE, *et al.* Safety of a systematic endoscopic biopsy protocol in patients with Barrett's esophagus. Am J Gastroenterol 2000;95:1152–7.

51 Reid BJ, Blount PL, Feng Z, *et al.* Optimizing endoscopic biopsy detection of early cancers in Barrett's high-grade dysplasia. Am J Gastroenterol 2000;95:3089–6.

52 Peters FP, Brakenhoff KP, Curvers WL, *et al.* Histologic evaluation of resection specimens obtained at 293 endoscopic resections in Barrett's esophagus. Gastrointest Endosc 2008;67:604–9.

53 Komanduri S, Swanson G, Keefer L, *et al.* Use of a new jumbo forceps improves tissue acquisition of Barrett's esophagus surveillance biopsies. Gastrointest Endosc 2009;70:1072–8.

54 Curvers WL, ten Kate FJ, Krishnadath KK, *et al.* Low-grade dysplasia in Barrett's esophagus: overdiagnosed and underestimated. Am J Gastroenterol 2010;105:1523–30.

55 Wani S, Falk GW, Post J, *et al.* Risk factors for progression of low-grade dysplasia in patients with Barrett's esophagus. Gastroenterology 2011;141:1179–86.

56 Buttar NS, Wang KK, Sebo TJ, *et al.* Extent of high-grade dysplasia in Barrett's esophagus correlates with risk of adenocarcinoma. Gastroenterology 2001;120:1630–9.

57 Tharavej C, Hagen JA, Peters JH, *et al.* Predictive factors of coexisting cancer in Barrett's high-grade dysplasia. Surg Endosc 2006;20:439–43.

58 Prasad GA, Wang KK, Buttar NS, *et al.* Long-term survival following endoscopic and surgical treatment of high-grade dysplasia in Barrett's esophagus. Gastroenterology 2007;132:1226–33.

59 Corley DA, Levin TR, Habel LA, *et al.* Surveillance and survival in Barrett's adenocarcinomas: a population-based study. Gastroenterology 2002;122:633–40.

60 Van Sandick JW, Lanschot JJ, Kuiken BW, *et al.* Impact of endoscopic biopsy surveillance of Barrett's esophagus on pathological stage and clinical outcome of Barrett's carcinoma. Gut 1998;43:216–22.

61 Das D, Ishaq S, Harrison R, *et al.* Management of Barrett's esophagus in the UK: overtreated and underbiopsied but improved by the introduction of a national randomized trial. Am J Gastroenterol 2008;103:1079–89.

62 Abrams JA, Kapel RC, Lindberg GM, *et al.* Adherence to biopsy guidelines for Barrett's esophagus surveillance in the community setting in the United States. Clin Gastroenterol Hepatol 2009;7:736–42.

63 Ngamruengphong S, Sharma VK, Das A. Diagnostic yield of methylene blue chromoendoscopy for detecting specialized intestinal metaplasia and dysplasia in Barrett's esophagus: a meta-analysis. Gastrointest Endosc 2009;69:1021–8.

64 Curvers W, Baak L, Kiesslich R, *et al.* Chromoendoscopy and narrow-band imaging compared with high-resolution magnification endoscopy in Barrett's esophagus. Gastroenterology 2008;134:670–9.

65 Song LM, Adler DG, Conway JD, *et al.* Narrow band imaging and multiband imaging. Gastrointest Endosc 2008;67:581–9.

66 Curvers WL, van den Broek FJ, Reitsma JB, *et al.* Systematic review of narrow-band imaging for the detection and differentiation of abnormalities in the esophagus and stomach. Gastrointest Endosc 2009;69:307–17.

67 Kantsevoy SV, Adler DG, Conway JD, *et al.* Confocal laser endomicroscopy. Gastrointest Endosc 2009;70:197–200.

68 Dunbar KB, Okolo P, Montgomery E, *et al.* Confocal laser endomicroscopy in Barrett's esophagus and endoscopically inapparent Barrett's neoplasia: a prospective, randomized, double-blind, controlled, crossover trial. Gastrointest Endosc 2009;70:645–54.

69 Sharma P, Meining A, Coron E, *et al.* Real-time increased detection of neoplastic tissue in Barrett's esophagus with probe-based confocal laser endomicroscopy: final

results of an international multicenter, prospective, randomized, controlled trial. Gastrointest Endosc 2011;74:465–72.

70 Falk GW. Risk factors for esophageal cancer development. Surg Oncol Clin North Am 2009;18:469–85.

71 Hameeteman W, Tytgat GN, Houthoff HJ, *et al.* Barrett's esophagus: development of dysplasia and adenocarcinoma. Gastroenterology 1989;96:1249–56.

72 Sharma P, Falk GW, Weston AP, *et al.* Dysplasia and cancer in a large multicenter cohort of patients with Barrett's esophagus. Clin Gastroenterol Hepatol 2006;4: 566–72.

73 Reid BJ, Haggitt RC, Rubin CE, *et al.* Barrett's esophagus. Correlation between flow cytometry and histology in detection of patients at risk for adenocarcinoma. Gastroenterology 1987;93:1–11.

74 Reid BJ, Blount PL, Rubin CE, *et al.* Flow-cytometric and histological progression to malignancy in Barrett's esophagus: prospective endoscopic surveillance of a cohort. Gastroenterology 1992;102:1212–19.

75 Reid BJ. P53 and neoplastic progression in Barrett's esophagus. Am J Gastroenterol 2001;96:1321–3.

76 Prevo LJ, Sanchez CA, Galipeau PC, *et al.* P53-mutant clones and field effects in Barrett's esophagus. Cancer Res 1999;59:4784–7.

77 Wong DJ, Barrett MT, Stoger R, *et al.* p16INK4a promoter is hypermethylated at a high frequency in esophageal adenocarcinomas. Cancer Res 1997; 57:2619–22.

78 Reid BJ, Levine DS, Longton G, *et al.* Predictors of progression to cancer in Barrett's esophagus: baseline histology and flow cytometry identify low- and high-risk patient subsets. Am J Gastroenterol 2000;95:1669–76.

79 Dunn JM, Mackenzie GD, Oukrif D, *et al.* Image cytometry accurately detects DNA ploidy abnormalities and predicts late relapse to high-grade dysplasia and adenocarcinoma in Barrett's oesophagus following photodynamic therapy. Br J Cancer 2010;102:1608–17.

80 Fritcher EG, Brankley SM, Kipp BR, *et al.* A comparison of conventional cytology, DNA ploidy analysis, and fluorescence in situ hybridization for the detection of dysplasia and adenocarcinoma in patients with Barrett's esophagus. Hum Pathol 2008;39:1128–35.

81 Reid BJ, Prevo LJ, Galipeau PC, *et al.* Predictors of progression in Barrett's esophagus II: baseline 17p (p53) loss of heterozygosity identifies a patient subset at increased risk for neoplastic progression. Am J Gastroenterol 2001;96:2839–48.

82 Wong DJ, Paulson TG, Prevo LJ, *et al.* p16INK4a lesions are common, early abnormalities that undergo clonal expansion in Barrett's metaplastic epithelium. Cancer Res 2001;61:8284–9.

83 Schulmann K, Sterian A, Berki A, *et al.* Inactivation of p16, RUNX3, and HPP1 occurs early in Barrett's-associated neoplastic progression and predicts progression risk. Oncogene 2005;24:4138–48.

84 Wang JS, Guo M, Montgomery EA, *et al.* DNA promoter hypermethylation of p16 and APC predicts neoplastic progression in Barrett's esophagus. Am J Gastroenterol 2009;104:2153–60.

85 Galipeau PC, Li X, Blount PL, *et al.* NSAIDs modulate CDKN2A, TP53, and DNA content risk for progression to esophageal adenocarcinoma. PLoS Med 2007;4:e67.

86 Sato F, Jin Z, Schulmann K, *et al.* Three-tiered risk stratification model to predict progression in Barrett's esophagus using epigenetic and clinical features. PLoS ONE 2008;3:e1890.

CHAPTER 18

Barrett's Esophagus: Treatment Options

Jianmin Tian and Kenneth K. Wang

Mayo Clinic, Rochester, MN, USA

Key point
- The key to successful ablation is patient selection. This begins with selecting patients with significant neoplastic lesions that might benefit from treatment. It is very important to emphasize patient compliance, with an esophagogastroduodenoscopy at scheduled intervals in the postablation period. The important step is to identify and eradicate cancer at an early stage (no more than T1a) while endoscopic treatment is still a good option. Recurrence usually does not affect overall outcomes.

Potential pitfall
- For a patient with visible lesions such as nodules, thickened folds, mass, ulcers, strictures, and/or high-grade dysplasia at multiple biopsy levels, it is essential to perform mucosal resection to obtain sufficient tissues for accurate diagnosis before any ablation.

Introduction

The prevalence of Barrett's esophagus (BE) in patients with gastroesophageal reflux disease (GERD) has been about 5.7% [1]. However, only about half of BE patients have symptoms. This has led to a situation where most patients are diagnosed either incidentally or with more advanced disease. Our current understanding is that non-dysplastic Barrett's esophagus (NDBE) progresses to low-grade dysplasia (LGD), then to high-grade dysplasia (HGD) and esophageal adenocarcinoma (EAC), although patients do not always progress in a step-wise fashion. It is uncertain whether this is due to sampling error and these mucosal changes are not discovered or, alternatively, there is rapid evolution to more advanced neoplasia. The

---

Practical Manual of Gastroesophageal Reflux Disease, First Edition.
Edited by Marcelo F. Vela, Joel E. Richter and John E. Pandolfino.
© 2013 John Wiley & Sons, Ltd. Published 2013 by John Wiley & Sons, Ltd.

currently held belief is that the primary target for treatment of BE is dysplastic mucosa. The estimated 10-year survival is similar in patients with non-dysplastic BE and in the general population [2]. Thus treatment of all patients with BE without dysplasia at this time may not ultimately lead to any survival benefit. If selected patients at higher risk of cancer can be identified in this group, for instance through use of biomarkers, treatment would likely prove to be useful.

There is consensus in current clinical practice on treating patients with high-grade dysplasia in Barrett's mucosa after this diagnosis is confirmed by two expert pathologists and concomitant invasive adenocarcinoma has been excluded [3]. As demonstrated in a recent metaanalysis and systematic review, endoscopic treatment reduces the incidence of esophageal adeno-carcinoma with most of the benefit of ablation being observed in patients with HGD [4]. It has been reported that the survival of HGD patients with endoscopic therapies is comparable to patients with esophagectomy. Postablation surveillance is very important regardless of types of endo-scopic treatment, because the rates of detecting EAC after ablation were 6.0% for HGD, 0.8% for LGD, and 0.03% for NDBE [5].

For more advanced neoplasia such as adenocarcinoma that is confined to the mucosa, mucosal resection techniques are recommended. Endoscopic mucosal resection (EMR) is suitable for T1a lesions (intramucosal EAC) because the percentage of lymph node metastasis (LNM) is low in this condition. However, any lesion that is more advanced than T1a should be managed by non-endoscopic approaches.

In this chapter, we will focus on the clinical indications, procedure details, efficacy, outcomes, and complications of each endoscopic modality.

Endoscopic mucosal resection

Since it was first described in 1984, EMR has been adopted into practice in diagnosis, staging and treatment for BE with dysplasia and early cancers in addition to its applications in the stomach and colon. Overall, it is a safe and effective method for managing most lesions less than 1.5 cm in diameter in the luminal gastrointestinal (GI) tract. For larger lesions, endoscopic submucosal dissection (ESD) is preferred over piecemeal EMR since this allows *en bloc* resection of the lesion. Circumferential EMR to eradicate the entire BE was reported in 2003 in 12 patients who had HGD or intramucosal EAC. Although no recurrence was observed, complica-tions occurred in six cases with four bleedings and two strictures [6]. Two subsequent studies in 2005 and 2006 [7,8] showed a high rate of stricture (up to one-third of the patients). Despite this radical treatment, the recurrence rate of Barrett's mucosa was up to 11%. Currently this circumferential EMR approach is being replaced by sequential targeted EMRs along with ablation for residual flat mucosa in the United States.

Patient selection

Patient selection is an important step to assure success and minimize complications such as bleeding, stricture and perforation.

- Thorough work-up to rule out distal metastatic lesions using positron emisson tomography (PET)/computed tomography (CT) scans should be performed for cancer patients, because those with advanced disease would not benefit from this procedure. Then endoscopic ultrasound (EUS) should be done primarily for nodal staging. EUS has been considered as the most accurate non-invasive method for staging but a recent metaanalysis of 12 EUS studies revealed that EUS found only 65% concordance for T-staging when compared to EMR or esophagectomy findings. High-frequency miniprobe EUS does provide more accurate T-staging though even this technique is still not accurate enough to exclude the use of EMR [9]. Nevertheless, locoregional lymph node positivity by EUS with fine needle aspiration (FNA) still adds significant value in patient management.

- The percentage of lymph node metastasis (LNM) has been estimated as 1–6% [10–13] for intramucosal cancer (T1a). But up to one-third of patients with submucosal esophageal cancer (T1b) lesions could have LNM at the time of esophagectomy. Thus any lesion that is more advanced than T1a should not be treated with EMR for curative intent. Lymphovascular invasion or high-grade malignancies are also felt to be contraindications for endoscopic treatment.

- Generally speaking, previous biopsies do not affect subsequent EMRs unless they are performed within a few days of attempted resection. However, previous EMRs can lead to tissue scarring, and subsequent EMRs at the same location are associated with higher risk of failure and complications. If a lesion is not lifted (i.e. non-lifting sign) after submucosal fluid injection, then EMR should be reconsidered to avoid perforation. Poor wound healing could also lead to difficulty after EMR.

Procedure

The main technique for EMR involves submucosal injection and lifting, followed by electrocautery and mechanical resection [14].

Preparation

American Society of Gastrointestinal Endoscopy guidelines [15] should be followed for the management of anti-platelet or anti-coagulation (APAC) medications. In a retrospective report, patients who underwent EMR while on or off APAC medications were studied. This study showed the rate of major GI bleeding was 0.23% for those on APAC versus 0.59% for those off APAC. However, ischemic events (myocardial or cerebral ischemia) happened in 6.25% of those who were off clopidogrel versus 0.22% of those on clopidogrel ($P=0.051$) [16].

Identify the lesions for endoscopic mucosal resection

If there is an obvious mass in the esophagus, then it is probably too advanced for curative EMR. If there are nodules and thickened folds, which are often associated with cancers [17], they should be targeted for EMR. For less apparent lesions, narrow band imaging (NBI) or chromo-endoscopy may aid the endoscopist in defining the margins. This step of lesion identification could be difficult in some cases. Even trimodal methods (high-resolution endoscopy followed by autofluorescence imaging (AFI) and NBI) did not improve the overall detection of dysplasia compared with standard video endoscopy and biopsies [18]. Dysplasia or even early EAC is still found in a significant number of patients by random biopsies in areas where no obvious target was identified for EMR.

Technique

Submucosal injection of saline is an important initial step to separate the mucosal layer from the muscular layer so that (a) the muscular layer will not be suctioned into the cap and (b) the deep margin will have fewer thermal effects when electrocautery is applied. This is important in avoiding perforation. Other solutions such as 1:200,000 epinephrine could also be used to achieve better homeostasis. For submucosal dissection, hypertonic glucose, glycerol, and hydroxypropylmethyl cellulose have been used to maintain a submucosal cushion. These agents are not useful with EMR since a persistent cushion makes suction of the lesion into the cap more difficult.

Endoscopic mucosal resection can be performed in several ways, with the common feature being the use of a snare to achieve tissue removal. Original methods include strip biopsy using a two-channel therapeutic endoscope but this is mostly obsolete since the technique is difficult to perform. The most commonly used current methods are cap- or band ligation-assisted EMR. For the cap method, a soft or hard, flat or oblique transparent cap, which comes in multiple diameters, is friction fitted firmly at the end of a regular esophagogastroduodenoscopy (EGD) scope. Although the manufacturer recommends using tape to secure the cap, this is usually not necessary as the friction fit is sufficient. The esophagus is intubated and submucosal injection is performed. A crescent snare is positioned on the internal circumference of the cap; the lesion is suctioned into the cap and then the snare is closed around the tissue. Prior to resection, it is beneficial to "tug" on the snare to observe the esophageal wall motion relative to the repeated traction by the snare. If the entire wall moves with traction, this suggests that the snare has captured the outer muscular wall of the esophageal wall and one should open the snare and recapture the mucosa to avoid perforation. Once the mucosa is appropriately captured, the snare is applied with a pure cautery current to resect the lesion.

Ligation-assisted EMR is very much like band ligation for esophageal varices. Once a band is placed over the lesion, a hexagonal snare is used to resect it either above or below the band, and the specimen can be collected using a Roth net or snare. These two methods (cap or ligation EMR) yield similar results [19,20]. Piecemeal EMRs can be performed for larger lesions, although ESD may be a better choice in such situations with a lower risk of recurrence [21].

Figure 18.1 depicts the EMR procedure.

Postprocedure care

After EMR patients usually do not require hospitalization unless there is a complication or their overall medical status is tenuous. Postprocedural instructions usually include clear liquid diet for 24 h, avoid crunchy food, aspirin or other non-steroidal anti-inflammatory drugs (NSAIDs) for an additional 2 weeks and temporarily holding clopidogrel (Plavix) or other platelet inhibitors for 2 days unless the patient has a high risk of cardiovascular events.

Patients should return for further EGD exam every 3 months in the first year after HGD or intramucosal esophageal adenocarcinoma (IM-EAC) has been resected with tumor-free margins (i.e. R0 resection), or return in 6–8 weeks if the margin is positive for tumor cells (i.e. R1 resection). If submucosal adenocarcinoma is found, then esophagectomy should be considered because of the higher risk of lymph node metastasis (LNM).

Complications

Overall, EMR for carefully selected patients is safe in experienced hands. Minor complications such as chest discomfort and nausea are usually short-lived. Serious complications including major bleeding, perforation, and stricture are fortunately rare.

The average complication rate of EMR is approximately 14% with a major complication rate of 10% (bleeding requiring blood transfusion (2%), perforation (0.5%) or stricture (7%)).

Bleeding

Clinically significant bleeding can be seen in up to 3.8% of patients after EMR [22]. The rate is influenced by the patient's medical conditions and the procedure itself. If suspicion of late bleeding is high, prophylactic hemostasis methods such as Hemoclips® should be used. Bleeding risk increases

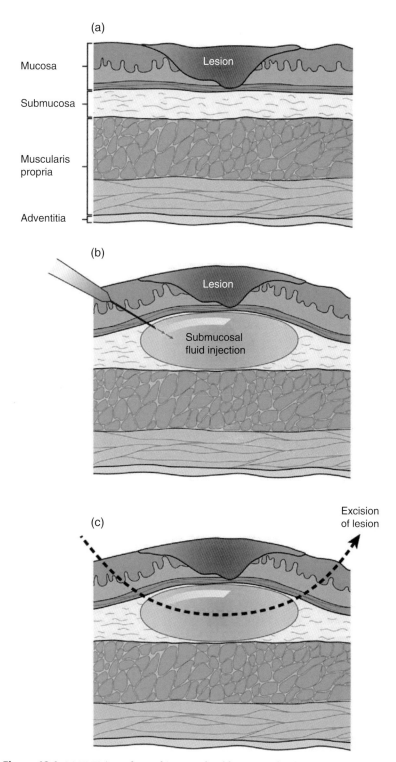

Figure 18.1 (a) EMR is performed in superficial lesions with a low risk of nodal metastases. (b) The submucosal injection of saline acts as a cushion separating the mucosa from the muscularis propria. The presence of a *lift sign* suggests the absence of deeper invasion. (c) The submucosal saline cushion mitigates the risk of deeper injury and perforation during resection. Reproduced from Namasivayam *et al.* [14], with permission from Elsevier.

with increased number of mucosal resections performed. Generally bleeding is treated with clipping to avoid further thermal injury to the mucosa.

Perforation
The rate of perforation has been described to be up to 2.5% [22–24]. The recommendation is to exam the EMR site carefully to identify perforation early. A "target sign" in which the pink muscularis propria layer is broken by a dark spot is a potential site of perforation. In such cases, stents and/or clips can be applied to seal the defects, and then followed by gastrografin contrast study to ensure no leakage. The over-the-scope clip has also been used in this situation. A nasogastric tube should be placed, and the patient should be hospitalized with fluid and nutrition support and treatment with antibiotics. If found and treated early, the majority of patients will have satisfactory recovery from perforation after a few days. Pneumomediastinum is a mild form of perforation and is usually managed by nil by mouth, supportive measures, and observation.

Stricture
This has been reported to occur in up to 23% of patients receiving EMR [25]. The risk of stricture appears to be related to multiple EMRs, circumferential EMRs, and EMRs with other modalities such as photodynamic therapy (PDT) or radiofrequency ablation (RFA). The risk of strictures is increased if EMR has removed 75% or more of the circumference of the esophagus. Most strictures can be managed by repeated dilation or stents.

Outcomes
Biopsies
Compared to regular biopsies, EMR obtains more tissue for diagnosis and staging with improved accuracy. Approximately 24% and 40% of patients who were initially diagnosed with HGD and IM-EAC) had their diagnoses changed to IM-EAC and submucosal EAC (SM-EAC) respectively based on EMR [26]. This was also supported by a metaanalysis based on 15 original articles and four abstracts which showed that EMR upstaged 16% of cases and downstaged 12%. Conversely, random biopsies also detected lesions in locations other than EMR sites. Given the patchy distribution of dysplastic and neoplastic tissues, EMRs and biopsies are actually complementary to each other.

Eradication and recurrence
All seven published studies regarding EMR have been case series. The largest one, from Pech et al., included 349 patients with HGD and T1 stage EAC [27]. Among these 349 patients, 279 were treated with EMR and 70 received PDT, EMR plus PDT, or argon plasma coagulation (APC). About

96% achieved complete response (margin-free resection plus one normal endoscopic follow-up examination) after an average of 2.1 EMRs per patient, and recurrence was found in 21.5% of patients during the median follow-up of 63 months. However, it should be noted that this case series included 30 submucosal EACs who were unfit for surgery, and 35.8% of the whole cohort had piecemeal resection. These two types of patients are usually at higher risk of recurrence. Independent risk factors for recurrence included long segment of BE, multifocal carcinoma, piecemeal EMRs and a longer period to achieve complete remission (>10 months). Among 13 (3.7%) patients who failed EMR and subsequently had esophagectomy, 11 had non-healing ulcers and/or scarring from previous endoscopic treatment.

Another study of 100 carefully selected low-risk IM-EAC patients showed that EMR was very successful in achieving complete remission in 99% of cases, and 5-year survival was 98%. However, metachronous cancer was observed in 11% of cases after 36.7 months of follow-up [28]. This underlined the importance of long-term surveillance and also suggested the need for combined therapies of EMR and other modalities such as RFA, PDT, and cryoablation. Generally, the mucosal resection techniques are used to eliminate areas of visible cancer while ablative therapies are used to eliminate the intestinalized mucosa that remains. In six studies in 2003–2007 (prior to Pech's study in 2008), recurrence of malignancy after achieving complete responses was observed in up to 26% of patients [27]. Usually these recurrences can be managed by further endoscopy to achieve another complete response.

Mortality

In a study of 178 patients with IM-EAC, the endoscopy (EMR with or without other modalities) group had a similar cumulative mortality rate as the esophagectomy group (17% versus 20%, $P=0.75$) after a mean follow-up of 43 and 64 months, respectively [22].

Radiofrequency ablation

Radiofrequency ablation (RFA) is a thermal ablation method that uses radiofrequency energy to destroy tissues with penetration depth of 0.5 mm when energy density is $12 J/cm^2$ [29, 30]. The RFA system was first cleared by the Food and Drug Administration (FDA) in 2001 for BE, among other cautery applications. The HALO[360] (BÂRRX Medical) has a balloon with 60 tightly spaced electrodes encircling it over 3 cm in length (Figure 18.2). The diameters of available balloons range from 18, 22, 25, 28, 31 to 34 mm. The HALO[90] is shown in Figure 18.3. The upper surface containing electrode

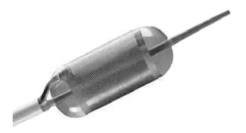

Figure 18.2 HALO[360] is a circumferential balloon with electrode array at the outside surface.

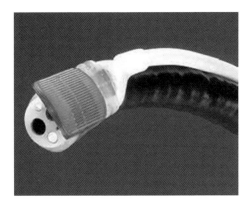

Figure 18.3 HALO[90] is not balloon based. It is used for segmental ablation of BE.

array is measured at 20 mm by 13 mm. It has the same electrode spacing and can deliver energy density of 15 J/cm² and power of 40 Watt/cm². The device is mounted on a pivot to allow opposition against the esophageal wall. This device is attached to the outside of the endoscope and positioned to contact the lesion by manipulation of the endoscope tip. The average patient needs approximately three sessions to achieve remission.

Patient selection

The efficacy and side-effect profile make RFA the intervention of choice for HGD. RFA for LGD may be of value in young patients and/or those with long segment or multifocal disease. However, the diagnosis of LGD itself has significant interobserver variability among pathologists. Additionally, since the risk of progression to esophageal cancer is lower than HGD, the cost-effectiveness of ablation versus surveillance EGD is yet to be established. The treatment of non-dysplastic BE is of uncertain value unless additional risk factors such as strong family history of adenocarcinoma are present [31].

At the time of writing (2012), there have been no human data on the use of RFA alone for IM-EAC. Since the device is designed to be superficial, treatment of cancers that may penetrate deeper into the mucosa is not recommended.

Procedure

First, the size of esophagus is determined to allow selection of the right balloon size if the HALO³⁶⁰ is to be used. To do this, a sizing balloon can be inserted over a 0.035 inch diameter guidewire to the esophageal lumen, and the generator attached to the end of the catheter which will automatically insufflate and deflate the sizing balloon to gauge the esophageal diameter. This measurement can be started from the proximal end of BE to the distal, with measurements made every centimeter. This can be done without direct endoscopic visualization but if there are strictures present, endoscopy is recommended to ensure that the measurements are accurate. The equipment will average the diameters over a 4 cm segment to provide the estimated balloon size to use.

A 1% N-acetylcysteine spray is usually used before ablation to remove excessive mucus for optimal contact between the device and the esophageal mucosa.

The HALO³⁶⁰ catheter can be inserted into the esophageal lumen over the guidewire, and an endoscope is placed alongside the HALO³⁶⁰ catheter for better visualization. Once the target BE area is selected, the treatment coils are aligned visually with the proximal most extent of the columnar mucosa balloon. First, the balloon is inflated and the air is suctioned from the lumen to ensure good contact. A preset amount of energy, 12 J per square centimeter, is then delivered by pressing a foot pedal. Multiple applications are needed for segments that are >3 cm in length. After the entire segment has been treated, the catheter is removed outside the patient and cleaned with water. The ablated esophageal surface is also cleaned by scraping off the coagulative debris with the small flexible cap at the end of the scope, followed by careful inspection of this area. Then the treatment balloon is reinserted to start the second pass by repeating the steps in the first pass.

There is usually some residual BE after initial RFA with the HALO³⁶⁰. The HALO⁹⁰ can be used to ablate this residual BE on a second EGD exam about 3 months later. Careful examination with white light and NBI is done first. Then the HALO⁹⁰ device is friction fitted to the exterior of the endoscope tip at the 12 o'clock position. Close contact with the esophageal lining can be achieved by manipulation of the endoscope tip. During the first pass, two applications can be done at the same location. After all the residual BE is treated, the ablated areas need to be carefully inspected, followed by gentle scraping of debris off the esophageal wall with the HALO⁹⁰ device and plain water flushes. Next, the device and scope are removed outside the patient to be washed and cleaned before the second pass.

Postprocedure management

Radiofrequency ablation is an outpatient procedure, and patients are observed in the recovery area until they meet discharge criteria. Patients should be instructed to expect some chest pain/discomfort. They should take a full liquid diet for 24h, then slowly advance the diet over the next couple of days but avoid crunchy food for 2 weeks. Meanwhile, they should not take NSAIDs for 2 weeks and clopidogrel (Plavix) for 2 days unless a high risk of cardiovascular events requires earlier reinstitution of these medications. Proton pump inhibitor therapy twice a day for a month and then daily afterwards with or without sucralfate should be recommended to control reflux. Sucralfate is added to provide additional mucosal protection.

The follow-up interval will be every 3 months for HGD patients in their first year after diagnosis. If no dysplastic tissue is found at the end of the first year, patients can be followed every 6 months and then yearly, and then at the intervals specified by available guidelines [3].

Complications

The most frequent side-effect is chest pain, which is seen more often when a long segment is ablated in one session and can be managed with oral analgesics. Fentanyl patches can be used to avoid the oral route with more severe pain. Stricture occurs in 0–6% and is amenable to endoscopic dilation. Bleeding (including minor ones without transfusion or hospitalization) is seen in up to 10%. Infrequent side-effects include major bleeding and perforation (<1%). In a study of 298 treatments from 84 patients [31], no perforation or procedure-related death occurred. One patient who received anti-platelet therapy for heart disease had GI bleeding, which was managed with endoscopy. A second patient had overnight hospitalization for new-onset chest pain 8 days after RFA. A third patient was hospitalized due to chest discomfort and nausea immediately after RFA.

Outcomes

There is only one reported randomized controlled trial (RCT) evaluating RFA for the treatment of dysplastic Barrett's mucosa. This study included 127 patients with LGD or HGD [5], and complete eradication of dysplasia (CE-D) occurred in 90.5% and 81.0% of patients in LGD and HGD groups respectively at 2-year follow-up. The rate of complete eradication of intestinal metaplasia (CE-IM) was 77% versus 2% for the RFA and sham groups respectively, based on an intention-to-treat analysis. Patients in the RFA group had less disease progression (3.6% versus 16.3%, $P=0.03$) and fewer cancers (1.2% versus 9.3%, $P=0.045$).

There are five case series of RFA experience on dysplastic Barrett's mucosa and three studies on NDBE. Overall, the complete eradication rates ranged from 70% to 100% for dysplastic or non-dysplastic tissues. During the follow-up (all studies had >12 months of follow-up), only one study showed that 2% of patients (1 of 44) had recurrence of a 1mm Barrett's island.

Photodynamic therapy

Photodynamic therapy (PDT) has been used since the 1980s to treat skin cancer, wet macular degeneration, bladder cancer, cholangiocarcinoma, esophageal dysplasia, and cancer. PDT has three key elements: the drug (photosensitizer), the light, and singlet oxygen that mediates cell death [25].

- *Drug.* The only one approved in the US for GI applications is sodium porfimer (Photofrin®), which is an intravenous (IV) injection given 48 h before photoradiation. Some centers in Europe use 5-aminolevulinic acid (5-ALA), which is an oral agent taken 4 h before the procedure. Currently, 2-[1-hexyloxyethyl]-2-devinyl pyropheophorbide (HPPH), a chlorine-type molecule derived from porphyrin, is being studied as an alternative drug in research trials to replace sodium porfimer. HPPH is likely to be a better agent for PDT because of its photophysical and pharmacological properties such as high plasma clearances (84.5 mL/h), selective and durable anti-tumor photodynamic activity, which means it might have similar efficacy and a more desirable side-effect profile than sodium porfimer.
- *Light.* Laser light at 630 nm wavelength is applied during the procedure from a very small cylindrical diffusing fiber that is placed through the regular endoscope channel.
- *Oxygen.* Once the light interacts with the drug in the presence of oxygen, a singlet oxygen state is created which causes cell death.

Patient selection

Most PDT experience comes from patients with HGD. However, PDT could also serve as palliative treatment for advanced esophageal cancer. One retrospective study revealed that symptomatic palliation rates from chemotherapy alone, PDT alone, and PDT plus chemotherapy combined were 60.0%, 85.2%, and 93.9% respective [32]. However, more complications after PDT were reported among those patients with prior chemoradiation therapy.

Procedure

Sodium porfimer IV at 2 mg/kg body weight is given over 3–5 min 48 h before the procedure. If 5-ALA (used in Europe) is chosen as the photosensitizer, it is given by mouth 4 h before the procedure.

Through the working channel of the endoscope, a cylindrical diffusing fiber is passed that can be 1, 2.5 or 5 cm in length and is positioned in the center of the lumen encompassing the length of the Barrett's esophagus segment. There can be overlap with the normal squamous tissue since squamous tissue is highly reflective and generally does not absorb much light. A centering balloon to more effectively deliver light has been used in Europe; this balloon system was available in the States but is no longer being manufactured.

Laser light at 630 nm is applied for a total energy dose of 200 J/cm. Usually no more than 7 cm of BE is treated in one session. This is applied at a power of 400 milliwatts per centimeter fiber to avoid heating of the tissue that occurs at higher light output powers. Some centers perform a second PDT 2 days after initial photoradiation to inspect the ablated field and perform a "touch up" for the skipped lesions using less energy (50 J/cm). Of note, it can be difficult to visualize the mucosa during photo-radiation; the use of NBI may be helpful to improve visualization as the filters applied for imaging attenuate light from the laser fiber.

It is essential to instruct the patient about avoiding bright lights (surgical lights, sunlight) for 30 days, continuing proton pump inhibitors (PPI), and taking medications if needed for nausea, vomiting, and chest pain.

Complications

Complications such as chest pain, nausea, and vomiting are transient in most cases. The perforation rate of approximately 1% is lower than that of EMR. Fistula or pleural effusion is also rare. However, strictures and photosensitivity have been the main drawbacks for PDT using Photofrin.

Photosensitivity

Up to 69% of patients may have skin reactions to light which may last for a month [33]. Other than light avoidance, there are currently available medical interventions that can mitigate this. Sodium porfimer is currently FDA approved for use in Barrett's esophagus. A newer agent, HPPH, might have less photosensitivity which is reported to be only a week in clinical trials [34].

Stricture

Stricture occurs in as many as 35% of PDT patients after an average of 2.2 applications [25]. Risk factors for stricture development after PDT include history of prior esophageal stricture, prior EMR, and more than one PDT application in a single treatment session. The use of centering balloons was not associated with significant reduction in stricture formation [35]. Only 1–2% of patients had strictures after PDT using 5-ALA in Europe, but hypotension and sudden death were reported. 5-ALA may produce hypotension in patients and it has been standard practice during its administration in Europe to provide the patient with preadministration IV hydration.

Outcomes
Mortality
Among patients with HGD treated with PDT and EMR, the mortality was similar to those who had esophagectomy (9% versus 8.5%) at 60-month follow-up. No patients in either group had esophageal cancer-related death [33].

Complete eradication
For dysplastic BE, there have been 19 studies and three of them were RCTs. One small RCT in 2005 by Ragunath compared PDT and APC mainly in LGD patients (13 in each arm). The results revealed that PDT was numerically but not statistically better in achieving complete eradication (77% versus 62%) [36]. Overholt *et al.* studied one cohort of 218 HGD patients and compared PDT (138 patients) with omeprazole (70 patients). During the initial 18 months of treatment and follow-up, complete ablation was achieved in 77% versus 39%, and progression to cancer occurred in 13% versus 28% for the PDT and omeprazole groups respectively. The benefit of PDT over omeprazole in 5 years was demonstrated by the follow-up data from this cohort: PDT was effective in eradication of HGD and slowing down the progression to cancer [37].

Recurrence
Photodynamic therapy was shown to be effective in eliminating HGD compared to PPI therapy alone (78% versus 39%), and it also decreased the risk of EAC by 50% after at least 48 months of follow-up [38]. Biomarkers using fluorescence *in situ* hybridization (FISH) can detect loss of 9p21 (p16 gene) and 17p3.1 (p 53 gene), gains of the 8q24(c-myc), 17q (HER2-neu), and 20q13 loci and multiple gains, which were found more often in patients with recurrence [39]. These markers reflect gene copy number alterations within the mucosa which is suggestive of chromosomal instability that is often found in cancer progression.

Endoscopic submucosal dissection

Endoscopic submucosal dissection was first introduced in 1998 for early gastric cancer. It was shown to reduce recurrence of larger (>1.5 cm) esophageal/gastric lesions because of the ability to perform *en bloc* resection [40–42]. Another advantage of ESD over EMR is that the specimen margins are less affected by electrocautery and the pathology assessment of margins is more accurate. ESD is a more lengthy procedure than EMR (2–3 times), has higher complication rates, is technically more challenging, and

Table 18.1 Studies on ESD use for esophageal lesions.

Author, year	Types of lesions	No. of patients (lesions)	En bloc resection rate	Major bleeding *	Stricture	Perforation [†]	Recurrence	Follow-up **
Oyama, 2005	ESCC (T1a)	102	95%	NA	7%	0	0	NA
Kakushima, 2006	EAC at GE junction	30	97%	0	3.3%	3.3%	0	14.6
Fujishiro, 2006	ESCC (Tis or T1a)	43	100%	0	16%	6.9%	2.3%	17
Hirasawa, 2007	GE junction EAC	58	100%	0	1.7%	0	0	36.6
Ishihara, 2008	168 ESCC and 3 EAC	EMR (140)	78.6%	0.8%	2.5%	0	1.7%	NA
		ESD (31)	100%	0	0	3.4%	0	–
Ono, 2009	ESCC	84 (14 SM lesions)	100%	0	18%	4.7%	1.2%	21
Mizuta, 2009	Superficial ESCC	33 (42)	NA	0	16.7%	11.9%	NA	NA
Chaves, 2010	Early EAC	5	83.3%	0	NA	0	NA	9.5
Teoh, 2010	ESCC and dysplasia	EMR 10	69.2%	10%	0	0	10%	22.2
		ESD 18	95.4%	0	11.1%	5.6%	0	–
Repici, 2010	Early ESCC	20	90%	0	5%	0	0	18
Nonaka, 2010	Superficial ESCC	25 (27)	89.9%	0	12%	4%	0	NA
Takahashi, 2010	ESCC (T1N0)	EMR 184	53.3%	0.5%	9.2%	1.6%	9.8%	65
		ESD 116	100%	0	17.2%	2.6%	0.9%	–
Ishii, 2010	Superficial ESCC	48 (53)	100%	0	22.9%	0	0	23
Yamashita, 2011	Superficial ESCC	EMR 56	44.6%	0	14.3%	7.1%	7.1%	39
		ESD 71	97.2%	0	8.5%	1.4%	0%	–

*Bleeding that required transfusion or hospitalization.

[†]Did not include mediastinal emphysema.

**Mean or median follow-up in months.

EAC, esophageal adenocarcinoma; EMR, endoscopic mucosal resection; ESCC, esophageal squamous cell carcinoma; ESD, endoscopic submucosal dissection; GE, gastro-esophageal; NA: not available; SM, submucosal.

A few case studies with very small sample sizes (<5 cases) from Saito (2008), Probst (2009) and Coda (2010) were not included in the table above.

reimbursement may be an issue. Therefore, ESD has not yet gained wide popularity in the US or Europe.

Patient selection

Endoscopic submucosal dissection is usually reserved for large (>1.5 cm), early esophageal cancer (no more advanced than T1aN0M0), flat (type 0–III) or ulcerated lesions that are unsuitable for conventional methods including EMR. However, ESD on a previous EMR site may present additional risks because tissue scarring at the submucosal layers makes it very difficult to separate them from the mucosal layers on top. Dissection of such esophageal lesions carries a high risk of perforation.

Procedure

With the aid of regular EGD, NBI or chromoendoscopy, the margins of the lesion are marked using electrocautery.

A mixed solution of saline, hyaluronic acid or hydroxypropylmethyl cellulose and indigo carmine is injected into the submucosal space to separate mucosal from muscular layers. Indigo carmine provides better visualization of submucosal layers than plain saline.

Then a special device, such as an insulated-tip knife, triangle-tip knife, flex knife, fork knife, flush knife or hook knife, is used to slowly and carefully make a circumferential incision, and then the lesion is dissected along the submucosal layer. None of these knives has been found to be superior. Visible vessels that are encountered during this process should be coagulated with pulse electrocautery.

Careful inspection of the area for bleeding or perforation is performed after dissection.

Complications and outcomes

Table 18.1 summarizes results of ESD studies. ESD devices are approved by the FDA for use in the United States.

Cryoablation

Cryoablation is a non-contact ablation procedure that uses medical grade $-196\,^{\circ}C$ liquid nitrogen or refrigerated gas (usually carbon dioxide, CO_2) administered by catheter through the endoscope's working channel. Its use for BE was first reported in 2005 by Johnston [43]. In 2007, it was officially approved by the FDA. Two devices are available commercially: truFreeze® cryospray ablation (CSA Medical Inc., Baltimore, MD) and the Polar Wand® (GI Supply, Camp Hill, PA). They use liquid nitrogen and CO_2 respectively.

Patient selection

Cryoablation is mainly for BE with HGD (or subgroups of LGD when indicated). Some studies have shown success in early cancers that either failed conventional ablation or when a patient is unfit for esophagectomy.

Procedure

A 16 Fr modified nasogastric tube is placed over a guidewire in the stomach and connected to continuous wall suction to decompress during the cryoablation procedure. It is essential to monitor for abdominal distension during the entire procedure to avoid perforation from excessive gas in the stomach.

Then a polyamide catheter is placed through the regular EGD channel, and positioned at 3–4 mm beyond the tip of the endoscope.

Gas flow can be initiated by pressing on the foot pedal. Treatment is usually twi cycles of 20 sec or four cycles of 10 sec. Usually an interval of 60 sec is allowed between cycles to allow tissue thawing.

Complications

A study of 77 patients showed that the most common complaint was chest pain (17.6%), followed by dysphagia (13.3%), odynophagia (12.1%), and sore throat (9.6%) [44]. Another study of 333 treatments among 98 patients showed no perforation, 3% stricture, and 2% severe chest pain [45].

Outcomes

In the largest study of cryoablation for dysplastic BE, 98 patients were retrospectively included. Only 60 completed the planned cryoablation therapy. Fifty-eight subjects (97%) had complete eradication of HGD; 52 (87%) had complete eradication of all dysplasia; and 34 (57%) had complete eradication of all intestinal metaplasia [45].

Endoscopic cryoablation could be an alternative for T1a cancer patients who have failed other conventional therapies such as EMR or chemoradiation, or those who are unfit for surgery. A recent study demonstrated that cryoablation yielded about 72% of complete endoscopic response for 36 patients with T1 cancer [46]. However, this study only had 11.5 months of follow-up and long-term information is lacking.

Multipolar electrocoagulation

Multipolar electrocoagulation (MPEC) is well known to most gastroenterologists as it has been widely used in coagulation for bleeding control. MPEC is performed with a 7 Fr or 10 Fr catheter that has two electrodes, which enables completion of an electrical circuit at the working end while in contact with the target tissue [47]. The electrical current passes through the target tissue and then causes desiccation and destruction, which leads to tissue injury.

Studies of MPEC for BE eradication are limited to NDBE and include three case series for MPEC and two RCT studies comparing APC with MPEC [48,49]. The overall complete eradication rate was approximately 60–75%. Currently the role of MPEC is limited to performing "touch-up" therapy for NDBE.

Argon plasma coagulation

Argon plasma coagulation (APC) is a non-contact technique performed by using a through-the-endoscope catheter that provides ionized argon via monopolar current to produce mucosal coagulation. The depth of injury is dependent on the flow of gas, power setting, distance of the catheter tip to epithelial surface, duration of application, etc. APC for esophageal therapy is usually performed at a lower power setting than for stomach therapy. Some studies have demonstrated that injury may reach the muscularis propria at usual settings of 20–40 W. APC has been used for many other GI indications such as treatment for gastric antral vascular ectasia and radiation proctopathy, etc. Overall, it is a safe, readily available, and easy-to-perform procedure.

However, the experience of APC for BE has mostly come from NDBE studies. There were 28 studies published between 1998 and 2008, including seven RCTs comparing APC to PDT, MPEC or surveillance [8]. Currently, as there is considerable debate about the need to treat NDBE, we will not review these studies here.

There are very few reports regarding the use of APC to treat LGD and HGD/EAC, most of which are case series with very small sample sizes. The largest case series included 29 HGD patients treated with APC; 25 (86%) patients responded (22 had complete regression to neosquamous esophageal mucosa) [47]. Four patients developed cancer in the mean follow-up of 37 months. Ragunath *et al.* compared the effectiveness of APC with PDT among dysplastic BE patients (mainly LGD) and concluded that PDT was slightly more effective in eradicating dysplastic tissue. The photosensitizer used in PDT preferentially accumulates in the dysplastic areas, resulting in selective destruction of dysplastic tissue [50]. The effect of PDT may be more than just physical tissue ablation and could be more advantageous than thermal ablation methods. Stricture rate was up to 3.2% of patients after APC.

Laser

When tissue absorbs laser light, thermal injury occurs in the superficial layers. This is the mechanism of laser treatment for BE. The depth of injury depends on the wavelength of laser light, the properties of target tissue, power setting, and duration of application. The types of lasers include neodymium (Nd):YAG, potassium titanium phosphate (KTP):YAG, carbon dioxide (CO_2), neodymium-holmium, and diode. It has been reported that the Nd:YAG laser could cause deeper tissue injury, up to 4–6 mm. The studies reporting the use of laser therapy for BE eradication are all case series from 1997 to 2003. The complete eradication rate varied from 67% to 100%, and some studies showed about 25% of recurrence of BE [51]. Stricture rate was up to 4.5%. The use of laser in the GI tract has largely been supplanted by other safer and more effective techniques.

Combination of endoscopic therapies

Studies on combined therapies are few and heterogeneous. One study in 2008 reported on 31 patients (16 EAC, 12 HGD, and three LGD) who were treated by EMR followed by RFA. All except one subject (98%) achieved complete eradication of dysplasia and intestinal metaplasia. In the study from Pech *et al.* (2008), after EMR resection of early EAC, ablative therapies using APC (136 patients) or PDT (64 patients) of remaining non-neoplastic Barrett's mucosa yielded lower recurrence of EAC than those patients without ablations (16.5% versus 29.9%, $P=0.001$) [24].

Surgery with or without chemoradiotherapy

Esophagectomy is no longer the standard treatment for HGD as outcomes of endoscopic treatments have been shown to be comparable to esophagectomy [3]. The vast majority of IM-EAC can be managed by endoscopic therapies. However, esophagectomy with or without chemoradiotherapy is usually recommended in the presence of LNM, which may be found in one-third of SM-EAC [52].

For patients with HGD or IM-EAC who have non-healing ulcers or extensive scars from previous endoscopic therapy, esophagectomy is also an option. Based on local expertise, a transhiatal or transthoracic, either standard open surgery or minimally invasive approach can be performed. Some studies showed similar outcomes between open versus minimally invasive approaches, but patients with the latter approach had shorter length of hospital stay and faster recovery. A population-based study of early non-squamous cell esophageal cancers (Tis, T1a and T1b) using Surveillance Epidemiology and End Results data showed that endoscopic therapy may have equivalent long-term survival compared to esophagectomy. However, the endoscopy group had fewer submucosal cancers and information about co-morbidities and chemoradiotherapy was not available in this analysis.

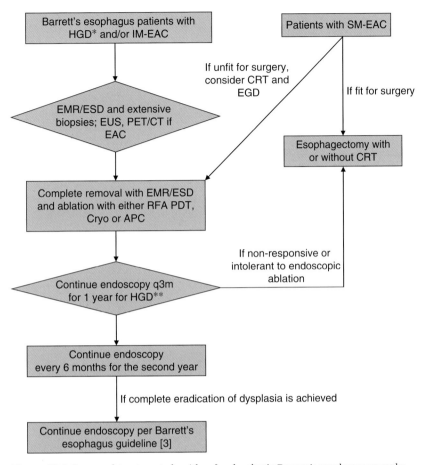

Figure 18.4 Proposed treatment algorithm for dysplastic Barrett's esophagus or early esophageal cancer.

*The benefit of LGD ablation is not established. Some authors advocate ablation for young patients or those with multiple levels of LGD.

**EGD every 2 months till all IM-EACs are resected if margins of EMR specimens are positive for tumor, or EGD every 3 months in the first year if margins are free of tumors, then every 6 months for the second year, and yearly from the third year or at intervals set by the guideline [3].

APC, argon plasma coagulation; CRT, chemoradiotherapy; cryo, cryoablation; CT, computed tomography; EGD, esophagogastroduodenoscopy; EMR, endoscopic mucosal resection; ESD, endoscopic submucosal dissection; EUS, endoscopic ultrasound; HGD, high-grade dysplasia; IM-EAC, intramucosal esophageal adenocarcinoma; PDT, photodynamic therapy; PET, positron emission tomography; RFA, radiofrequency ablation; SM-EAC, submucosal esophageal adenocarcinoma.

Management algorithm

The management schema for patients with Barrett's esophagus with high-grade dysplasia or cancer is shown in Figure 18.4.

CASE STUDY

A 75-year-old Caucasian man had a 20-year history of frequent heartburn currently controlled with a daily PPI. EGD 1 year ago for work-up of iron deficiency anemia revealed a 4 cm hiatus hernia and a long segment of Barrett's mucosa (C5M7 by Prague criteria). White light endoscope and NBI exam showed a small (3–4 mm) nodular lesion in the distal esophagus. Random biopsies from every 2 cm of BE showed LGD and focal HGD; biopsies from the nodule showed HGD. These findings were confirmed by two GI pathologists.

What is the most reasonable next step in management?
Studies showed that visible lesions such as nodules, mass, ulcers, and strictures are high-risk findings indicative of cancers. The recommended management before any ablative therapy is to perform EMR in addition to EUS exam. According to the pooled analysis by Konda *et al.* [30], about 40% of patients who underwent esophagectomy for HGD were found to have occult cancer. They also pointed out that 11% of patients with visible lesions were found to have invasive adenocarcinoma versus 3% of patients with no visible lesion. Certainly, the roles of EMR and random biopsies are complementary in diagnosing occult cancers.

How do you counsel patients regarding the endoscopic mucosal resection procedure?
It should be explained that EMR is a low-risk outpatient procedure that is useful to search for hidden cancers that may be missed by biopsies. After EMR, the patient could experience some chest discomfort, nausea, and minor bleeding.

What is the long-term plan?
Sequential EMRs should be performed until all visible lesions have been removed. After a review of the pathology, an ablation method is chosen, which may include RFA, PDT or cryoablation. For patients with difficult-to-heal ulcers or excessive scarring that leads to non-lifting after submucosal injection, further endoscopic therapy may be difficult or ineffective, and esophagectomy should be discussed as an alternative.

What is the overall follow-up plan?
The patient should have endoscopic evaluation every 3 months for the first year after the diagnosis of HGD, and follow-up every 6 months during the second year, then annually if complete eradication is achieved. Patients should return every 3 months if IM-EAC is removed via EMR and the margins are free of tumor. If margins are positive, then the patient can take 6–8 weeks to heal, and return for further resection until all visible lesions are gone.

References

1 Rex DK, Cummings OW, Shaw M. Screening for Barrett's esophagus in colonoscopy patients with and without heartburn. Gastroenterology 2003;125(6):1670–7.
2 Eckardt VF, Kanzler G, Bernhard G. Life expectancy and cancer risk in patients with Barrett's esophagus: a prospective controlled investigation. Am J Med 2001;111(1):33–7.

3 Wang KK, Sampliner RE. Updated guidelines 2008 for the diagnosis, surveillance and therapy of barrett's esophagus. Am J Gastroenterol 2008;103:788–97.

4 Menon D, Stafinski T, Wu H, Lau D, Wong C. Endoscopic treatments for Barrett's esophagus: a systematic review of safety and effectiveness compared to esophagectomy. BMC Gastroenterology 2010;10:111.

5 Shaheen NJ, Sharma P, Overholt BF, et al. Radiofrequency ablation in Barrett's esophagus with dysplasia. N Engl J Med 2009;360(22):2277–88.

6 Seewald S, Akaraviputh T, Seitz U, et al. Circumferential EMR and complete removal of Barrett's epithelium: a new approach to management of Barrett's esophagus containing high-grade intraepithelial neoplasia and intramucosal carcinoma. Gastrointest Endosc 2003;57:854–9.

7 Peters FP, Kara MA, Rosmolen WD, et al. Stepwise radical endoscopic resection is effective for complete removal of Barrett's esophagus with early neoplasia: a prospective study. Am J Gastroenterol 2006;101:1449–57.

8 Wani S, Sayana H, Sharma P. Endoscopic eradication of Barrett's esophagus. Gastrointest Endosc 2010;71(1):147–66.

9 Attil T, Faigel DO. Role of endoscopic ultrasound in superficial esophageal cancer. Dis Esophagus 2009;22(2):104–12.

10 Stein HJ, Feith M, Bruecher BL, et al. Early esophageal cancer: pattern of lymphatic spread and prognostic factors for long-term survival after surgical resection. Ann Surg 2005;242:566–75.

11 Altorki NK, Lee PC, Liss Y, et al. Multifocal neoplasia and nodal metastases in T1 esophageal carcinoma: implications for endoscopic treatment. Ann Surg 2008;247:434–9.

12 Pennathur A, Farkas A, Krasinskas AM, et al. Esophagectomy for T1 esophageal cancer: outcomes in 100 patients and implications for endoscopic therapy. Ann Thorac Surg 2009;87:1048–55.

13 Buskens CJ, Westerterp M, Lagarde SM, et al. Prediction of appropriateness of local endoscopic treatment for high-grade dysplasia and early adenocarcinoma by EUS and histopathologic features. Gastrointest Endosc 2004;60:703–10.

14 Namasivayam V, Wang KK, Prasad GA. Endoscopic mucosal resection in the management of esophageal neoplasia: current status and future directions. Clin Gastroenterol Hepatol 2010;8(9):743–54.

15 Zuckerman MJ, Hirota WK, Adler DG, et al. ASGE guideline: the management of low-molecular-weight heparin and nonaspirin antiplatelet agents for endoscopic procedures. Gastrointest Endosc 2005;61:189–94.

16 Vikneswaran N, Lutzke LS, Prasad GA, et al. Bleeding and thrombotic risk in endoscopic mucosal resection (EMR) with clopidogrel. Gastrointest Endosc 2010;71:AB126.

17 Buttar NS, Wang KK, Sebo TJ, et al. Extent of high-grade dysplasia in Barrett's esophagus correlates with risk of adenocarcinoma. Gastroenterology 2001;120(7):1630–9.

18 Curvers WL, Herrero LA, Wallace MB, et al. Endoscopic tri-modal imaging is more effective than standard endoscopy in identifying early-stage neoplasia in Barrett's esophagus. Gastroenterology 2010;139(4):1106–14.

19 May A, Gossner L, Behrens A, et al. A prospective randomized trial of two different endoscopic resection techniques for early stage cancer of the esophagus. Gastrointest Endosc 2003;58:167–75.

20 Abrams JA, Fedi P, Vakiani E, et al. Depth of resection using two different endoscopic mucosal resection techniques. Endoscopy 2008;40:395–9.

21 Esaki M, Matsumoto T, Hirakawa K, et al. Risk factors for local recurrence of superficial esophageal cancer after treatment by endoscopic mucosal resection. Endoscopy 2007;39:41–5.

22 Prasad GA, Wu TT, Wigle DA, *et al.* Endoscopic and surgical treatment of mucosal (T1a) esophageal adenocarcinoma in Barrett's esophagus. Gastroenterology 2009;137:815–23.

23 Kodama M, Kakegawa T. Treatment of superficial cancer of the esophagus: a summary of responses to a questionnaire on superficial cancer of the esophagus in Japan. Surgery 1998;123:432–9.

24 Pech O, Behrens A, May A, *et al.* Long-term results and risk factor analysis for recurrence after curative endoscopic therapy in 349 patients with high-grade intraepithelial neoplasia and mucosal adenocarcinoma in Barrett's oesophagus. Gut 2008;57:1200–6.

25 Wang KK, Lutzke L, Borkenhagen L, *et al.* Photodynamic therapy for Barrett's esophagus: does light still have a role? Endoscopy 2008;40(12):1021–5.

26 Nijhawan PK, Wang KK. Endoscopic mucosal resection for lesions with endoscopic features suggestive of malignancy and high-grade dysplasia within Barrett's esophagus. Gastrointest Endosc 2000;52(3):328–32.

27 Pech O, May A, Rabenstein T, Ell C. Endoscopic resection of early oesophageal cancer. Gut 2007;56(11):1625–34.

28 Ell C, May A, Pech O, *et al.* Curative endoscopic resection of early esophageal adenocarcinomas (Barrett's cancer). Gastrointest Endosc 2007;65(1):3–10.

29 Van Vilsteren FG, Bergman JJ. Endoscopic therapy using radiofrequency ablation for esophageal dysplasia and carcinoma in Barrett's esophagus. Gastrointest Endosc Clin North Am 2010;20(1):55–74.

30 Konda VJ, Ross AS, Ferguson MK, *et al.* Is the risk of concomitant invasive esophageal cancer in high-grade dysplasia in Barrett's esophagus overestimated? Clin Gastroenterol Hepatol 2008;6(2):159–64.

31 Shaheen NJ, Frantz DJ. When to consider endoscopic ablation therapy for Barrett's esophagus. Curr Opin Gastroenterol 2010;26(4):361–6.

32 Li LB, Xie JM, Zhang XN, *et al.* Retrospective study of photodynamic therapy vs photodynamic therapy combined with chemotherapy and chemotherapy alone on advanced esophageal cancer. Photodiagn Photodynam Ther 2010;7(3):139–43.

33 Prasad GA, Wang KK, Buttar NS, *et al.* Long term survival following endoscopic and surgical treatment of high grade dysplasia in Barrett's esophagus. Gastroenterology 2007;132:1226–33.

34 Bellnier DA, Greco WR, Loewen GM, *et al.* Population pharmacokinetics of the photodynamic therapy agent 2-1-hexyloxyethyl -2-devinyl pyropheophorbide-a in cancer patients. Cancer Res 2003;63(8):1806–13.

35 Prasad GA, Wang KK, Buttar NS, Wongkeesong LM, Lutzke LS, Borkenhagen LS. Predictors of stricture formation after photodynamic therapy for high-grade dysplasia in Barrett's esophagus. Gastrointest Endosc 2007;65(1):60–6.

36 Ragunath K, Krasner N, Raman VS, Haqqani MT, Phillips CJ, Cheung I. Endoscopic ablation of dysplastic Barrett's oesophagus comparing argon plasma coagulation and photodynamic therapy: a randomized prospective trial assessing efficacy and cost-effectiveness. Scand J Gastroenterol 2005;40(7):750–8.

37 Overholt BF, Wang KK, Burdick JS, *et al.* Five-year efficacy and safety of photodynamic therapy with Photofrin in Barrett's high-grade dysplasia. [see comment]. Gastrointest Endosc 2007;66(3):460–8.

38 Overholt B, Lightdale C, Wang K, *et al.* Photodynamic therapy (PDT) with porfimer sodium for the ablation of highgrade dysplasia in Barrett's esophagus (BE): international, partially blinded randomized phase III trial. Gastrointest Endosc 2005;62:488–98.

39 Prasad GA, Wang KK, Halling KC, *et al.* Correlation of histology with biomarker status after photodynamic therapy in Barrett esophagus. Cancer 2008;113(3):470–6.

40 Ishihara R, Iishi H, Uedo N, *et al.* Comparison of EMR and endoscopic submucosal dissection for en bloc resection of early esophageal cancers in Japan. Gastrointest Endosc 2008;68(6):1066–72.

41 Muto M, Miyamoto S, Hosokawa A. Endoscopic mucosal resection in the stomach using the insulated-tip needle-knife. Endoscopy 2005;37(2):178–82.

42 Oka S, Tanaka S, Kaneko I, *et al.* Advantage of endoscopic submucosal dissection compared with EMR for early gastric cancer. Gastrointest Endosc 2006;64(6): 877–83.

43 Johnston MH, Eastone JA, Horwhat JD. Cryoablation of Barrett's esophagus: a pilot study. Gastrointest Endosc 2005;62(6):842–8.

44 Greenwald BD, Dumot JA, Abrams JA, *et al.* Endoscopic spray cryoablation for esophageal cancer: safety and efficacy. Gastrointest Endosc 2010;71(4):686–93.

45 Shaheen NJ, Greenwald BD, Peery AF, *et al.* Safety and efficacy of endoscopic spray cryoablation for Barrett's esophagus with high-grade dysplasia. Gastrointest Endosc 2010;71(4):680–5.

46 Greenwald BD, Dumot JA, Horwhat JD. Safety, tolerability, and efficacy of endoscopic low-pressure liquid nitrogen spray cryoablation in the esophagus. Dis Esophagus 2010;23(1):13–19.

47 Attwood SE, Lewis CJ, Caplin S, Hemming K, Armstrong G. Argon beam plasma coagulation as therapy for high-grade dysplasia in Barrett's esophagus. Clin Gastroenterol Hepatol 2003;1:258–63.

48 Dulai GS, Jensen DM, Cortina G, Fontana L, Ippoliti A. Randomized trial of argon plasma coagulation vs. multipolar electrocoagulation for ablation of Barrett's esophagus. Gastrointest Endosc 2005;61(2):232–40.

49 Sharma P, Wani S, Weston AP, *et al.* A randomised controlled trial of ablation of Barrett's oesophagus with multipolar electrocoagulation versus argon plasma coagulation in combination with acid suppression: long term results. Gut 2006;55(9): 1233–9.

50 Stewart F, Baas P, Star W. What does photodynamic therapy have to offer radiation oncologists (or their cancer patients)? Radiat Oncol 1998;48:233–48.

51 Pech O, Gossner L, May A, Ell C. Management of Barrett's oesophagus, dysplasia and early adenocarcinoma. Best Pract Res Clin Gastroenterol 2001;15(2):267–84.

52 Wang KK, Prasad G, Tian J. Endoscopic mucosal resection and endoscopic submucosal dissection in esophageal and gastric cancers. Curr Opin Gastroenterol 2010;26(5):453–8.

Index

Page references in *italics*; those in **bold** refer to Tables

Practical Manual of Gastroesophageal Reflux Disease, First Edition.
Edited by Marcelo F. Vela, Joel E. Richter and John E. Pandolfino.
© 2013 John Wiley & Sons, Ltd. Published 2013 by John Wiley & Sons, Ltd.